Trying to Give Ease

Trying to Give Ease

Tommie Bass and the
Story of Herbal Medicine

John K. Crellin and Jane Philpott

DUKE UNIVERSITY PRESS

Durham and London, 1990

This work is not intended as a field guide or
formulary. The information from Bass and from
the historical record is to be read in the context
of traditional wisdom and practices and is not a
recommendation for using herbs in the changed
conditions of today's health care. Herbs can be
toxic or interfere with other medications.

© 1989 Duke University Press
First printing in paperback, 1997
All rights reserved
Printed in the United States of America
on acid-free paper ∞
Library of Congress Cataloging-in-Publication
Data appear on the last printed page of this book.
This volume was previously published under the
title *Herbal Medicine Past and Present, Volume 1:
Trying to Give Ease.* The companion volume,
*A Reference Guide to Medicinal Plants: Herbal
Medicine Past and Present,* was previously
published under the title *Herbal Medicine Past
and Present, Volume 2: A Reference Guide to
Medicinal Plants.*

Dedicated to the spirit of the World Health Organization's call for health for all by the year 2000.

Contents

A. L. Tommie Bass died in August 1996, about eight years after the original manuscript of this volume was completed. He had seen a remarkable growth of interest in herbal medicine during that time. As one reflection of this interest, Peggy Brevoort, in a 1996 discussion on the U.S. botanical market, stated that the size and intensity of consumer interest in botanicals was "exemplified in 1994 when this small [herb] industry successfully lobbied to pass legislation which dramatically changed the way botanicals are regulated. Congress received more mail on the Dietary Supplement Health and Education Act of 1994 than on any subject since the Vietnam War."

Tommie Bass began to promote commercially prepared herb capsules in 1983, even though this countered his long-standing recommendations of using teas and salves. Moreover, commercialism contrasted sharply with his own service to patients, which was mentioned in his *New York Times* obituary: "[Bass] spent much of his life treating the people of Cherokee County and surrounding areas without taking payment."

Since 1988, various approaches to the use of herbs in health care have become more conspicuous. For some people, nutritional herbalism has come of age as a result of the 1994 Dietary Supplement Health and Education Act, which legislates that herbs can be marketed as "safe" unless proven otherwise by the government. In addition, given certain criteria, labels can include dosage recommendations and warnings about particular uses without dooming the herb or product to be branded as a drug or food additive.

Nutritional herbalism often shades into what can be described as eclectic herbalism, which embraces an interweaving of concepts that are called on to rationalize recommended uses of a particular herb. Concepts are drawn from traditional systems — for example, aboriginal medicine of North America and China — as well as from new ideas about energy medicine.

In contrast to such eclecticism is so-called rational herbalism. Its proponents will only accept the effectiveness of an herb on the basis of western science. The reputation of an herb is, or tends to be, dismissed if it cannot be explained by modern pharmacological studies and clinical trials. The exclusive emphasis on science makes this approach a favorite among many health care professionals and government regulatory bodies, as well as a few practitioners of alternative medicine. In fact, a noticeable feature of herbal medicine in recent years has been renewed interest in the chemical and pharmacological investigation of herbal medicines as part of the search for new drugs. Specialist volumes such as *Phytochemistry of Plants Used in Traditional Medicine* (Oxford: Clarendon, 1995) reflect this search, as well as the emergence of such sociopolitical issues as the intellectual property rights of indigenous peoples and the urgent need for plant conservation.

The recent growth of diverse approaches to herbal medicine, along with limited legislative controls, has allowed questionable practices to emerge; some, in fact, appear to be downright fraudulent. There is, we believe, a greater need now than in 1988 to investigate many of the current recommendations. Because society only has limited scientific resources for such studies, we must judiciously use other means to assess herbal medicine. The experience and knowledge of "old-timers," like Tommie Bass, is one. New uses, or those unknown to Bass, are not necessarily invalid; however, if they have no scientific basis, and if they are absent from the historical record (and here we include Bass) or if they have not been generally mainstream in the past when herbs were in everyday use, we must be extra cautious before accepting them. This volume pursues these issues as they describe and contextualize the practice of a unique individual.

John K. Crellin
Jane Philpott
1997

Acknowledgments

This book emerged out of an invitation from Allen Tullos to evaluate the reputation of the herbs known to and used by A. L. Tommie Bass. Once we saw that Mr. Bass's practice was both extensive and a significant social force in his area, it became clear that the project had to be expanded in order to avoid an overly superficial review. Although Allen Tullos did not remain with the project because of his own schedule, many thanks are due to him for his seminal role in initiating an intriguing journey.

Many people have responded to queries or provided general support. In the early years of the project, many students in a medicinal plant course led by Philpott and Crellin in the botany department at Duke University provided enthusiasm that encouraged a broad study. Later, Professors Robert Kral and Robert L. Wilbur helped enormously with various questions about identification and current botanical nomenclature. Invaluable for specific queries have been Janus Antonovics, Richard Bell, Lincoln Constance, J. A. Duke, Frances Hammersand, James Harden, J. T. Kartesz, Jim Massy, Mildred Mathias, Donald E. Stone, Philip Teigen, Sue Thompson, Rytas Vilgalys, and Norman Farnsworth. The latter also provided some monetary savings by providing free copies of NAPRALERT bibliographies. General support in the form of secretarial services and office supplies has come from the Medical History Program and the Mary Duke Biddle Foundation, and (including word-processing help) from the Department of Botany and, personally, from Jane Philpott. Library support has been crucial and three librarians at Duke University and their staffs deserve special gratitude: Bert Livingstone, Biology-Forestry Library; Warren Bird, Duke University Medical Center Library; and G. R. T. Cavanagh, Trent Collection, Duke University Medical Center Library. Some travel money for the collection of specimens has been provided by the Duke University Research Fund.

Above all, the project has been dependent on the patience of A. L. Tommie Bass, who has responded to endless queries for eight years. Moreover, he has encouraged visitors to be candid in talking about their use of herbal remedies. It is invidious to single out particular visitors to Bass, many of whom have patiently spent much time imparting ideas and information, but Judy and Barry James deserve thanks for facilitating many introductions, especially in the nutritional product phase of Mr. Bass's practice; additionally, they have provided insights into aspects of southern Appalachian life. Another person who has been patient during much of the gestation of the book, even while easing its birth in many ways, has been Joanne Ferguson, editor-in-chief at Duke University Press. Not only have her quiet, penetrating questions helped enormously but she also has never appeared overly daunted by the substantial size of the manuscript. Particular thanks are also due to the keen eye of copyeditor Mindy Conner, and to the many courtesies of the staff of Duke University Press.

Jane Philpott's ill health throughout much of the project and vision problems since 1984 have meant that an overwhelming portion of the work and the authorship of the book is that of John Crellin. Her personal thanks go to many friends, including colleagues who, through sustained high interest in the project, have been personally helpful in many ways, especially to long-time friend Jane Elchlepp. Thanks, too, to those who helped with transport after driving became unsafe, especially to Mel Turner and others he recruited. For computer related services and advice appreciation is due to Robert Chau, Molly Mcmullen, Cleo Robertson, Susan Garbeth Jones and the Computation Center at Duke University.

Introduction

P eople today face a bewildering choice of medical treatments
supplemental or alternative (some say complementary) to orthodox medicine, including osteopathy, chiropractic, Christian Science and other forms of faith healing, herbal medicine,
over-the-counter pharmacy, and many more. Most people retain a
basic confidence in orthodox medicine, but many are intrigued by
alternative practices and sample or use them regularly, notwithstanding much perplexity about the reliability and safety of alternative
approaches and questions about the honesty and qualifications of the
practitioners. A vast array of advocacy literature dealing with alternative health care exists, but, unfortunately, few balanced and analytical approaches are available. The present account aims to describe
and evaluate impartially one alternative practice in an Anglo-Saxon
setting.

Studies of traditional herbal practices have followed many overlapping directions. Prior to the 1930s, accounts for the most part focused
on charms and magical recipes, suggesting analogies to the beginnings of Western medicine. Other studies were Baconian in approach,
compiling lists of folk beliefs to preserve information in order to trace
the spread of ideas or to illuminate thought processes. Recent investigations tend to focus more on the context in which folk medicine
is practiced, its contribution to local health care, and its relation-

ship to regular Western medicine. Another approach, mostly used by ethnobotanists, chemists, and pharmacologists, rather than folk-lorists and anthropologists, examines the possible pharmacological effectiveness of plants for use in Western medicine. These studies garner information on remedies used by folk practitioners and lay-people, screen plants for active principles, and follow up leads from chemical or cross-cultural comparisons. Whatever the approach to traditional medicine, basic questions arise as to why people turn to it rather than to scientific medicine, and whether or not it is effective.

The present account is broader than most, even though it is based largely on our study of a single herbalist in the southern Appala-chians, A. L. Tommie Bass. We have omitted descriptions of herb uses by such practitioners as root doctors and spiritualists, and do not cover recent trends in herbal medicine embracing vitalist ideas. In fact, during the early stages of the study, its scope quickly grew as attention was given to relevant social factors, popular ideas about dis-ease, and analyses of historical roots and background. In many ways information on the matrix of relevant factors grew in topsy-turvy fash-ion as Mr. Bass's memory was prompted in different ways, and we constantly witnessed new aspects of his practice. Taken together, the diverse material illustrates the complexity of people's attitudes and behavior as a consequence of innumerable cultural and genetic con-siderations. Of course, not all considerations are relevant all the time for explaining particular practices, because individual patients "se-lect" consciously or unconsciously (sometimes to reinforce notions already held) factors congenial to their needs.

II

Individual readers will find different parts of the study of special in-terest according to their own attitudes and interests. Some physicians may conclude that the study reinforces their concerns over the dan-gers of traditional medicine, while others can appreciate that most remedies are analogous to over-the-counter medicines available from drugstores and elsewhere. They may also see this account, or at least certain aspects of it, as contributing to discussions about primary health care and community medicine. In fact, much of the discussion shows that physicians, pharmacists, and other health professionals should become better acquainted with herbal remedies as part of self-care, and that herbal medicine need not be viewed as confrontational to regular practice.[1]

The ready availability of herbal remedies raises as many issues for consumers as for health professionals. Although a profusion of books, pamphlets, and articles have appeared on herbal remedies, most are uncritical compilations. The discussions on the apparent success of herbal remedies and on the dangers of taking some of them are of interest to all. Among the variety of reasons for success are confidence in the biological activity of plants, a positive attitude toward or faith in the practitioner (whose ability may have been acquired by "gift," apprenticeship, or formal or self-education), personal involvement in the treatment, a sense of tradition, and a common cultural background and knowledge of herbs between patients and practitioners.

While social and cultural factors are undeniably important, how much they contribute to the success of herbal practitioners occasions much debate and disagreement. Certainly the outcome of each meeting between practitioner and patient reflects individual personalities and idiosyncrasies, the nature of the medical problem, and the patient's reasons for seeking the consultation. Some people visit herbal practitioners hesitantly after disillusionment with orthodox medicine, while others always employ herbal practitioners for second opinions. It seems clear that the concerns and needs of individuals when they are ill are variable and that the flexibility of herbal practice accommodates the needs of a variety of people.

Two questions arise for all readers. Is the local study that is central to this book relevant to the American scene in general? Does the American experience have anything to offer to an understanding of herbal medicine in other countries? After all, Appalachia is generally viewed as a unique region in an advanced Western country.[2]

The answer to both questions is surely yes, for the study raises many general issues ranging from concerns for an individual's medical problems to the dynamic relationship between alternative and professional practices. Furthermore, aspects of the American herbal story have had a direct impact on practices elsewhere, notably in Britain. Although alternative medical practices are probably no more conspicuous today than at many times in the past, more studies are needed on reasons for the present high level of interest in many

Western countries. This includes Britain, where the National Health Service generally ensures that no economic barriers stand in the way of seeking medical care, as is often the case elsewhere, and where the upper classes are turning to alternative therapies in significant numbers.[3]

Generally accepted reasons for the recent widespread growth of Western interest in marginal medicine are considered. These include disquiet with regular practices, such as side effects of drugs, high hospital costs, and the frequently impersonal approach of many physicians and allied health personnel. Factors generally given less attention include a general suspicion of technology and nostalgia for the "old days." It has been implied that nostalgia contributed to the success of the practice of Dr. Jarvis, a licensed physician who attracted widespread attention in the 1950s and 1960s by promoting the medicinal value of honey and apple cider vinegar. Jarvis's views were presented as an alternative to orthodox medicine and provided a pastoral view that seemed to reinforce differences between an urbanized, cultured society and a rural one.[4]

The World Health Organization recognizes that traditional medicine remains the major source of health care for more than two-thirds of the world's population.[5] Conclusions to the present study note a number of points linked to the widely asked question: "Whither traditional medicine?" We consider, for instance, attempts at integrating traditional and Western medical systems and approaches to understanding traditional pharmacology.[6] This account can be seen as a description of the persistence of traditional practice in a modern, industrialized nation committed to scientific medicine. In turn, this raises questions about the future of traditional practices in developing countries as they become more industrialized.

III

Among the academic disciplines that find common ground in the themes and issues of traditional medicine are anthropology and sociology (especially the "applied" areas of medical anthropology and medical sociology), folk-life studies, ethnobotany, and ethnopharmacology. The study of traditional medicine has been more the preserve of anthropology, with its in-depth interviews, than of sociology, with its tendency to elicit information by questionnaires. Even so, as anthropologists have vigorously pursued analytical frameworks for their observations, the flavor of more and more studies of traditional medicine has become sociological.

The present study has an anthropological approach insofar as it is based on participant observation and interviews over a long period of time. We also relied on the approaches—common in folk-life studies —of recording and endeavoring to distinguish the oral and popular traditions, mostly through the extraordinarily acute memory and narrative talents of Mr. Bass.

Some anthropologists may consider that the findings are not adequately placed in an overall theoretical framework (including attention to symbolism), as many studies on cultures in Africa and elsewhere have been. Two factors have shaped a direction away from a single theoretical position. One is the deep disagreements within anthropology on how best to understand cultural groups; the second, that during the last twenty years or so Bass's practice (like others observed) has developed an increasingly broad clientele crossing all social classes. For this reason, too, we take a cautious attitude toward sociological views that see an association between many forms of healing and new religious movements. Theories about the multiple reasons that exist for using herbal remedies can too easily impose an order, a neatness, which does not do justice to the whims of fancy, coincidence of events, and complex interplay of factors uncovered by our study.

Much of the analysis is based on historical perspectives. This highlights a close similarity between much present-day herbal practice and therapies prescribed within regular medicine until around the 1940s. The term herbal medicine has been used in the title both because it embraces the folk and professional sectors of health care and because the terms "traditional" and "folk" medicine imply developments long distinct from regular medicine rather than the dynamic relationships that exist between the two.[7]

Reasons for placing emphasis on the history of medicinal plants perhaps merit additional comment, because it is commonplace knowledge that herbs have a long history; indeed, it is so well known that many people see herbal medicine as merely a quaint legacy of the past. However, an emphasis on the history of medicinal plants reveals that the conceptual framework of modern herbal practice rests on theories and notions that have long been part of regular medicine and have acquired a cultural force, though often in modified form.

A number of issues are highlighted by our approach. They include the perennial questions, Why there is a persistence of folk beliefs? and Can making decisions to research the chemistry and pharmacology of a plant be helped by historical perspectives? Precise documentation contributes to both issues because it is necessary to make adequate assessments of a plant's historical popularity and whether or not a reputation rests on sound testimony and critical sources or is the consequence of hearsay or doubtful theory. Folklorists often have been fascinated more by geographical relationships than by common historical origins. Diffusion, rather than origins, has been the main concern; yet historical accounts can explain, or at least suggest, why plants are used for similar purposes in diverse, apparently unrelated cultures.[8]

The oral history we recorded—mostly from Mr. Bass, who has garnered and synthesized a community's knowledge—is an important part of the volume; it can be seen as contributing to folk-life studies which preserve information on bygone and rustic ways of life. However, this is no longer the thrust of most folk-life studies, and while perspectives and knowledge generally unrecorded from a working practice and now disappearing from Anglo-Saxon traditions are preserved, the material also contributes to an understanding of many popular ideas about disease and treatment, people's foibles and concerns, and the relations between academic and popular knowledge. All of this is a reminder of the value of understanding the scope of a society's stock of knowledge.[9] Furthermore, the oral accounts (plus commentary) illuminate perceptions about twentieth-century social change and contribute to understanding the impacts of changes in medicine, not so much in terms of medical science and the medical profession, but in the context of minor and chronic illnesses, which impinge on everyone and exact a major economic toll everywhere.

Considerations of botany—plant identification and distribution— are also essential in assessing traditional medicine. Exact identification of plants raises many questions, especially when allied or analogous species are found to be used rather than those commonly reported in the literature. This suggests that regional differences in traditional medicine are often the direct outcome of plant distributions rather than the result of different levels of knowledge about plants from one region to another. Undoubtedly the richness of Appalachian flora has been an important factor in shaping Bass's practice. We give some attention to false identifications of plants by herbalists and the significance of this for herbal medicine. Hopefully, the way botany and history are combined in the account helps to establish the herbal pedigree of many plants. Amid current concerns over the safety and effectiveness of herbs, some health authorities are increasingly relying on a plant's past reputation in their assessments of herbs. Unfortunately, there is a paucity of information that sifts advocatory from other positions.

IV

Details on how the practical part of the study was undertaken need comment. The project started in 1980 after Allen Tullos, who had reviewed aspects of Mr. Bass's life in a master's thesis in the curriculum in folklore at the University of North Carolina, Chapel Hill (1976), suggested that the story of Tommie Bass as herbalist be written. The authors visited Mr. Bass frequently, collecting information about his life and knowledge of herbs. During field trips, voucher specimens were acquired for the Duke University herbarium.

John Crellin gathered information about the plants and about Bass's practice from Mr. Bass and his visitors, friends, and acquaintances, as well as from people in his community who have never sought his advice. This resulted in hundreds of hours of discussions, generally recorded on tape. The use of questionnaires proved to be a serious disruption to the relationship between Mr. Bass and his visitors, and they were rarely used. However, specific questions were asked during lengthy informal and semistructured chats with visitors.

All the activities with Mr. Bass prompted his memory in various directions. Bass also cooperated by tape-recording a diary for an eight-month period, listing the daily number of visitors and many of the reasons for their visits. He also has supplemented this information with innumerable tapes on special topics and with many telephone conversations.

Complementing visits to Leesburg, Mr. Bass has been to North Carolina on eight occasions for week-long visits. On such trips his memory was further triggered in different ways by visits to medical and pharmaceutical museums, and by repeated conversations about each remedy that he knows. The latter approach included detailed discussions on such works as Jane Bolyard's *Medicinal Plants and Home Remedies of Appalachia* (1981), R. B. Browne's *Popular Beliefs and Practices from Alabama* (1958), and V. E. Tyler's *The Honest Herbal* (1982).

As the study proceeded, some of Bass's friends, neighbors, and visitors became principal sources of information, not only about him and his herbal practice but about their own attitudes toward herbs and their effectiveness. Bass and his friends and acquaintances have shown a great deal of interest in self-treatment through the use of herbs now commercially marketed in capsules, a trend we discuss in chapter 6.

Unlike some traditional healers, Mr. Bass has been especially forthright in sharing information. Indeed, in recent years it has become his mission to spread knowledge about the identity of herbs. It is a mark of Bass's knowledge and integrity that he is consistent in the information he has given over a period of years.

An inevitable concern is how much our attention has altered Bass's practice. He once said, "I don't want to be telling something I can't back up. I know I'm not connected with your college, but I don't want people to get the impression I'm talking out of my head. All we're trying to do is to teach you people. A preacher said at a talk of mine, 'Ladies and gentlemen, black and white, we're glad to have Mr. Bass. He has given his time. He has been to the University of North Carolina and to Duke. He's not connected with the universities in no way, but you know they're a lot of help to him.'"

It seems clear that our attention has added an aura of authority to his practice and encouraged interest in it in the minds of many who know Mr. Bass. However, the growth of his practice up to 1982, when he was offering advice to about two thousand people a year, is due more to the local newspaper publicity he has received and the widespread revival of interest in herbal remedies. Likewise, while it is clear that Mr. Bass has imbibed some knowledge and ideas from us, the impact has been miniscule compared to the recent influence of the health food movement and its promotional strategies.

V

The decision to begin this account with an extended historical perspective was made not only because this sets a general scene, but also because we introduce many points considered later in the specific context of Bass's practice. Some readers may prefer to start with the voice of Mr. Bass (chapter 2) and return to chapter 1 prior to beginning an analysis of his practice (chapter 7). Chapter 2 illustrates Bass's oral talents and patterns of thinking, and also gives a clear sense of his geographical and social environment. Chapters 3, 4, and 5 focus on specific aspects of his life which relate to his development as an herbalist. Chapter 6 describes the extent of the practice in terms of the numbers and attitudes of his visitors. Details of his advice and herbal recommendations are covered in chapter 7, although much specific information is also found in the second volume,* which is a guide to medicinal plants. Chapter 8 serves as a summary and also reinforces and develops various points to show how Bass's practice helps illuminate traditional herbal medicine in general.

---

*Volume 2 is *A Reference Guide to Medicinal Plants: Herbal Medicine Past and Present,* which was previously published under the title *Herbal Medicine Past and Present Volume 2: A Reference Guide to Medicinal Plants.*

CHAPTER 1

Medicinal Plants and Their Traditions: A Complex of Ideas

This plant has given ease ever since time.

Much of the faith Mr. Bass and his visitors place in herbs rests on longtime beliefs as well as on such concepts as the role of sensory characteristics in determining medicinal properties. By illuminating such features, the historical perspective given in this volume provides a sense of why herbal knowledge persists with a strong cultural presence, if not force, within a popular tradition. The account as a whole also provides some explanation for the uneven persistence of knowledge about certain herbs by covering many factors ranging from changing opinions about physiological effects to the changing influence of such symbolism as life-giving properties "seen" in certain evergreen plants.

"DISCOVERING" MEDICINAL PROPERTIES

One of the most perplexing features of traditional—and regular—therapy is why so many seemingly diverse uses have been recorded for medicinal plants. Confusion arises not only because of the effects of changing theories and the introduction from time to time of new uses and regimens, but also because the same use is sometimes described from a variety of viewpoints. For example, a plant may be listed as a diuretic (function), a kidney cleanser (action), or a cure (e.g., for kidney stones). In other words, functions, actions, and uses, all closely related, may be listed together as distinct entities.[1] This has to be constantly borne in mind whenever medicinal properties are listed either in present or past use.

The beginnings of Western therapy as recorded on Mesopotamian clay tablets and Egyptian papyri, and the Greek and Roman writings by Theophrastus, Galen, Pliny, and Dioscorides are not considered here, except to note that they pose questions that are pertinent to the story of therapy in many eras. How has man learned about the medicinal properties of plants? How does he view the relations between empiricism and theory, and between popular and scientific knowledge?

Most considerations of the origins of knowledge about medicinal plants tend to stress the importance of instinct, psychological needs, and empirical observation working together over long periods of time.[2] Pertinent to this are observations on the use of plants by sick animals (a source of information Bass still believes to be very valuable) and the use of sensory properties, as discussed below.[3] Perhaps, too, man's employment of many medicinal plants for a variety of nonmedical uses has been important, for the consequent familiarity aided in learning and spreading information about medicinal properties. Nowadays, many herbalists believe that they have an almost intuitive sense of whether or not a plant is "medical."

A fascinating question about medicinal plants is why, out of the thousands that have been introduced, has only a core group of a few hundred been used within any given culture? Perhaps 200 or so plants formed the basis of the ancient materia medica; 68 made up the core of three late medieval herbals; the 680 simples included in the May edition of the celebrated 1618 London *Pharmacopoeia* are generally considered more representative of everyday practice than the 1,190 in the December issue of the same year; and about 600 medicinal plants were known or used in the United States in the 1830s. A recent survey of herbal medicines currently sold in Britain indicates that the 5,500 or so products available are derived from about 550 plants.[4]

Undoubtedly many factors contribute to the introduction of drugs, their popularity, and the length of time they remain in general use. Many botanical remedies were seemingly overenthusiastically introduced. Aside from entrepreneurship, this fervor sometimes rested on empirical grounds and sometimes on theoretical considerations, although the latter two factors are often so closely intertwined that it is commonly difficult to discern which contributes most to the acceptance or rejection of a new medicine or of a new use for an existing one.

Empiricism—observations and information gathered supposedly without theoretical presuppositions—is conspicuous in all areas of medicine. The discussion of self-treatment in chapter 4 illustrates the willingness of laypersons to try out new remedies, an attitude that seems almost timeless.[5] Laypeople have not been alone in empirically trying out recipes new to them. Countless physicians, conspicuously from the late seventeenth century onward, have stressed that the "best" medical practice rests on experience, not theory. Disputes have long been waged over the relative values of theory ("Dr. Reason," or rational medicine) and empiricism ("Dr. Tradition," or clinical experience), but even some who felt intellectually uncomfortable with empiricism have argued that, "though pregnant with evils," empirical approaches have provided many "benefits to the science of medicine."[6] Empiricism has frequently been valued on the basis that the data collected was in accord with nature, especially if it was garnered from perceptive native peoples, a viewpoint still commonplace today.

The empirical thrust—the constant search for new remedies so conspicuous in the history of medicine—is prominent in many current herbal practices. Bass, for instance, is always ready to try out a new remedy, as reflected in periodic enthusiasms. In 1981, on the advice of a Cherokee Indian, he started to use goldenrod regularly in one of his medicines for rheumatism, and in 1983 he employed wild yam for rheumatism on the basis of a newspaper article. Many of his visitors are likewise eclectic, some—even in Bass's mind—to the point of gullibility when they use certain herbs such as Solomon's seal in a "magical" way.

Empiricism in therapy relies a great deal on personal testimony that a medicine has worked. Since the late eighteenth century, and especially in recent decades, the misinterpretations that can arise from a single or relatively few instances of usage with favorable outcome have been emphasized by physicians, but commonly this has made little impression on laypeople. The notion of rigorous scientific thought is difficult for many to grasp; it seems only natural to link two closely related events as cause and effect, rather than wonder whether or not a coincidence exists. This is often seen in Bass's practice.[7]

Although empiricism and a readiness to extrapolate from one or a few positive therapeutic experiences is central to Bass's thinking, he continually draws upon theoretical concepts. In fact, when the "rampant empiricism"—as it is often called—in medicine at any time is examined closely, it is often seen to be sustained by theoretical or cultural notions. As some of the monographs in volume 2 make clear, the apparently inexplicable reputation of various plant remedies may rest more on theoretical than on empirical grounds. It is clear, too, that shifts in theories can occur without altering therapeutic practice, which sometimes suggests fundamental confidence in empiricism, sometimes excessive faith, and sometimes an inertia to change.[8]

There is no doubt that theory has played a considerable role in the enlargement of the materia medica over time within both domestic and professional medicine; indeed, it has often been the case that some new remedies that were found empirically or introduced through an erroneous concept became established only if they were theoretically acceptable to many physicians.[9]

One of the most pervasive concepts of all time, and still current today, is the humoral theory. Established in classical times, it has unquestionably shaped not only the choice of medicines but also just how they were employed for particular ailments.[10] Early humoral theory postulated that every living body was composed of four basic qualities or principles: hot, cold, moist, and dry. By a combination of these, in pairs, four humors were formed: blood (moist and hot), black bile (dry and cold), yellow bile (dry and hot), and phlegm (moist and cold). Ill health and disease were thought to rest on a lack of equilibrium of the humors, an idea which provided the basis for the employment of numerous medicaments believed to act either by possessing opposite qualities or by removing humors via, for example, urine or sweat. By the Middle Ages quantification of drug action based on degrees of qualities led to sophisticated compounded medicinal preparations with many ingredients.[11] After the seventeenth century specific references to such drug qualities as "hot," "dry," "cold," and "moist" tended to disappear from Western scientific medicine. Even so, many ideas, certainly the notions of hot and cold, persisted and can be found today in traditional medicine in many parts of the world, including Appalachia.[12]

Central to the humoral theory—and to most approaches to therapy over time—is the constant comparison of one treatment with another. Conclusions drawn from analogy always have been a key feature of medical and scientific thinking. At times these conclusions have been accepted at face value rather than serving as sources of scientific and medical hypotheses, as has generally been the case since the eighteenth century.[13]

One persistent example of the employment of analogy is the doctrine of signatures. Pervasive by the sixteenth century, this doctrine explained that the "inner virtues" of a plant (or animal) stand out if the "signature," or outer appearance, is observed carefully.[14] Some signatures are easy to discern: the yellow color of saffron suggests usefulness for jaundice, and the brainlike surface of a walnut indicates its value for head ailments. It is not easy to say how influential the doctrine actually has been. It certainly did not excite the curiosity of mankind, as is sometimes said,[15] especially after it disappeared from regular medicine during the eighteenth century, yet the doctrine is still pervasive. Viewed in either the context that God left a signature on remedies, or the context of what is called sympathetic magic ("like cures like"), examples of its use today are easy to find both in published herbals and in oral testimony ("wild ginger is good for the heart, since it looks like one").[16] Bass employs the concept more to suggest possible new uses (yellow plants can be tried for jaundice) than to rationalize existing practices.

The fully developed doctrine of signatures embraced various levels of complexity, including astrological explanations. The stars, for instance, were said to represent way stations, a sort of "halfway house," which aided virtues and powers from the ineffable, spiritual, divine being entering into material objects on Earth. In consequence, close relationships were postulated between various healing powers and the motions and activities of the stars.[17]

Although astrology plays a negligible part in Bass's thinking, he and many visitors—especially those who see unity in nature—keep an open mind about its role in herbal medicine. After all, astrology still has a pervasive influence in nonmedical facets of life (even if not openly admitted) such as knowledge and use of the signs for planting and sowing. Furthermore, the astrology widely disseminated by Culpeper's famed herbal (for example, that herbs under Venus cure, by sympathy, infirmities under Jupiter), which is known to Bass, is still commonplace in many recently published herbals.[18]

For similar reasons associated with cultural influences, nonnatural (magical) explanations probably influence Bass's practice more than is immediately apparent. Bass's visitors were often reluctant—at least initially—to discuss magical beliefs, not so much because they run counter to modern medicine, but more because many are considered "old-fashioned" and have overtones of being antireligious. Yet it became clear that magical associations, obvious with such plants as black snakeroot, Solomon's seal, and five-finger grass, are pervasive.[19] Nonnatural folk beliefs remain in people's systems; even if belief is muted, some feel—especially if "granny knew them and she lived to a ripe old age"—that it is prudent to use them, thus contributing to persistent usage.

Another long-standing concept conspicuous in Bass's thinking—more so than the doctrine of signatures—is the employment of sensory properties to determine medicinal uses. This is considered below as part of the discussion of plants naturalized in North America and used by Mr. Bass.

NATURALIZED REMEDIES: CONSTANCY AND CHANGE

Bass is well aware that many of the plants he knows have a history extending "back to the Bible" (especially "biblical hyssop") or were brought over by colonists or immigrants. In one sense, numerous naturalized remedies have the special pedigree of exotic drugs (like the Chinese rhubarb he knows), a term generally used for plants from the "East and faraway places." There is no doubt that colonial physicians relied mainly on cultivated or naturalized (i.e., introduced) plants and imported remedies (sometimes of plants already naturalized), and used only a few plants indigenous to North America.[20] The rich eighteenth-century records, such as the letters written between 1710 and 1717 by London merchant Joseph Cruttendon to customers in the New World, reveal an abundant trade in many drugs and preparations—clearly subject to seasonal problems of supply and consequent high prices—that remained popular until the late nineteenth century; others faded from general usage in consequence of revisions of the materia medica in the eighteenth century (for example, salt of vipers, surfeit water, and spirit of cockle purge).[21]

Around six hundred crude drugs and prepared medicines were generally available to eighteenth-century colonial physicians.[22] Of the principal imported medicines of that time, Bass knows or uses only a few, such as anise, asafetida, calamus, camphor, peppermint, turpentine, and storax, as well as three New World plants well established early in European medicine: sarsaparilla, sassafras, and Virginia snakeroot. During the eighteenth century, naturalized remedies already in domestic practice in the Colonies crept into regular colonial medicine rather than being imported. Of these, Bass uses apple, beech, bramble (blackberry and raspberry), catnip, clover, comfrey, dandelion, elder, ground-ivy, hyssop, mullein, oak, wild carrot, and willow. Bass knows but does not use other items employed in colonial times like calomel, cinchona bark, cinnamon, lavender water, paregoric (a preparation of opium), saffron, and sulfur.

Illustrating both late colonial reliance on European remedies and a sense of change is a serialized herbal in Christopher Sauer's Pennsylvania German almanacs published from 1762 to 1778. Two hundred and sixty-six plants, essentially selected from Theodor Zwinger's *Theatrum Botanicum*, were described. Sauer, who recognized the needs of Pennsylvania readers, did not slavishly copy Zwinger. Although he rarely cited indigenous American drugs—a few were mentioned, like Indian turnip, in the belief that they were essentially the same as European plants—Sauer recognized the availability of naturalized plants. He also indicated that some exotics could be obtained at local apothecaries' shops. It has been suggested that Sauer's selection of plants (only 19 percent of 1,418 in Zwinger's *Theatrum*) reflected those especially helpful for the diseases facing the Pennsylvanians.[23]

Other German almanac publishers—Heinrich Miller (1769–77) and Bailey (1778–89)—also included herbs. Nine plants were recorded by all three publishers, suggesting that considerable importance was attached to them. These plants (some of which are considered in the monographs in volume 2) are celery, elderberry, elecampane, fennel, greater celendine, mallow, parsley, rue, and spoonwort.[24] In fact, these were not viewed as important medicines in a first-aid sense.

They were simply alternative choices to medicines widely used in the eighteenth century. Representative of major categories popular at the time are: aloes (purgative), antimony (diaphoretic), calomel (for biliary problems), cinchona bark (a tonic and for fevers), hartshorn drops (stimulant), ipecacuanha (emetic), jalap (purgative), opium (an-algesic and for diarrhea), senna (purgative), tarter emetic (emetic and purgative), and valerian (for nerves).[25]

Many of the monographs in volume 2 illustrate the long history of naturalized plants, the changing concepts behind their use, and the waxing and waning of their popularity. Many uses listed for such "hot and dry" plants as calamus, catnip, and wild carrot were described as "deobstruent"; for instance, diuretic, emmenagogue, carminative, and for removal of humors. During the eighteenth century, many medical uses, physiologically efficacious or otherwise, of countless "hot" plants were scrutinized and reevaluated as part of a general revision of therapy motivated by a sense of professional responsibility on the part of many physicians. Some plants fell by the wayside, some disappeared from the prescriptions of doctors but remained domestic remedies, and others persisted in regular medicine, generally with a reduced range of recommended uses and made into a smaller range of medicinal preparations.[26]

The revision movement embraced a rhetoric of criticism of all "old" practices, changing fashions (for example, fading interest in distilled waters),[27] and "scientific" attitudes (or at least a basis of experience). Critical-minded and influential William Cullen (1775) said that since calamus—to give one example—is not remarkable for *aromatic* and *bitter* virtues "it has been, of late, neglected."[28] Such attitudes led another influential author, William Lewis (1791), to write: "This root is generally looked upon as a carminative and stomachic medicine, and as such is sometimes made use of in practice. . . . It was formerly an ingredient in the mithridate and theriaca of the London pharmacopoeia; and in the aromatic and stomachic tinctures, and compound arum powder of the *Edinburgh Pharmacopoeia*; but it is now rejected from these, and it does not at present enter any official preparation."[29]

Despite its decline in popularity, calamus persisted in use into this century, and many continued to emphasize its effectiveness. An occasional commentator, at least early in the nineteenth century, was enthusiastic. American William Barton (1818) said that "it is one of the most efficacious stomachics" for "dyspeptic, flatulancy, and other disorders of the stomach, and in colic," and that it deserved the attention of physicians.[30] Most American works were more circumspect, mentioning only carminative properties with occasional reference to sudorific and tonic actions.[31] Calamus is still used, despite a ban on its sale by the U.S. Food and Drug Administration (FDA). Mr. Bass employs it modestly as a carminative, in contrast to the smorgasbord of uses with little historical pedigree often found in today's herbal advocacy literature, generally the result of indiscriminate garnering of all reputed uses—some theoretical—from past literature.

Many naturalized plants employed by Bass were once considered "cold and dry" (e.g., oak) and, less frequently, as "temperate and dry" (e.g., mullein) rather than hot and dry. Such properties as cold, dry, and temperate were correlated with certain uses, often binding or astringent. Uses like treating sore throats with astringent botanicals are accepted today as having an empirical basis, whereas such other actions as the management of menorrhagia apparently had a justification based primarily on theory or analogy.[32] The practices of today's herbalists still reflect a mixture of empiricism and theory, the latter accounting for both the origin and continuance of certain uses. Bass generally is far more in line with empirical usage than many herbalists who have acquired much of their knowledge through schools of herbal medicine.

THE ROLE OF SENSORY PROPERTIES

Mullein (temperate and dry) is relatively bland, with no overt sensory properties apart from a mucilaginous chewing gum-like quality. Plants with bland properties, like the almost tasteless chickweed, became less widely used in the eighteenth and nineteenth centuries and generally declined in popularity more quickly than such aromatic plants as catnip. In suggesting why the mildness of the plant contributed to its decline in popularity, some comments are appropriate on the plant qualities of hot, dry, cold, and moist—so conspicuous in Gerard's *Herball* and other discussions on medicinal plants at the time—and how these were thought to correlate with medical properties, ideas very pertinent to Mr. Bass's practice today.

There is some debate on whether the four qualities are based on observable sensory properties (e.g., the hotness of mustard) or primarily on theoretical ideas in accord with the general concept of humors described above. One commentator has argued recently, largely based on a study of sixteenth-century herbals, that the qualities were empirically derived from the taste of a plant: hot from a bitter taste, dry from sourness, and moist from sweetness, while cold was a theoretical concept or perhaps linked with an appreciation of poison causing death.[33] Such a viewpoint has much to offer but may give insufficient attention to the fact that a considerable matrix of factors has been at play in characterizing medicinal plants, including smell.

While the study of the effects of sensory properties on the body is, in many ways, in its infancy, one can speculate that plants produce physiological effects through stimulation of the taste buds. Any understanding of the past use of sensory properties has to consider that observations on the range of tastes were probably interpreted to fit prevailing theory. We suggest that since there were only four components of matter—earth, air, fire, and water—only four taste categories emerged. Different shades of taste, more than the well-known sweet, sour, salt, and bitter (all of which perhaps form a continuum), were therefore accommodated into the four qualities hot, cold, dry, and moist.[34] Additionally, observed pharmacological actions were often rationalized in the same manner. John Gerard and others associated particular qualities with specific medicinal effects (see, for example, "Mustard" and "Puffball" in volume 2).

A discussion of the early story of sensory properties and associated medical uses in classical times is unnecessary here, but it is important to understand that the employment of sensory characteristics to ascertain or rationalize medical actions continued within the framework of regular medicine until well into the nineteenth century, and persists within alternative medicine today.

In terms of colonial medicine, John Floyer's *Touchstones of Medicines* is an appropriate starting point among many others, including ideas on the most effective odors—sweet or sharp—to purify the air. Floyer, who subsequently established a considerable medical reputation, saw himself building on past knowledge found in the writings of Hippocrates, Dioscorides, and Galen. But, no longer bound by Galenic concepts of four humors and four basic elements of matter, he consciously went beyond describing plant properties solely in terms of hot, cold, moist, and dry.[35] From his own experiences he widened the sensory categories to be considered in determining medicinal properties and included compound tastes to identify the constituents, and hence properties, of plants. ("The most simple principles of plants [do not have] one simple mode or affection [e.g., watery, earthy, oily, and acid] but two or more depending on their motion and texture.") Floyer focused on the acerbic, acrid, aromatic, astringent, austere, bitter, fetid, mucilaginous, nauseous, nitrose, pungent, and sweet.[36] He once wrote:

> God has given us our senses whereby, with the help of experiments we can discern the virtues of all our medicines. By their tastes and smells we know their qualities: hot medicines which accelerate our circulations, and all the cold tastes which stop the velocity of it and the secretions. . . . Plants which have mixed tastes have mixed principles. We cure diseases by contrary tastes. The watery, acid, styptic and mucilaginous tastes correct the bitter, salt and acrid humours, by cooling and diluting them; and the acrid, bitter, salt and sweet correct mucilaginous humour by fermenting, incising and attenuating of them.[37]

In many ways Floyer's approach provides merely another way of explaining uses recorded in Gerard's *Herball*. For instance, Floyer's comments on calamus echo Gerard's views on deobstruent action: "The aromatick weed: The roots taste bitterish, with an aromatick taste and smell, by which it discusses wind. It is cordial and provokes urine and works as an aromatick. It favours something of balsamick turpentine." [38] Even if Floyer's work essentially reexplained existing practices, his influence and enthusiasm must not be underestimated.

One of the most influential eighteenth-century writers on materia medica, both for Europeans and Americans, was Edinburgh's William Cullen (1710–1783). When discussing his own belief in the value of ascertaining sensory properties, he made clear his indebtedness to Floyer as well as to "David Abercrombie, Hoffman and several others." He did not specifically mention the celebrated Linnaeus, whose confidence in sensory properties unquestionably influenced him.[39] Cullen referred to sensory properties throughout his writings on materia medica. He wrote, for instance, that, "in general, a stimulant virtue is discovered by a strong impression on our senses." [40] On the other hand, he wrote explicitly that "the want of odor or taste" suggests the absence of medicinal virtue. The difficulty, he said, "is to ascertain the degree," and he added that substances which did not affect or hardly affected taste or smell should be considered "inert and useless," and thus be rejected from the materia medica. (Exceptions were a few "of a nourishing, emollient or demulcent quality.")[41] When Cullen described chickweed as a mild, "insipid plant," he added that it is ranked "sometimes as astringent, sometimes as emollient, but in either intention its virtues are inconsiderable."[42]

Interestingly, "neutral" plants have never been conspicuous in medicine, and they declined in numbers during the eighteenth century. The relatively small number of such plants (commonly foods) in present-day traditional medicine in certain regions has occasioned considerable discussion—often without historical context—on how much acculturation has occurred in particular societies.[43]

Although J. Schoepf included plants he supposed, judging by smell or taste, to have medical properties in his influential *Materia Medica Americana* (1787), doubts over identifying properties through sensory characteristics were emerging. This was partly a result of numerous eighteenth-century studies on the effects of drugs on the body and partly due to a growing appreciation that the sensory properties did not always correlate with new information on constituents.[44] James Murray in 1815 indicated that many instances of "obscurity and error" undermined any extensive application of the idea: "The different tastes and odors are so little reducible to precise definition or description, that few general rules can be formed by them."[45]

Emphasis on the value of taste and smell was pushed to one side as more and more active principles of plants and new chemical remedies, characterized on chemical rather than sensory grounds, were introduced after the 1820s. Indeed, the enthusiasm associated with the discovery of many alkaloids in the 1820s, along with new concepts in physiology and pharmacology, served to focus much interest on plant remedies, but from new viewpoints.[46] Even so, significant interest in sensory properties persisted for a while. C. S. Rafinesque, for instance, in his *Medical Flora, or Manual of Medical Botany of the United States of North America* (1828–30) said that the most obvious indication of medicinal properties of plants arose from the evidence of sensible properties. For example: (1) nauseous-tasting plants are narcotics, emetics, cathartics, and antispasmodics; (2) acrid-tasting plants are salivatories and stimulants; (3) bitter-tasting plants are tonic and corroborant; (4) acerbic plants are astringents and diuretics; and (5) insipid plants are emollients, demulcents, and diluents. He also advocated the helpfulness of the sense of feeling, such as coolness (refrigerants), heat (stimulant and rubefacient), and stinging (external stimulants).[47]

Although the importance placed on sensory properties diminished in the nineteenth century, it remains conspicuous in Bass's practice, both in his own thinking and among those who visit him. In fact, he appreciates clearly the following associations listed by Murray in 1815,[48] some, from today's perspective, based more on theory than on an empirical basis:

Property	Taste
astringency	styptic
tonic	bitter
stimulants	aromatics
narcotics	fetid

Bass has an acute sense of smell, and he describes many plants by their odor (mayapple "has a medicinal powerful odor," and pokeroot "an obnoxious odor"). He also readily employs sensory characteristics to suggest that a plant he has not seen before might have medicinal properties, just as he believes a local physician, Dr. Matthews, did in the 1920s.[49] Above all, Bass employs sensory properties to rationalize the existing reputations of many plants. For example, "all bitter medicines are tonics"; "bitter medicines are good for the liver"; "all astringent medicines are good for rheumatism" and as styptics and to control diarrhea; "all fetid medicines are good for the nerves"; and the "stronger the smell, the stronger the medicine." Bass also argues that plant analysis helps us to understand why sensory properties are so important; he gives the example (one accepted as correct) that all barks have an astringent taste because of their tannin content.[50]

INDIGENOUS REMEDIES

The pervasive role of analogy in Bass's thinking serves as an appropriate bridge to comment on North American indigenous plants—

how they entered therapy, how they arose to popularity (commonly within regular medicine), and why many had lost or were losing favor by the end of the nineteenth century, although they remain the core of much herbal practice today. The story of indigenous remedies is of special interest because only a few established a place in medical practice overseas, and these provide a distinctive picture of medicine in the United States, at least throughout the nineteenth century.[51] The following comments do not raise new concepts that lie behind Bass's practice, but instead bring a better appreciation of botanical medicine of the recent past and how it reached and influenced modern herbal practice with overtones of nationalism and the special value placed on native remedies.

The extensive employment of indigenous remedies in the nineteenth century has two interrelated origins: usage by American Indians and usage by colonists, who sometimes incorporated (perhaps with some modifications) Indian knowledge. Early colonial writings and other evidence suggest that most Indian tribes had a substantial knowledge of indigenous medicinal plants before colonization —knowledge acquired through instinct, empirical observation, and concepts of disease based on sorcery, breach of taboo, disease object intrusion, spirit intrusion, and soul loss.[52] Nevertheless, the extent of the early impact of Indian knowledge on settlers remains uncertain.[53]

Two considerations prevent a precise understanding of Indian influence. One is whether or not drugs were always used for their pharmacological actions; certainly, on occasion, magical concepts had a hand in determining drug use. Second, even assuming physiological effectiveness behind reputed uses, the generally late recording of Indian knowledge in any substantial amount—mostly during the nineteenth and twentieth centuries—probably includes much information already transmitted from colonists to Indians.[54] Even early writers such as John Josselyn (1672) and John Clayton (1687) implied transmission when they referred to plantain as Englishman's foot: "As to our plantain . . . it was never known before the English came into this country."[55] Furthermore, the many uses commonplace in white medicine which were listed in well-known nineteenth-century root and herb "Indian doctor" literature suggest white influence rather than basic Indian knowledge or even separate discoveries. Regular medical writings, from the nineteenth century and other times, which attribute early knowledge of medicinal plants to Indians generally provide no documented evidence and frequently reflect an uncritical attitude toward Indian knowledge.

Questions about the extent of Indian influence have to consider that colonists were not so dependent on Indian knowledge of plants as is frequently supposed. Immigrants, for instance, even found a few species of medicinal plants common to North America and Britain (e.g., *Geum rivale, Viburnum triloba,* and *Cerastium alpinum*)[56] alongside a larger number of indigenous species closely allied or analogous to those in Europe. Furthermore, plants brought by early colonists often naturalized quickly in the absence of competition from American flora in the disturbed and cultivable ground left after woodland vegetation was cleared.

In learning about indigenous plants, colonists often "determined" their medicinal value on the basis of physical appearance, sensory properties, and analogies to those already known in Europe. Then, experiences of using the indigenous plants (e.g., tag-alder) might confirm the presumed medical properties. Insight from analogy appears in the writings of Josselyn (1672) and James Petiver (1699).[57] Petiver did not mention sensory characters, but they are implicit in his conjecture that botanical characteristics provide clues to medicinal properties.

While the overall impact of Indian knowledge is, we believe, often overrated, undoubtedly a few drugs were introduced into regular medicine, and more into domestic practice. Depending on their attitudes toward Indians, some whites were attracted to Indian remedies more than others and expressed their interest in print or personally. George Swain, writing from Asheville, North Carolina, on 26 January 1810 about how he acquired medical skills, commented:

> I never intended to do anything in respect to venereal complaints as there was a poor man in the Country who had sufficient skill in roots and plants to treat slight infections very well and as I had fortunately procur'd a knowledge of a useful plant from the Indians (*Veronica virginiana*), which I added to his stock of knowledge. I flatter'd myself that his specifics would be competent to almost any case. But I miscalculated on the efficacy of these plants and have been oblig'd to assist him in a number of instances of gonnorhoea with mercurials.[58]

Amid many such episodes, it has been suggested that no more than about seventeen remedies were adopted from Indian practice into mainstream regular medical use; these include bloodroot, boneset, cascara, lobelia, pinkroot, sassafras, senega, Virginia snakeroot, wintergreen, and witch hazel.[59] Some less-popular plants and Indian regimens entered domestic medicine, especially for difficult-to-manage ailments. The problem of treating wounds (doing more than merely applying plants externally) was one area where Indian success was often mentioned. But this was sometimes no more than reinforcing employment of some plants already understood within the framework of Western medicine (e.g., tulip tree); sometimes the reinforcement seems to rest on common interest in sensory characters to determine medicinal value and notions akin to the doctrine of signatures.

The extent of black influence on white medicine is no more certain than Indian contributions. Bass does not believe that he has learned much from blacks, which seemingly reflects little general impact on white medicine, despite some specific influences. Bloodroot is still popular among blacks who visit Bass, as are Virginia snakeroot, Jerusalem artichoke, boneset, and cotton root, all discussed in the monographs in volume 2.[60]

EMERGING POPULARITY OF INDIGENOUS REMEDIES

Interest in indigenous North American plants is part of the early pioneer story. Certainly it was part of the sixteenth-century exploration of what is now the Virginia and North Carolina coasts. French efforts at colonization (including early Canada) are also part of the story, which involves the possible role of French apothecary Louis Hébert, who sent North American plants to Paris at the beginning of the seventeenth century. Although the use of some indigenous remedies became commonplace in the late seventeenth and early eighteenth centuries, a more general enthusiasm did not emerge until after 1750.[61] Many instances of this deepening interest can be cited.[62] In 1761 a survey of native medicinal plants was undertaken at the Moravian settlement at Bethabara, North Carolina, where European plants were dominant in the medical garden. Among the plants and their effects noted were squashweed for rheumatism, milkweed for pleurisy, Indian physic for fevers, and Robin's plantain, a snakeroot, and marsh holly as valuable antidotes.[63]

Over the next few decades momentum emerged as more and more writers described American indigenous plants. Jefferson, Schoepf, and others at the time both encouraged and reflected a growing sense of nationalism that helped shape interest in American remedies.[64] This was sharpened by such writings as William Currie's *Historical Account of the Climates and Remedies and Methods of Treatment* (1793), which focused attention on the view that the environment produced diseases unknown in Europe. Belief was growing in a sentiment, succinctly expressed later, that "our young practioners [should] be made acquainted with the diseases of our country, and not rely altogether upon foreign authors."[65]

A distinctive feature of American therapy that was emerging around 1800, fostered by nationalist sentiments, was "heroic" treatment. This is especially significant in the story of plant remedies, because botanical movements owed some of their success to their use as alternative approaches. Benjamin Rush—a prime figure in establishing heroic treatment—decided, during the yellow fever outbreaks in Philadelphia during the 1790s, that letting massive amounts of blood and administering large doses of calomel and jalap was an effective treatment. This interventionist approach ultimately received considerable support, and it was applied to manage many other medical problems.

Concurrent with heroic therapy, interest in indigenous plant remedies mushroomed within regular medicine. Benjamin Smith Barton's influential short work entitled *Collections for an Essay towards a Materia Medica of the United-States* (1798) accomplished much of his intention to extend knowledge of the medicinal properties of the "indigenous vegetables of the United States . . . beyond the labours of the Bartrams, Colden, Kalm and Schoepf." It listed eighty-nine plants, of which more than sixty found an established place in practice. By the time of the last edition of Barton's essay (1810), the many component threads of the nationalistic interest in indigenous remedies were each shaping the preferences of certain physicians. These components included: (1) patriotic sentiments for the new nation; (2) the wish to be economically independent of the large quantities of drugs imported from Europe; (3) the belief that valuable new drugs were to be found in the American flora (perhaps already discovered by the Indians), reflecting the view that God had planted medicinal plants for American diseases in America; and (4) the general concern for improving medicine, sometimes allied with the opinion that much of the European literature was redundant for the American scene.[66]

Although the nationalist thrust of interest in indigenous remedies was cemented by a blossoming of texts written between 1812 and 1824 by W. P. C. Barton, Jacob Bigelow, N. Chapman, and others, evidence from prescriptions and other sources suggests that the popular European remedies mentioned earlier were still commonplace within regular medical practice. However, estimates of interest have to take into account patients' demands not always registered in prescriptions. When physician James Mease reported in 1806 on the effective use of *Geranium maculatum* for hemorrhage, he noted that a patient's father had suggested its use after having learned about it from "one of the aborigenes of our country."[67] The eclectic approach to therapy of many laypeople unquestionably influenced the practice of many physicians, as illustrated in some of the plant monographs in volume 2.[68]

Apart from interest in Indian remedies, other forces encouraged popular interest in native plants. Influential in the first half of the nineteenth century was Samuel Thomson (1769–1843), the founder of the Thomsonian botanic practice of medicine. The influence of Thomsonianism—for example, Thomson's learning about herbs from the oral tradition (reminiscent of Mr. Bass) and the use of a core of remedies of which the most popular were lobelia, cayenne pepper, and steam baths—is well known. Undoubtedly Thomsonianism, which can be seen as a grass-roots movement reflective of many social, religious, and medical currents, contributed to a close questioning and criticism of many regular medical practices (including heroic therapy) as well as reinforcing the usage of many botanicals then being established as medicines in professional and lay practice.[69]

Other less conspicuous botanical movements existed concurrent with Thomsonianism. One unorganized group of practitioners was "Indian root and herb doctors." While little is known of these practitioners—even whether or not most of them were Indians or how many had itinerant practices—a collective influence emerged through publications. Notable was Peter Smith's *Indian Doctor's Dispensatory* (1813). Smith was somewhat eclectic in his sources of information (they included, for instance, Indians and Culpeper's seventeenth-century herbal), and he took exception to current usage of calomel. He focused on simples (e.g., "the home ipecacuanha," or "Indian physic," and scurvy grass root) rather than the "medicine of the shops." While just how much original Indian knowledge such publications contained is not clear, they encouraged the view that much could be learned from the Indians—a view still widely held in modern herbalism.[70]

THE HEYDAY AND DECLINE OF
INDIGENOUS REMEDIES

It is appropriate to consider the first *United States Pharmacopoeia*, published in 1820, not only as a milestone in the institutionalization of American medicine and pharmacy but also as a culmination of the initial period of enthusiasm for indigenous remedies.[71] The philosophy of the *Pharmacopoeia* and its subsequent revisions cemented the twin approaches of critically appraising the materia medica and paying special attention to indigenous remedies as part of the overall search for new remedies. A secondary list in the early pharmacopoeias included indigenous botanicals of uncertain reputation. The editors "preferred to swell the subordinate rather than the primary catalogue, especially as this arrangement will most likely prompt further investigations into the character of the substances in question."[72]

The number of overseas and indigenous botanicals included in nineteenth-century editions of the *U.S. Pharmacopeia* (and the "companion" dispensatories) was on the order of five hundred. Much of the ongoing investigations into these plants—by physician-naturalists and a growing number of pharmacists—can be seen as part of a Baconian thrust, the gathering of large amounts of data with the hope of advancing American science and medicine. This approach helped to show that assessing the activity of medicines from effects on a single or a few patients only can be misleading. In consequence, doubts —reflected in many spirited debates—were raised over the value of many remedies and existing therapeutic regimens; doubts also were fostered by the introduction of countless new remedies such as iodine, iron salts, bromides, organic analgesics, antitoxins, and vaccines with the argument that they were superior to existing drugs.

Also contributing to lessening confidence in botanical remedies were physiological theories which sharpened critical thinking by raising disagreement between those practitioners who placed their greatest confidence in an empirical approach to medicine and those who felt strongly that therapy had to rest on a "rational" approach. H. E. Wood (1874) expressed the sense of confusion in therapy with only a little exaggeration, saying that scarcely anything had been established beyond the "primary facts that quinine will arrest an intermittent, that salts will purge and that opium will quiet pain or lull to sleep." He complained too that the profession "clings to established therapeutic facts as with the heart and hand of one man, clings with a desperation and unanimity whose intensity is the measure of the unsatisfied desire for something fixed."[73]

Wood's remarks on rheumatism—one of his examples of therapeutic discord—are pertinent to our discussion of the ailment in chapter 7. "In this disease, bleeding, nitrate of potash, quinine, mercurials, flying blisters, purgation, opium, the bromides, veratria, and a host of other remedies, all have their advocates clamorous of a hearing, and above all the tumult are to be heard the trumpet-tones of a Chambers, 'Wrap your patients in blankets and let them alone.' "

Amidst a milieu of rapid change during the last decades of the nineteenth century—which embraced an emphasis on "scientific" medicine—and partly in response to the therapeutic confusion and hopes for a "new" therapeutics based on evaluations from animal studies, an emerging defensiveness over employing botanical remedies—indigenous and foreign—can be sensed; or at least a difference in views between older physicians and the younger ones reared on the newer chemical remedies becomes apparent. Thomas Hill, for instance, when talking to the Medical Society of North Carolina in 1894 on the indigenous materia medica, said that as an old physician who had practiced medicine for forty years, he was advising the younger members of the profession to pay more attention to the study of botany and to keep their eyes and ears open in order to "frequently get some valuable hints from humble and unexpected sources."[74]

Revision of the 1890 *United States Pharmacopoeia* illustrates the debate and tension of the time. Generally well-regarded remedies such as cimicifuga, dogwood, and magnolia were retained or discarded according to a vote of members of the revision committee, which was far from unanimous.[75] Defensiveness toward existing therapies was, as it still is, generally interpreted as medical conservatism or the inertia of tradition. While this was undoubtedly true at times, many practitioners preferred to continue to rely on experience and the tried-and-tested remedies.

Yet the attitudes toward herbal remedies and their uses at the end of the nineteenth century were not entirely negative. Many factors were working to sustain an interest in botanical remedies among some physicians. There were regional considerations encouraging interest, such as the nationalist spirit and interest in local remedies generated in the South during the Civil War and postbellum period, but more general influences were probably of greater significance. The Thomsonian movement had been in eclipse since the 1850s, although threads of its practice persisted through the century (indeed, it is still noticeable at the present time) to sustain much herbal practice.[76] As Thomsonianism declined from its heyday, two other groups of botanic practitioners emerged, the neo-Thomsonsians and the Eclectics. Both groups arose from disillusioned members of the largely uneducated and evangelical Thomsonian practice who sought survival in "scientific respectability."

While some neo-Thomsonian botanical works published during the transition in the 1840s and 1850s influenced later writers, the long-lasting Eclectic Reform movement had the greatest influence.[77] It is, in fact, still a force in certain facets of herbal medicine today, particularly among practitioners of naturopathy. Mr. Bass recollects hearing about Eclectic doctors during the 1920s, a time when Eclectic practice was still noticeably active with an institutional backbone of books, journals, medical colleges, and state organizations in place. Eclectic practitioners were always relatively small in numbers compared with regular physicians—in 1900 there were perhaps 9,500 Eclectics, versus 73,000 regular physicians. Although these figures have to be treated cautiously, the Eclectics' influence was pervasive.[78]

Eclectics, who accepted many aspects of regular medical practice but maintained a botanical emphasis in treatments, viewed themselves as reformers who aimed to create a "distinctively American practice of medicine."[79] John Uri Lloyd, the widely respected pharmacist and promoter of Eclectic medicine, said in 1924 that "eclecticism . . . made a specialty of introducing American drugs to replace the foreign equivalents and this stand [of] the Eclectic school, to which I have stood committed for over forty years, has [been] maintained ever since that day." Other facets of eclecticism, which combined traditionalism with its nationalism, were its antinarcotic and wholistic approaches. According to Lloyd, "Prescriptions are not made for the name of the disease, but . . . for the patient, according to the conditions and symptoms he presents. They deal directly with the individual affected. We make no specific cures for named diseases." "The action of a drug, in disease, is often very different to what it is in health." Also noteworthy is the Eclectics' emphasis on empiricism. Various Eclectic leaders reminded practitioners of the role of Indians in establishing the importance of indigenous remedies.

While the precise impact on the general public and on regular medicine of a hundred years or so of Eclecticism is difficult to assess, it was hardly negligible. Many Eclectic practitioners established cordial relationships with regular practitioners and forged fruitful and influential community roles. All this helped to retain some focus on indigenous remedies, which were still conspicuous in the early twentieth century when over two hundred botanicals still had some place in medical practice.[80] Significant, too, was the impetus to research that Eclectic practice provoked; this contributed to the widespread employment of such plants as *Mahonia aquifolium, Eriodictyon* spp., and *Rhamnus purshiana* within regular medical practice.[81] Eclectic publications were also important. While the numerous editions of John King's *American Eclectic Dispensatory* carried essentially the same information on particular plants as did textbooks of regular medicine, Eclectic writers were less prone than regular physicians to revise existing information, while some twentieth-century Eclectic textbooks promoted new concepts and uses unacceptable to regular physicians. The Eclectic influence remains today in some popular herbals, including Meyer's *The Herbalist*, a favorite with Mr. Bass. On the other hand, some Eclectic publications contribute to differences between Bass's practice and those of some naturopathic practitioners who use Eclectic publications as basic texts.[82]

Other factors contributing to the popularity of indigenous remedies during the nineteenth century also merit mention. Herb dealers were still a significant force. Shaker communities, which gathered, cultivated, and vigorously marketed herbs and medicines, were a major influence. A nationalistic spirit was often present, as proclaimed on the cover of an 1830 herb catalog:[83] "Why send to Europe's bloody shores / For plants which grow by our own doors?" Notes from Shaker catalogs and from herb dealers who both competed with and did business with the Shakers are included in relevant monographs in volume 2. One of these dealers was C. J. Cowle, who developed a substantial business in the North Carolina Appalachians between the 1840s and 1870s. Among the indigenous botanicals he often promoted was Bowman's root (see volume 2), following a favorable article in the *American Journal of Pharmacy*; "Can such a valuable medicine be longer neglected?"[84]

Much more influential in the last decades of the last century and into the present one were budding pharmaceutical manufacturing companies such as the Detroit firm of Parke-Davis and Eli Lilly of Indianapolis. They marketed considerable numbers of indigenous herbs and the medicines prepared from them. These were used within Eclectic and regular practices, and reached country stores like the Mackey store in Leesburg, which served the Bass family. Both companies did a great deal to promote interest in botanicals in general. Parke-Davis provided support for the botanist-explorer H. H. Rusby, and Eli Lilly hired the company's first botanist and established the Lilly Botanical Department in 1890. As a start in developing a reference collection of drugs, six thousand botanicals were obtained from a North Carolina collector.[85] Both companies published invaluable catalogs. Though these were oriented to the medical and pharmaceutical professions, it seems clear that the use of the products contributed to the popular tradition.

Yet another thread in the story of botanical medicines is the practice of homeopathic medicine. Developed largely by Austrian physician Samuel Hahnemann (1755–1843), homeopathy, which employs minute quantities of drugs in treatment, is rationalized on vitalistic concepts of physiology. Homeopathic practice achieved considerable popularity in nineteenth-century America, and a number of indigenous remedies became incorporated into its practice. How much this helped to popularize indigenous plants in general is very difficult to say, especially as opinions supporting the influence of homeopathy generally go beyond accepted scientific evidence.

The last decades of the nineteenth century thus witnessed contradictory trends in therapy, but overall there was a decline in the reputation of many botanicals. Even by 1870 discussions appeared in medical journals on "obsolete materia medica," which included "many
trivial medicines which survive among the vulgar."[86] In the twentieth
century this trend has included an increasingly clear distinction between regular medicine and many facets of self-care, a topic discussed
later.

REGULAR THERAPY AND HERBAL MEDICINE

Because of the distinction seen nowadays between regular medicine
and much self-care, we must avoid the danger of seeing herbs and the
issues raised by their use as exclusive to the popular tradition. This
account can be viewed as part of the growing interest in seeing how
therapeutics has shaped medicine as a whole. One recent writer, for
instance, interprets trends in nineteenth-century therapeutic practices among American physicians as a way for physicians to define the
boundaries of their profession in an era before regulation existed.[87]
This is not the place to debate this intriguing interpretation, which
has to be considered in the context of the overall roles of physicians
(making diagnoses, treating, and offering prognoses and support) and
the value placed by the public on physicians' general experience. Just
as relevant is a consideration of therapies practiced by physicians
and those undertaken by laypeople. In fact, despite some obvious differences (particularly in certain hospitals), there was much overlap,
especially as treatment embraced much more than drugs (diet, for instance), and patients often had much input into their treatment as a
whole.

Many of the details in the present account illustrate various characteristics of therapeutics undertaken within the framework of professional and sectarian medical care as well as self-care. These include
persistence of concepts amid apparent change (historical antecedents
for most of Bass's opinions can be found) as well as numerous contradictory views. The story of therapy is beset by conflict—especially
noticeable in times of fairly rapid change in medical thinking such
as occurred during the last decades of the nineteenth century and

the early twentieth century—and various examples of seemingly idiosyncratic usage are indicated in volume 2 amid consensus opinions about principal uses. But, above all, this account provides a constant reminder that in any consideration of therapeutic effectiveness, personal attitudes may be no less significant than science and its concern with theory and standardized medicines.

CHAPTER 2

"I've Always Got By": The Voice
of a Modern Herbalist

INTRODUCTION

F olks have called me a backwoodsman or a mountain man, and
I tell them I'm a hillbilly without a guitar," says Mr. A. L.
Tommie Bass of Leesburg in Cherokee County, northeast Alabama. As he stands on the stoop of his homemade shack in the
southern reaches of the Appalachians, it is easy for him to recall his
memories. His rural setting—the woods and fields that he considers
his own big garden—is much the same as when he was a young man
living in Mackey, long since a rural route of the Leesburg post office.
The western view is one of variety and contrasts. A mile away, across
cultivated fields in the broad Coosa Valley, are the bluffs and escarp-
ment of Lookout Mountain overlooking Shinbone Ridge. The valley
is a patchwork of cotton, corn, and sorghum fields, wooded creeks,
roads, and a few scattered buildings. Before 1961 the Coosa River
meandered through the valley. Since then, Lake Weiss, which was
created by damming the river near Leesburg, dominates the scene.
The lake comes within half a mile of Mr. Bass's home and covers the
lowlands and the broad bends of the riverbed.

If, in his late seventies (he was born in 1908), memories form a
large part of Bass's life, he also remains an active herbalist. Although
since 1983 he has gathered and dug fewer plants from the woods and
fields than he once did, he still is constantly asked for advice and is
always ready to share the accumulated knowledge of his lifetime.

This chapter outlines facets of Bass's life, using extensive verbatim quotations from his recollections which reveal many insights into his background and character. We have omitted much from his story, giving precedence to topics that help with an understanding of his success as an herbal practitioner.

Tommie Bass's story raises questions about how some of his views and his reputation as an herbalist have been shaped by his innate character, his upbringing as the eldest son in a large family, his surroundings, and various social factors. Unfortunately, determining the relative importance of each factor in what can be called his socialization as an herbalist is impossible, although some obviously are more significant than others. Bass's personality is marked by thriftiness, skills at story telling, a tendency to demean himself which borders on an inferiority complex, a transparent honesty and uncritical readiness to accept a person's word (sometimes to the point of gullibility), and a readiness to offer a helping hand to all who need it. Although they reflect his personality, these traits have been shaped, directed, and reinforced by his family and social circumstances.

Along with three brothers and two sisters (born between 1911 and 1924), Bass had an upbringing full of hard times and constant chores. Both parents left an indelible imprint on him. His father, an undoubted patriarch and strict disciplinarian, taught him to earn a livelihood by working at a variety of jobs. Mrs. Bass tempered the strict discipline and, although constantly at work feeding and clothing the family, always made time for the children. She is remembered as almost flawless, able to run a large family without fuss and to organize the children's household and outside jobs. That children's games and festivities are not especially well remembered reflects, Bass says, hard times.

Bass relates that the family was viewed as different from others in the Mackey-Leesburg community. As recent arrivals from Tennessee, they were unlike the long-settled Coosa Valley planters, the third- and fourth-renters (who paid a third or fourth of their crop for rent), or the sharecroppers, who owed half of their crops to the landlord. Furthermore, the Basses did not depend on cotton for their livelihood; and certainly, unlike many, they were not bootleggers. They relied on truck farming, trapping, timbering, and a range of selling and buying activities. This ensured not only developing many acquaintances, but also avoiding poverty amid the difficult social and economic circumstances of the 1920s and 1930s.

Many of Bass's characteristics and habits of self-sufficiency (embracing a fear of dependence, a spirit of nationalism, and belief in the right to carry a gun), a strong work ethic, and a sense of fatalism reflect not only Appalachian mountain culture but also the self-sufficient lives of small farmers in the upland South. In many ways people in the area, a geographic overlap of Appalachian and deep southern cultures, were neither mountaineers nor lowland southerners because they were not isolated. They depended largely on small farms and a credit system dominated by cotton.

Bass's recollections highlight change in the region and how he sidestepped much of it. His many skills, developed by the time he was a young man, ensured his ready integration into the community, and he did not leave the area in 1937 when the rest of the family were enticed into Georgia by industrial wages. By staying and exercising his variety of skills, Bass has been an onlooker to the dissolution of many customs and habits in the face of "industrial progress."

Social and economic struggles and changes in the southern Appalachians have been subject to scrutiny in recent years, and conflicting opinions exist about the causes and their impacts. Issues that have vexed commentators include the extent of modernization amid traditionalism, the supposed inability of the Appalachian people to understand modern society, impoverishment, and class conflicts. These issues are not dealt with directly here, but such considerations as the amount of discernible stress caused by these conditions are grist to the discussions.

Whatever the influences these factors have had on Bass, much of the fascination he arouses lies in the differences people see in him compared with others in his community. In addition to his herbal activities, other factors contribute to his appeal and distinctiveness. His personal habits, often mentioned by those who know him, include a spartan life-style—extending to teetotalism—his cluttered shack and yard, his oral talents, by which he weaves lengthy monologues around jokes and local stories, and his rich storehouse of information. A more diligent observer also notes his ability and willingness to undertake a wide range of jobs such as sharpening saws and skinning animals, skills which have allowed him to stay outside the main sources of employment in his community—light industry and full-time farming.

People ask Mr. Bass if he has special powers of healing. Strenuously denying this, he claims that the help he gives people rests solely on the herbs. Not everyone agrees, if only because of the charisma they see in him. The charisma, for some, lies in finding so many diverse features in a single individual whose life-style is such a contrast to their own. For other people, however, Bass's charisma is indefinable and more than the sum of his complex personality and his range of talents. People see him differently according to their backgrounds, attitudes to health professions, and, perhaps most important of all, their relations with him and just how much of himself he reveals to them. Some consider that just listening to him is therapeutic. Many verbatim quotations are included throughout the present account, but here his voice is given free rein, as Bass so often does for visitors.

"I CAN'T QUIT JABBERING": RECOLLECTIONS

Bass loves to talk about his early years. He relates how in 1917 his family, after many homes in previous years, moved to the Lookout Mountain area of Cherokee County, where he has lived ever since. His father had been told that, with its wooded creeks, it was a good area for fur dealing. The Basses settled first near Slackland, where they grew vegetables in the narrow Owl's Hollow between Lookout Mountain and Shinbone Ridge. After less than a year they had to move because they resisted the landlord's requirement for growing cotton. However, after moving to the side of Lookout Mountain, they found once again that they had to grow cotton to rent a house. Eventually they homesteaded on the side of Lookout Mountain, where young Tommie spent more and more time clearing land and utilizing its resources as well as truck farming and peddling. Bass was introduced to herbs early, at a time "when nearly everyone used them."

> Back in my boyhood days, when I was growing up, back to somewhere along 1918, nearly everybody used herbs, the common people, sharecroppers—black and white—and the old doctors. One doctor here in Cherokee County, Alabama, a famous old-time doctor, gathered medicines from all over. One of his main medicines was black snakeroot.

Mother didn't make many medicines, but the one I remember most was the cough remedy. She used wild cherry bark, mullein, honey or sorghum molasses or sugar, and a little lemon and pepper. And it didn't tear up your stomach.

My great-grandparents brought a recipe for salve from England. Mother would make it for the family and a few neighbors. Sometimes she'd sell it at fifty cents a jar. She'd make it by boiling the jimsonweed leaves to cook out the fluid. Then she'd add the hog lard, yellow sulfur, and sometimes a bit of homemade tobacco. I use the formula in making my salve, but I've added several more ingredients which make it much better. People didn't like the greasiness and odor.

I remember going in the woods in 1914 or 1915 with my father and mother. Went on a north slope of Lookout Mountain, looking for herbs. There was a big slippery elm tree there. Peeled off some of the bark and was chewing it. Walking around, I found a stalk of ginseng. I never will forget how surprised Dad and Mother was. I can just barely remember being in the woods, and them saying, "Tommie, it is ginseng!" Dad didn't hardly believe it. He thought it was angelico. It was growing near a lot of rattlesnake master and other things that looked like sang.

As far as being an herb doctor around in this area back when I was growing up, I don't remember who he was. We used to have several faith doctors who would lay their hands on you if you put your faith in them. They claimed to be born with a veil, just handed down from one generation to another. And some people swore they did them good. There was one named Mr. Alexander. People would come from far and near to him for all kind of diseases, especially mothers with children that had the hives.

We didn't have a big-time herbist. People got their own herbs from the field or the store. There was Aunt Molly Kirby, they called her, a great big black woman. She made herb medicines and hoodoos. Lots of men went to her when they had social diseases. She was also a midwife, delivered worlds of babies. She'd go out on the mountain and deliver babies. They didn't allow colored people out there much, but they'd allow her.

I'm the only old-timer herbist around here now, although lots of folks are selling herbs in capsules.

Many early memories are graphically etched in Bass's mind.

> When my sister, Lucy, was about three months old, we moved to
> Trenton, Georgia, because a man told Dad he would really buy
> the furs over there. Which he did. We moved in an ox wagon. The
> driver had a whip across his shoulder. Ox drivers wouldn't use
> the whip much, they'd just motion with it to get the oxen to go
> where they wanted. I remember walking along behind the wagon
> and seeing that whip dragging like a snake. It's just the same as
> if it was yesterday. Dad done well there at Trenton. He bought
> five or six houses and lots between Trenton and Chattanooga. We
> stayed there two or three years until about 1913.
>
> Dad would run into the hoboes who were walking the railroad
> track and they would tell him things. One of them told him he
> saw a man come out of the mountain down there in Alabama at
> Fort Payne with a whole sack of ginseng. Well, I don't doubt it,
> they're digging it there now. So we come on back to Alabama, in
> a two-horse wagon.
>
> I'd help my dad trap. We'd trap on Little Wills Creek. I first
> learned about trapping by catching rats in the old houses Dad
> was renting. I recollect the first muskrat I ever caught. Dad let
> me set a little number 1 Victor's jump trap. They had just started
> to making them—cost about a dime. I was so small, I laid down
> on my stomach at the creek bank and Dad held my legs. I set the
> trap right where the rat went in the water, the "slide" we called
> it. Muskrats make a slick place, just like we kids did sliding up
> and down that creek bank. Sometimes there'll be half a dozen of
> them that go down the same place. You set your trap about an
> inch under the water and fix it where he'll drown. I set the trap
> all right, but it come a big rain and the creek got up, so we didn't
> get to go back to the trap for a couple of days. When we got back
> we found that a mud turtle had eat the muskrat's head pretty bad,
> but Dad paid me fifty cents for the fur. Dad made pretty good
> money, when we lived near Keener.

Mr. Bass has very different memories of his mother, who unquestionably had a far-reaching influence on him.

> My mother didn't tell nobody how to do; she just went ahead and
> lived it, right down to the gnat's heel. She didn't have much to

say. She was a person that never told a joke, didn't use no kind of bad language, and if she told anything she actually had to see it.

She was firm. If she whipped one of us, we really did need it. She didn't get mad or nothing like that. Once she whipped my older brother worse than she should have. She always did hate that. He went and throwed a cat in the fire. What she whipped him for, though, he ran, run up a tree. She waited for him and really tore him up when he came down.

By 1917 the Bass family had moved to Lookout Mountain in Cherokee County.

Out on Lookout Mountain, and back in those in little valleys, people cut timber, and made some cotton, had their own gardens, had milk cows, and hogs. And there wasn't hardly a place up there that wasn't moonshining. They'd grow corn and make it up in whiskey. At one time, before my day, they rafted logs down the Coosa River.

Down in the valley in these bends of the Coosa River around Centre, and all down along the river between here and Gadsden, a few people owned most of the land and the common people worked for them—made sharecrops. The biggest part of the common people, especially the black people, worked on halfs, share-cropping for half the corn and half the cotton. The man that owned the land furnished the mules, the fertilizer—which they didn't use too much back in them days—seeds, and everything, and a house for them to live in. A third-and-fourth man was a little better off. He had his own mules and horses and paid the landowner a third of the corn and a fourth of the cotton.

About the only income folks had back in them days, unless they had a job on the railroad or in a sawmill, came in the fall of the year, when you picked cotton. Some farmers would have a few cows and maybe sell a yearling now and then, but they didn't have a regular market like we do today.

The only reason that we ever raised cotton was because we couldn't rent land any other way. In fact, we never made a dime off the cotton. We always made our money outside of that. Lots of times we'd have to pay for the cotton out of something else, because we didn't make it in a big enough way.

Bass enjoys describing everyday chores and activities after the family homesteaded on Lookout Mountain around 1925.

> We homesteaded on the mountain and had three plots. Forty acres in section three near the top of the mountain and two other forties down the side. Each family, each man or woman, could get as much as 160 acres of land. You lived on it three years, cleared up 5 acres to the 40 to put it in cultivation, and built your house and barn. When you filed your claim, it was fifty or sixty dollars, and you had witnesses to come look over your land to see if as much was cleared as was supposed to be. An old man, Minah Grogan, built a one-room house for us on the lower 40 acres. We remodeled it and built more to it. It was just a common shack.
>
> We cleared at least 15 acres and growed crops to prove the claim. In clearing the land, that's where I started digging herbs. We had to make everything we could.
>
> We cut timber all over the side of the mountain, and had a logging trail where we snaked logs. We had lines, and me and the mule, him or her, would snake logs on down to the valley. And I trapped all through there. I put my hands on might near every tree.
>
> When we lived on the mountain, we traded down in the valley at the big white store owned by the Mackeys, not far from where I live now. The post office was there until 1925. Back in them days, when they put up a store along the railroad, the government generally always would put a post office in there. The whole community was called Mackey—still is, but the nearest post office was Leesburg after 1925. We traded at the store and got our corn ground at the gristmill, and so we got acquainted with the old Mr. Mackey that run the store. The rest of the Mackeys run the gristmill. The first thing you know their family got to working for us, and we got to working for them, and the fact of the business is, we got like one big family—but not kinfolks. Old Mr. Mackey died in 1924.
>
> We got along fine with the Mackeys in the valley, but generally speaking, as recent as twenty years ago people down in the valley didn't associate with people on the mountain. A bunch of

young people from the valley who would go up the mountain for a dance were going to get into a fight in spite of the world. When the young folks from the mountain come down to the valley—the same way. Now you can't tell the difference.

Several families we knew on the mountain made whiskey, but we didn't have anything to do with the whiskey business. These folks that made it didn't have much other way to make a living. Take the Duncan boys. They were all born in North Carolina—came here with their father and mother. He was a real tall fellow and there was a young woman with them. He claimed that she was his daughter, but then he left his wife, and this young woman and him went over on the Big Tennessee River and lived in a houseboat. Well, that left Mrs. Duncan with Joe, Charlie, Troy, and George, and I believe there was another one—five boys. They were fishermen; they never did trap much. And eventually they got into making whiskey. Whiskey and fish would sell when nothing else did.

When they were still boys, they'd come visit us, and we'd hunt bees and cut bee trees together. Find a yellow-jackets' nest or a hornets' nest, and we'd all gang up—the Gentry boys and the Duncan boys, and we'd whip them things out. Some of us got stung. Just something like that to wear away the time.

After his father left, the oldest boy, Joe Duncan, got into making whiskey. The law came to the still, and he outrun the officers. He got away, went to Birmingham, Alabama, and started to work at Woodward Iron.

They was good people. They just had to get a little money, so they would make that whiskey. They made the yellow corn whiskey and the white corn.

Our family all worked together. Bought all the timber around us; cut that out for crossties and logs. My mother picked cotton and worked in the home. My sisters worked in the fields.

There was always something to do like making lye soap or buttermilk. I made I don't know how much buttermilk. A lot of it was drunk but it was also used for treating skin. The milk from the cow was, of course, sweet milk. Sweet cream was used for the diaper rash, or you could put it with plantain to bring out risens.

We drank a lot of buttermilk in the summer because we didn't have ice. In my boyhood days, I didn't even know what ice was, only in the wintertime. Had plenty of it then.

Me and my brothers and sisters never did go to school. We was learning at home. My mother had gone to school in Tennessee, up to about the tenth grade, and she started us all to reading. I remember reading the letters on goods boxes. Dad was in the produce business some, and he'd bring those boxes in that would be addressed to Keener or Gadsden, Alabama. I'd read newspapers, the Bible. We had an old blue-back speller and some magazines.

All of us children was born without doctors, with just the help of some neighborhood women. Mrs. Gentry helped with two of us over on the mountain. And when she had several children, Mother would go over there. That's the way mountain people—country people—used to do. That's why a lot of them never could get a birth certificate.

The worst sick spell I remember was during 1918, when we had the flu epidemic. My daddy—it like to have got him and one of my brothers. My mother and me never did get down with the flu. We got awful sick, but we could wait on the rest of them. Lot of people didn't pull through. Lots of people died here in Alabama.

If we couldn't make a living at one thing, some of us was doing another. Dad's byword was "play for what you see on the boards." And if he'd see something where we could make more money than we could on the farm, we'd go and do it—cut timber, pick blueberries, fish. We never even thought of making a dishonest dollar.

I've actually been working ever since I was eight years old. I've done everything. On the farm, picking cotton, cutting cordwood, making crossties, trapping, taking care of the stock.

The first commercial work that I remember doing was around ten years old. I started peeling crossties with my daddy. I peeled the bark off of them and he'd score and hew them. We'd make the ties in the times when it was too wet to plow or work in the fields. After I got on up, I'd say twelve years old, I went to cutting timber for sawmills. We worked from sun to sun, from daylight to dark, just according to how pushing the job was. There wasn't no hours; didn't know anything about hours.

A great deal of the Basses' activities, including the nature of their peddling, was seasonally determined.

In the late spring, anywhere from I'll say May on up, we'd get different kinds of berries to eat and wild plums and crab apples.

Now, dewberries, they start getting ripe along in about the middle of May. They make real good eating, and good jelly and pies. Mother had a half-gallon crock that she made by sawing off an old whiskey jug, and she'd make that full of dewberry jelly. Now that was for medicine. Nobody got it until they had diarrhea.

And then comes the serviceberry, and then the huckleberry or blueberry. And then the blackberry. And so the berry crop comes on from the middle of May to the last of July. I have picked blackberries in August.

We would generally buy a pig, or maybe two pigs, in the spring of the year, and put them in a pen. We'd give them what we called slop—which now we throw down the drain. But then we had a bucket, everybody did, in the kitchen, and when the women washed the dishes—they didn't use no detergent like we do now —they'd use lye soap. Of course, you can't poison a hog! Anyway, Mother'd put all that dishwater and scraps and leftovers in the slop bucket. Then we'd put the slop in a trough in the hog pen for the hogs to drink. We would feed them wild primrose by the armful, and careless weed from the garden and burweed and purslane that grows everywhere in the garden. It's a pest, but it really would fatten the hogs. We would keep the hogs like that till along in September or October.

Along in March and April it was garden-planting time. Set out onions and plant potatoes. Lot of times we'd plant corn in March. Back in those days we went according to nature. Mother Nature's got her way and she's going to have it. We always said that anything that grows above the ground, like beans, watermelons, cucumbers, and cantaloupes, and cotton, and okra, and butter beans, lima beans, and soya beans is planted when the sign is in what they call the twins or the arms. It shows up on the calendars with two little children with their arms wrapped around one another. And then another good time to plant is when the sign is in the balances. That's a real good time to plant most anything. And the best time to plant anything like beets, carrots, and turnips, and potatoes is when the sign is in the feet, anywhere from the knees down. You'll make a better crop by doing that. Now, a lot of people just hoots at you for thinking there are signs to plant under. But the Bible tells us that there is a time to plant and a time to pluck up that which is already planted. I don't always follow these signs anymore, but it can help. I know about tame plants from experience. I've always fooled with them.

Back then we didn't use fertilizer. We went in where we kept the cows, hogs, and mules and hauled out that compost. Putting out that manure was one of the jobs I dreaded. But it was there and you had to do it every spring. You had to take a bucket and go along and drop a handful every four feet in rows, and then you come along and dropped two grains of corn, and then come along with a hoe or plow and cover it.

The next thing we had to do was save all the wood ashes, and when the corn got up two or three inches, we'd go back and put a handful of ashes by each hill of corn, and come back and hoe it or plow it. If you made twenty bushels to the acre like that, you thought you were making real corn. Twenty-five was a top crop. Now, they don't think anything about making two or three hundred bushels. To keep the weeds out we had to keep hoeing or plowing until it was time to get a mess of roasting ears.

In the fall of the year it was cotton-picking time—any cotton we had and cotton in the valley. We'd get out in the field before day, put the sack on our shoulders. You try to keep picking and dragging that sack, until you get a big weigh-in, maybe seventy-five pounds at a time. Picking cotton is like running a race; just a few minutes will cause you to lose a lot of pounds.

The maypops would be ripe about cotton-picking time. You'd find them between the rows. Pick you a maypop and eat it as you go along; that'd sometimes keep you from having to stop and eat lunch.

The late fall was hog-killing time—in November—and to cut wood: oak and hickory for firewood, and pine for stove wood.

You had to cut wood for days and days, getting ready for winter. You could gather hickory nuts and acorns. They don't taste like chestnuts, but the hickory nuts is real good. We could gather winter huckleberries and black-haw berries and have something good to eat all the time. It's a way to live off the fat of the land.

One thing we did in the winter was trapping. It was from trapping that I got to know the woods. You could make good money catching wild animals for furs. You could make more at that than you could at digging herbs, unless you could actually get the ginseng.

Lots of things we did depended upon the weather—planting, trapping, fishing. Me and Dad fished some in the Coosa River. There was lots of sayings used before we had the weatherman. We still use a lot of them, they're as accurate as he is. There's one folks don't generally know about. When we saw what they called a sundog, why, we looked for rain or stormy weather. The fact of the business is, there's no dog to it. But you see two suns. What it is, is the rainwater in the clouds, and the sun reflects back and causes something similar to a sun or a faded-out rainbow to appear. If it is in the wintertime, we looked for cold, snowy weather; and in the summertime, we looked for stormy weather, within anywhere from eight hours up to three days.

We went by sayings to forecast mild or cold winters, too. If trees started to shed leaves from the top, we'd look for the worst weather before Christmas; if they started shedding from the bottom, we looked for the worst weather the last part. If it stayed pretty up to Thanksgiving, we looked for a cold winter afterwards.

If there was a big shuck on roasting ears and dry corn, a big crop of persimmons, hickory nuts, acorns, or pecans, and if there was an unusual amount of leaves that you had to rake up, we looked for a severe winter.

A lot of folks was superstitious, and a good many still are. Some of the superstition is more religion. My daddy could blow out fire; that is, if you got your hand burned, he would blow his breath on it, and he said something; of course you couldn't understand what he said. I had him blow on me one time and it did quit burning. He claimed he could teach a woman and a woman could teach a man. They could never teach the same sex.

My daddy was superstitious in many ways. He would never take a hoe into the house, why it's bad luck and someone will die within a year in your family. But I don't know. I never have checked it out. But it's been someone at some time has died, you know, during the time of it, and he figured that the hoe was a warning or something.

The year 1937 was a turning point in Bass's life. It was the year that his parents and sisters left to go to Trion, Georgia, where they hoped to find jobs. Looking back to the time, he still remembers vividly a dream that he felt was an omen:

I dreamed I was working in the new ground on the mountain. There was a big gulch, or holler, down below this new ground. I just happened to look across this place and saw a beautiful young lady. I thought she had the prettiest long hair; and of course, girls back them days bobbed their hair. This girl was leading the prettiest white horse and she came up to where I was, I started to . . . seemed like I wanted to say something, and I just froze. She just stood there and looked at me and disappeared.

The dream worried me for quite a while. It was the most unusual dream that I ever had in my life. My family broke up just after that; they left. I was down in Gadsden one day and when I came back, Mr. Mackey said, "Tom, your folks moved today." Well, of course they'd been talking about moving, but I didn't know they were going to move that day.

Bass moved in with the Mackey family and continued much the same life, working at a variety of jobs, many seasonal. Life was interrupted by wartime service in 1942, but a bout of arthritis led to a medical discharge after six months.

When I was discharged, I came back to Leesburg and stayed on with the Mackeys. I never have wanted to work in the city. I like to go to the city, but I want to come back to the country. You get out close to nature and you're close to where things are growing and living. You get in the city and everybody's in a rush and a push and a jar.

In the last forty years I've raised sweet potato slips, tomato plants, cabbage, onion, and pepper plants for the market. I went to work laying field tile and putting in septic tanks and helping to plumb houses. I've filed saws, skinned animals, sold insurance, dealt with fruit trees and shrubs—I was an agent and I grew them—and I've been pretty active handling herbs on the market —shipping them to dealers, and, of course, I try to give ease to folks with the herb remedies.

The last few years have seen a growing recognition of Bass as an herbalist.

I got to becoming famous in the sixties. Mr. Butler of the *Gadsden Times* started to write on me. I got to knowing him in 1962 or 1963. Butler started coming to see me because he was interested in herbs. He kept coming for ten or twelve years on Sundays and holidays. We roamed the woods around my place, and up on Lookout Mountain where I used to live, and up to Rock City. Then he took me to places in his car that I'd never been before. Butler wanted to learn about the herbs, but he was more interested in making teas and soups than medicines. He'd try anything for a tea—just to drink.

I remember especially that we went up to Yellow River Canyon, before the park was ever developed. Everybody said there was rattlesnakes up there. Well, I wore my boots, but there wasn't anything like snakes in there. It was the moonshiners making whiskey that got that out. They wanted to keep the people away. Mr. Butler just went with his low-cut shoes, and made it fine. We didn't see but one little snake, and it was a little old rattlesnake pilot.

Several times, Mr. Butler run a story about me and the herbs in the *Gadsden Times*. Every time there was a story, more and more people would come to my place for herbs and remedies, or just to talk. I would try to get them to gather their own herbs, if they would. I began to grow samples of the herbs on my place to teach the people how to identify them.

The papers in other towns began to run stories, and people from far and near would come or write to me. It like to drove me crazy. That was the time I was still collecting herbs under contract for Doc Sanders. I was working at a job, and in the evening

I'd gather the herbs and dry them in the loft of the big Mackey barn, where we used to dry the hay. I just had the son-of-a-gun full. I had all kinds of herbs in there; wild cherry—I shipped him hundreds of pounds of that.

Bass's conversation often harks back to changes that have taken place—"the way change is"—sometimes with nostalgia, but just as often with a matter-of-fact acceptance.

The biggest change that has happened around here after I got back from the army was when the Alabama Power Company came in here and built a dam and Lake Weiss.

They set stakes right near the Mackey place where the water might come—and it has. The next thing we knew, they was coming in buying land. They started around Centre and Cedar Bluff, and up and down the Coosa River and branches. Some people would sell, and others they made sell. Some people held their feet to the fire and got rich. The company bought up some other people's land for something like fifty dollars an acre. When they had so much land, they forced other people to sell. The government condemned their land, on the basis it was necessary for society. So folks had to take what they could get.

Course, Weiss Lake has brought a heap of retired people here and rich people—lawyers and doctors and bankers and preachers and teachers. Lots of young people, too. They live in trailers and work in factories, on the highway, with the REA [Rural Electrification Association]—in Centre and Gadsden and Rome and Sand Mountain, and in Boas and Albertville, and some all the way to Chattanooga.

There is ten houses now to where there was just one. The towns haven't growed; it's the areas out of town that's growed. It used to be that I could tell you everybody's name in the whole settlement.

In the way of herbs, the lake has been a disaster, and in farming it has been a disaster, but it has put fish here. They claim it's the best crappie fishing in the United States. And they've got a lot of bass and brim and catfish. Flooding the land has covered a lot of the best farmland, and wiped out the biggest part of lowland plants—like mayapple, bloodroot, chill-grass, and Sampson snakeroot. The water has done away with slippery elm and done away with a lot of the willows and also poplars. A lot of these things won't come back because most of the land around the lake is in cultivation, and a lot of that they keep poisoned with insecticides and so on. And the water flops up in waves and keeps it so some plants can't grow. But course other herbs comes washing in.

When it all happened, lots of people went off crying, and lots of people died from being shocked so bad about having to move out of their homes. Some people stood up and forced them to build up the land so they could keep their homes. But a lot of people had their houses condemned, and had to tear them down.

The churches have changed too. They're mostly brick now. Most of the churches forty or fifty years ago in the country was built just one-room outfits, and real tall. I never did know why they built them so tall, cause a storm would tear a church up when it wouldn't tear up nothing else.

I don't go to just one church; I go to a lot of churches around here. One or two of the churches I used to go to has got a little too ahead of me. They got plush seats—sits real good; carpet— you go way down in it. In Centre the two big churches are the Baptist church and the Methodist church. They have to take in several thousand dollars a week, or they go in the hole.

Back in my day, if the preacher got three dollars a week in money, why he thought he was doing fine. People paid him in chickens, eggs, canned fruit—things like that. Give him clothes that maybe they had used. But Lord, now they drive fine automobiles, most of them, and get fifteen, twenty, or thirty thousand dollars a year.

The old preachers would preach, and work regular jobs to make a living. Some of these preachers wasn't called. It was a bullfrog they heard.

Bass constantly expresses surprise that he has lived beyond three score and ten—"I'm on borrowed time." If wistfulness sometimes creeps into his conversation, his entrepreneurial instincts still make him open to new activities. But, above all, he is happy with his role as a teacher about herbs.

I still live on the old Mackey property. The house and a acre of land was willed to me. I built me a shack on the land. It's not a home but it's where I live. I use the big house for some things, but I like my shack. I am still active in the herb business in one way or another, but times have changed.

I don't ship herbs to dealers anymore, because shipping costs too much. I don't sell fruit trees and shrubs anymore for the same reason. It pays to go to K-Mart or Sears or somewhere to buy your trees. And people are not as quick to put out fruit trees now as they were at one time. One thing about it is it's easy to buy the fruits, you know. A lot of people used to have a strawberry patch and things like that. Well, now they go down to the supermarket and buy them.

The biggest part of the herb business now is in these capsules herb companies puts out. Most everything I dig and gather is now sold in these capsules. It's so convenient for people; it's all dosed out. I sell some of the capsules myself, but, mostly, I help my friends who are in this business by gathering the herbs and roots to show them what they look like, and tell them what they're good for. I keep busy just telling people about the herbs at meetings in all the towns around here, and even on the radio and television. Course, I still make a salve, and the rub, and some cough medicine, and some teas for some people when they need it. But, for the most part, nowadays, when folks come, I tell them about the capsules.

Well, I've done enough of this jabbering. Kind of like my daddy was, at least they told it on him. He was a big talker and interesting to talk with. They said that him and a fellow started talking one morning and Mother got their dinner and they was still talking, talked on till supper, and ate supper and talked on till breakfast.

The fellow finally said to my daddy, "John, if we didn't talk all day yesterday and last night and here we are talking this morning, and I don't know what we're talking about."

Dad said, "That's all right, Bill. Just sit back down there and we'll tell it all again."

CHAPTER 3

Health Matters in a Changing
Community

*'Twas a healthy place. It had a feeling in
general for fellow men.*

M r. Bass's character, life as a backwoodsman, and relations
with family and friends, all interwoven with community
activities, highlight his sharp recollections. It is clear that,
unlike many traditional practitioners, no single medical
problem, either personal or among family, friends, and acquaintances,
has been pivotal in his life. He denies that episodes of minor illness
during childhood and adolescence directed him toward herbalism,
although virtual freedom from ailments occurred only after an army
medical discharge for "arthritis." "I was stronger at sixty-seven than at
twenty-one."[1] His only longtime concern has been a "weak stomach,"
which makes him selective in what he eats. If minor ailments did not
encourage Bass to become an herbalist, this chapter shows that, along
with living conditions, they contributed to his medical socialization
and awareness, as they did to others in the community, especially
married women concerned with looking after their families.

Minor ailments are a conspicuous part of traditional herbal medical
practice everywhere. Unfortunately, determining the extent of sickness and morbidity—especially from noncommunicable diseases—
in any community is not easy, if only because individuals respond
to problems in different ways. We have used many quotations from
Mr. Bass's memories and those of his contemporaries. Admittedly
they reflect much of Bass's way of life (and his bachelorhood) and are
also tinted with a nostalgia that plays down the unhappy features of
times past; thus generalizations have to be drawn with caution. On

the other hand, his introspection and narration of the events that have shaped his life help us to deepen our understanding of one herbalist's life-style, and we see an intriguing mix of the past and present.

A feature of Bass's practice is that he sees people as individuals with different needs in health and illness. Many factors, some glimpsed in his recollections, have shaped this outlook. He respects individualism and is intrigued by differences in his own family. He certainly remembers that during the 1920s and 1930s there was some feeling that the mountain was healthier than the valley, at least those low areas near the Coosa River and along creeks where the specter of malaria still existed. However, his community—spread over nine or so square miles between Slackland and Bristow in the valley and on the side of Lookout Mountain—was considered a fairly "healthy place." In fact, the differences between mountain and valley were becoming less clear-cut than they once had been. More and more mountain people availed themselves of the market economy in the valley, supported as it was by railroads, even to purchasing more over-the-counter medicines. Interaction grew in many other ways, especially as local schools were consolidated. Eventually, according to Mr. Bass, "it got to where the boys on the mountain married the girls from the valley, and girls on the mountain married the boys from the valley." Nevertheless, for a long time, and perhaps even now, such factors as plantation farming in the valley and family kinships continued to sustain some sense of difference.

In the 1920s and 1930s about 150 people with incomes derived from farming or working at the sawmill or the railroad created, says Bass, a "friendly place." It had a "feeling in general for fellow men," although half-renters and the somewhat more affluent third-and-fourth renters came and went. Half-renters, or sharecroppers, had no equipment, mules, or horses of their own, and hence were dependent entirely on the landowners. Often living in "bad homes," some showed "no energy to help themselves and keep themselves clean." Bass considers, however, that the Mackey-Leesburg area had some of the more industrious half-renters, and, indeed, that the community was generally better off than others, especially those "over the mountain."[2]

A few families who owned most of the land in the area—creating a community with many close kinships—had "modern" houses with handsome porches. Railroad section men lived in "comfortable" houses belonging to the TAG (Tennessee, Alabama, Georgia) company, while renters lived in one- or two-room houses little better than shacks. Rooms generally looked untidy because there were few cupboards. Mr. Bass agrees with a description of mountain homes published in 1924: "A dried gourd hung on the nail will hold salt; another, sugar; a shelf or two forms the kitchen cabinet. Pegs or spikes are driven into the logs for the family wardrobe, beside which there is a large box and, sometimes a home-made chest of drawers."[3] Bass adds that the floors shook so much when the children ran across them that his mother's rising dough often fell flat.

Many believed that their living conditions encouraged "rheumatism," something Tommie Bass endured as a child and young adult. Drafts were common through bare plank walls and floorboards, which left cracks as they dried, and in some homes "stars could be seen through the roof." Rain sometimes came in, although, beginning in the 1930s, tin roofs provided a considerable improvement. Not only were drafts linked to rheumatism, but some people also blamed stuffiness, especially common at night if the house was occupied by many people. The Bass home, which had newspapers over the walls to keep drafts out, was often stuffy.

Writers describing the Appalachians in the 1920s often indicated that common cleanliness was "impossible" in the poor housing. Bass disagrees, as he does with the view that even in clean homes there was seldom any knowledge of what constituted sanitary cleanliness.[4] Certainly there were some awful conditions, as when his father stayed at a place where the chickens roosted above a meal bin without a cover: "If the chickens roosted in the wrong direction, the droppings fell into the meal." But Tommie Bass does not think living conditions and lack of cleanliness produced much sickness.

Although Bass remembers neither special concerns with keeping fit nor any noticeable preoccupation with public health up to the 1940s, he believes that most people followed long-standing "rules" of health which, from ancient times, centered on paying careful attention to fresh air, sleep, exercise, rest, passions, and diet.[5] It was "common sense," he says. Not everyone heeded the rules, but personal cleanliness was generally widespread. Baths in galvanized washtubs were common, though spring- or wellwater had to be carried in and heated on a stove: "If you worked outside all day, you needed a bath." "Most everyone had soap," commonly the "rough lye soap made in the home"; if the soap was "medicated" with sassafras, it was considered a good preventive against skin ailments.

While sassafras (or other additives like peppermint) did little to scent the lye soap, the odor bore no comparison to the obnoxious-smelling asafetida commonly hung around necks, especially children's, when illness—from colds to measles—was in the house. This falls in the long tradition of counteracting "pestilential matter" carried in the air, for which vinegar was also used in the Bass and other homes. Some people preferred suspending camphor around the neck. It was well known for such antipestilential use during the nineteenth century and earlier, and Bass has used camphor to counteract that "dangerous smell imprinted on my mind": the putrefaction of dead bodies. "I have been sitting up with them when the smell was so bad it made you sick. I used to bathe the body's forehead by rubbing camphor on it."[6]

Another well-remembered practice is rubbing turpentine around the neck or under the shirt. "One old family doctor would take a newspaper and saturate it real good with turpentine, and he'd put it under his shirt." Nutmeg also was employed at times, but its pleasant smell gave it an inferior reputation as a preventive. The disappearance of such practices after World War II was linked to more widespread use of commercial disinfectants and the availability of new treatments like antibiotics.

Commercial tooth powder and toothbrushes were readily available by the 1920s, but "chewing sticks"—usually black gum twigs or, less often, prickly ash—were commonly employed, and have still not disappeared entirely.[7] Bass notes that snuff takers also used black gum sticks (chewing exposed the fibrous "bristles") to spread snuff inside the lower gums, as well as for cleaning teeth. Bass has always used manufactured toothbrushes, which until the 1940s he dipped into soda water. Unfortunately, he began to lose his teeth early, at least fifteen were lost by the time he was forty; as he says, dental care was not readily available, apart from someone in the community always ready to pull a tooth. Like others of his generation in the area, Bass has never worn false teeth.[8]

Such vermin as rats, commonplace during the 1920s and 1930s, were feared more for bites than for spreading disease. Flies and roaches, on the other hand, were universally considered carriers of germs, and much time and effort was spent on controlling them. Local stores stocked growing numbers of commercial items. B-Brand was especially popular to supplement the homemade "shoofly," a piece of paper torn into tails that dangled from a smooth sourwood stick ("it was real pretty when it was finished"). Yet only after screens became common during the 1940s was there general escape from flies.[9]

Disinfectants were employed liberally. Many people recall carbolic acid (phenol), used in most homes for sanitation purposes and for various medical uses such as in salves employed "when infections set in." With regard to overall health, Bass believes that the introduction of DDT in the 1940s was far more significant than disinfectants. He remembers vividly that the problem of myriad roaches, chinch bugs, and so on, common in even the cleanest homes, was all "done away with by DDT."

A few ailments linked in the public mind with uncleanliness are widely remembered as commonplace. Two were "itch" (almost certainly scabies, for which Bass recommends pokeroot baths), and head lice, treated with a tea made from sassafras, white or red oak, or pennyroyal. Many people in the region remember family fusses when either complaint appeared, since it was likely to spread to everyone. Bass recalls that infections of the skin such as "erysipelas" sometimes followed scratching the skin. Interestingly, bedbugs have left few memories apart from many remedies to treat the bites.[10]

It is not easy to generalize on the quality of diet and its effect on health, despite the widespread incidence of the vitamin-deficiency disease pellagra in the South prior to the 1930s.[11] The epidemiological patterns of this disease were complex, and on looking back to the 1920s and 1930s, Mr. Bass now thinks that in his community "bad" cooking that destroyed vitamins was more of a problem than a reliance on "meat, meal, and molasses." He says that there is some truth in the comments made in 1924 about Appalachian food: "The average cooking is bad and renders the food unwholesome. The frying pan is the most common weapon, though the stew pot is a close second. Combined with old-time southern over-cooking, the restricted diet is also responsible for a depleted physical condition."[12] However, while Bass accepts that meals were often "cooked down real good and done," he thinks they were tasty and the "vitamins were cooked back in," particularly so for soup, turnip tops, and collard greens. Remembered well is the old iron pot into which went one vegetable or another—butter beans, polecat and whip-poor-will peas, turnip greens, onions, carrots—to be "cooked forever." Tommie Bass recalls preparing collard greens in his youth: "Say you're going to cook a mess for a noon meal. After an hour or so of boiling in a little water they'll be done but they're not so good, but you can eat them. Then you put them back on—and cook them for what we calls supper, some calls it dinner, and boy they're better. And then the next morning you put them back on—you cook them again. Just leave them in the pot. Just about the time all of them is gone, if you have enough for two or three days, boy they're out of this world." He adds that it was not until "vitamins came along in the 1930s" that folks thought more about cooking and health.[13]

Mr. Bass also confirms a view published in the 1930s that, despite many families keeping chickens, eggs were only eaten if they were surplus to those bartered for "groceries, patent medicines, or feminine trinkets such as needles, buttons, and thread; and snuff and tobacco." In contrast, another dairy product, buttermilk, was "taken by everyone" for its nutritious qualities, and for "breaking outs," prickly heat, and by young girls wanting to improve their complexions. Bass considers the "acid makes it good. The acid gets into the skin." The ready availability of buttermilk and its preparation is fixed firmly in his memory, which helps him recall the many milk and buttermilk cures once generally well known;[14] in a similar way, the key role hogs played in the local economy reinforces his enthusiasm for the medicinal properties of hog lard.

Bass does not feel that his family or those of close acquaintance had an especially limited diet, even during hard times, or that it contributed to ill health. With industry and ingenuity, he says, it was possible to live well off a "spot of land" through subsistence farming, borrowing, and bartering, although many did not. His recollections note how he acquired an extensive knowledge of "tame" and "wild" plants. The latter, including lambs-quarter, peppergrass, shepherd's purse, sour dock, poke salat, watercress, and others, often graced the Bass table.[15]

Such fruits as blueberry, dewberry, serviceberry, black-haw, and persimmon also were gathered. Occasionally, game meat—squirrel, turtle, and raccoon—was added to the diet. Many women, including Bass's mother, were imaginative cooks given the economic conditions they faced. Bass's wide knowledge of plain southern cooking includes memories of his mother's notable cobbler pies and hoecake, made at a time when the family often ate cornbread three times a day.[16]

In the early decades of this century such major health problems as hookworm, pellagra, tuberculosis, and typhoid were commonplace throughout the Appalachians and elsewhere, although except for pellagra their heyday was passing when Tommie Bass was in his teens. In fact, the low incidence of these diseases in his local population of a few hundred has left only fleeting memories, even of the 1918 influenza epidemic. He recollects only one or two cases of pellagra but remembers that people started to talk about nutrition for it in the 1920s. Bass recalls relatively little of the scourges of hookworm and tuberculosis; of smallpox he remembers only that several families caught the disease and were quarantined. Typhoid is remembered well, though some confusion with other acute intestinal ailments is probably at play. Bass has little recollection of the countless publications on personal hygiene and health, or the nationwide public health movements of the time, except for seeing posters in the railroad depot and post office reminding sufferers from tuberculosis to use spittoons with a lid instead of open-mouth floor types or the floor itself. An interesting anecdote concerns a postmaster who was murdered after he angered a family by insisting that the father use a spittoon when he was in the post office. Bass's only other recollection of tuberculosis in the 1920s and 1930s is the financial aid the army provided for one family after World War I.[17]

Mr. Bass's unawareness of the public health movement is undoubtedly linked with the rural nature of his community, his failure to attend school, and his never having been married. It was in the 1920s that a noticeable thrust to improve child health care became widespread. The provision of federal funds for states to support child health services, and especially the 1921 Sheppard-Towner Act for the Promotion of the Welfare of Maternity and Infancy were particularly relevant.[18] Some other area residents, all in their seventies or older, remember a feeling that everything was being "taken care of" during the 1930s.[19] Though this view is largely a recollection of the New Deal, it also reflects a sense that, for the first time, "everything was being treated," from bacteria to the mind. Mr. Bass and other informants believe that the trend was part of a "constitutional" approach to treating everything. Now, in a rather nebulous way, they feel that medicine only takes care of parts of our bodies, just as they hold that people do not take as much responsibility for their illnesses as they did in the past.[20]

While major illnesses in the community during the 1920s and 1930s left only incidental memories—perhaps best remembered is fear of a mad dog and catching rabies—memories indicate that relatively minor ailments and chronic problems, including infectious diseases and malaria, were rife; "it took three frogs to live and two of them had to be doctors." Many of Bass's recollections of minor and chronic problems are recorded in the monographs on herbs in volume 2.

An especially noteworthy chronic problem was alcohol consumption, though it was viewed as a social rather than medical issue. Bass believes that Mackey-Leesburg was one of the "drinkinest" places in the United States in the 1920s and 1930s, a world of moonshiners, bootleggers, and home brew makers. Around 1917–23,

> you could walk down the railroad, or down any road, after dark and see the little fires of whiskey stills twinkling in the mountains. They tried to put them out, but they showed up once in a while. They burnt hickory wood until they started to use gas. Hickory wood didn't make smoke, but it had a disadvantage; it smelt so good it would give them away to the officers. No telling how many bootleggers there were. Just as fast as they put them in jail and sent them off, another took his place. Just like if you kill one fly there's two or three that came back in their place.

Bass remembers that up to the 1940s many landowners and others were "sot" drunkards—"they now call them alcoholics"—who often drank whiskey in spells of weeks at a time. If whiskey was not available, rubbing alcohol, vanilla, shoe polish, or the Cordial Ennui of the Chattanooga Medical Company ("with 40 percent alcohol") were alternatives. Alcohol abuse accentuated many social problems: beaten wives and children, damaged homes, chronic ill health, and even fatalities from exposure in cold weather.

The many ailments—minor and chronic—led to a wide array of

self-care and visits to herbalists, faith healers, granny midwives, and others. In his valley and mountainside community—although not throughout the Appalachians in general—unlicensed medical practitioners were often as well known as country doctors, of whom no shortage existed. Three doctors were available in the thirty-square-mile area up to the 1940s, but Bass has relatively few recollections of them: "We did not need a doctor so I didn't know any of them. You only used a doctor when it was serious. If you didn't have the money, you waited as long as you could. Anyhow, the doctors gave you the same medications you had."[21] He remembers that in the 1920s Dr. John Matthews collected local roots and herbs such as black snakeroot, which he made into medicines in his office.

Memories of old "docs" in the Leesburg area are generally favorable. "They were doing it for the humanity, not for the money. I'm sorry to say a lot of these young doctors nowadays are more interested in money than anything." Mr. Bass remembers that in Dr. White's practice during the 1950s, when the nurse-secretary was asked about a bill, she sometimes replied: "We'll let you know when we need it." Adds Bass: "It's more like they were neighbors than doctors. You felt comfortable seeing them; now they scare you with this, that, and the other." Old-time doctors, like old Dr. Will White, who rode horseback, carried medicines and prepared their prescriptions in the home. They would come "any time of day or night with the medicine for three dollars." Two doctors in Centre, who lived in two of the finest houses in the town and ran offices and small clinics or hospitals in their homes, are remembered for always finding time to sit and talk; one allowed patients' families to bring in food. Close questioning of many informants suggests that self-care and doctors' care worked well together up to the 1930s, and that everyone generally recognized when it was necessary to call in professional help.

Dr. White's clinic became well known in the area, in fact almost a source of civic pride. In 1949 it was reported to be as "well equipped as any small hospital" (*Coosa River News*, 27 May 1949). For Mr. Bass the clinic reflected changing times. Others, too, felt that the 1940s was a pivotal period in the provision of health care services. For instance, a writer for the *Coosa River News* in June 1949 noted the growing impact of the public health movement, particularly the way it worked through children:

> Where once 34 doctors served, now only three medical doctors, counting a health officer, serve Cherokee County, and two chiropractic doctors. A lot of work has been taken off the doctors by our health officers' work. This has been accomplished by the cooperation of the parents, schools and the officials of the schools. We've learned to accept vaccinations, better standards of living and cleanliness. Now a visit from the health officer and nurse is welcomed at the schools. And a nurse does do a big work in the county, too. All families that are reached by the health department realize the importance of this department. And we've learned the health doctor and his assistants are interested in our children's welfare and our health as well.

Although such a view suggests a sense of self-satisfaction that was not felt by everyone, Bass and many elderly members of the community believe that it heralded the great medical strides of the past thirty years. While they are uncertain of details to document the changes— except perhaps treatment of cancer and "if you caught 'double pneumonia' you no longer had to start to dig your grave"—developments that have shaped their thinking are reported in local newspapers. Representative are "New TB Drug" and a report on a mobile chest X-ray unit (*Cherokee County Herald*, 23 February 1955) and the visit of the bloodmobile (*Cherokee County Herald*, 3 September 1955).[22]

Bass and others of his generation find it difficult to describe the impact of social change on medicine, largely because they have not tried to analyze it. However, most feel the greatest change has been toward a greater use of doctors brought about by a wider range of opportunities for employment, easier communication by telephone, better roads and more autos, and the advent of Medicare and Medicaid, all of which changed the pattern of people's lives.

Many, too, think that although the incidence of some diseases has declined dramatically (e.g., double pneumonia), newer ailments have come along requiring people to seek out doctors. Some of these are associated with a trend to a looser moral climate and more open sexual behavior. Male informants of Bass's generation focus on changing mores among women, including trends in clothes from dresses to trousers.[23] These changes are thought to create unsettled situations, a by-product of which is more widespread sexually transmitted disease.

Changing morals are also linked to the rapid influx of outsiders coming into the region around the new Lake Weiss and the nearby towns of Centre and Gadsden. Many newcomers—"retired and rich people, lawyers and doctors and bankers and preachers and teachers" —are more affluent than those long established in the area, have goal-oriented values, and are more aware of the notion that symptoms may herald serious disease.[24] Whether such factors translate into stress and more visits to doctors cannot be said with certainty, but they lie behind Bass's view that, nowadays, unnecessary visits are made to doctors.

When senior citizens are asked if the old days were better, the answer is invariably a clear "no."[25] All see vastly improved living conditions. On the other hand, elements of nostalgia or wistfulness frequently creep into conversations about the greater neighborliness that once existed and the challenge to live as comfortably as possible in the absence of running water and other utilities. Nostalgia for the past, for the "world we have lost," undoubtedly colors some comments made by Mr. Bass. Yet, notwithstanding his life in a culture with much poverty and his wistful air of pathos when reminiscing over some features of times past, he sees strengths in the past which offer disquieting comparisons with fashions in life today. Nostalgia, as noted below, is almost certainly one factor sustaining Bass's practice.[26]

Mr. Bass is no more conscious of widespread ill health in the community before the 1950s than in recent times, with their improved living conditions, though he believes more stoicism toward illness existed before than at present: "People had sicknesses that would keep them in bed for days and days. They didn't have shots like we have now to revive them." Sometimes, too, economics mandated the type and extent of care. "In those days there was no way of getting medical attention unless they paid for it themselves and therefore they'd go as long as they could without going for a doctor." Often the difference between being healthy and being ill in Bass's younger days was whether or not one could get up and go to work. His own ill health as a child and young man perhaps encouraged a degree of stoicism.

There were ever-present reminders of ill health and minor complaints in advertisements for patent medicines and news items about sick members of the community in the *Coosa River News*, especially up to the 1950s.[27] Nevertheless, these suggest neither a magnitude of concern with medical ailments greater than other communities outside Appalachia nor elements of hypochondria, as has been suggested for Appalachian people.

How much the community has been subject to overt strains or tensions, commonly considered to be caused by social change, is not clear. Although it does not appear to be a conscious factor, we have not undertaken exhaustive studies in this subjective and difficult-to-investigate area. Certainly it is clear that changes over the years such as the advent of Lake Weiss have produced personal distress for many individuals, but many close kinships exist, which, as Bass recognizes, "often help one to get through life."

Whatever the extent of the impact of stress and living conditions on health, no doubt exists that minor and self-limiting problems have always been commonplace. These provided Bass with innumerable opportunities in his early years, before he acquired the authority of an herbalist, to try out information on herbs. Since then they have remained the backbone of his practice.

Opinions about Bass's community raise general considerations. People tend to see their communities in different ways depending on how they view change. Those with middle-class values may view it positively; for instance, they may strongly support more facilities for "modern" medicine like health clinics and disavow the "obsolete" medicine of the old-time doctors. Others, particularly among the older generation, tend to focus on constant features of rural life and kinship, and to be less preoccupied with new comforts. Certainly Bass's practice as an herbalist over many years has been conspicuous for constant elements, despite growth and changing details. Even his present living conditions—a shack which he prefers to the once-handsome 1920s house left to him a few years ago—mirrors his earlier style of life, while his ability to perform many jobs, his rural ingenuity, and his longtime service to one family have allowed him to avoid the need to change his life in any substantial way. For many people this milieu both evokes and harnesses a great deal of nostalgia, even for "Granny's nasty-tasting medicines"; it also encourages a favorable disposition toward traditional medicine and an ethos in which specific criticisms of and frustrations with present-day regular medicine are voiced.

Bass's sharp recollections of the community suggest that he has always been able to put his finger on its pulse and monitor its concerns, or at least the concerns of individual members. His range of activities has aided him in this, as has his gift for humorous narrative and the use of his oral talents in many ways—as part-time auctioneer; rising in rural Baptist and Methodist churches to tell a story or give a testimony; and weaving humor into his daily dealings with workmates, customers, and visitors. Further, his skills, knowledge, and generosity have constantly helped and served people in the community in many ways—helping to lay out people (before burial insurance); pruning trees; sharpening saws; skinning animals for furs; giving away dried apples, green vegetables, and plants from his yard; visiting sick people in hospitals, nursing homes, and in their own homes; generosity with floral tributes and personal visits on the death of a friend or acquaintance (even those not close to him); and, not least, his herbal practice.

Examination of the community and Mr. Bass shows symbiotic relationships between him and many neighbors and friends, particularly those of his generation who hold the same values. Younger people are commonly intrigued by his knowledge, idiosyncracies, and seemingly simple life. Some see him as the last of a line of frontiersmen. Others see him as a bastion of values now disappearing.[28]

While, so far, we have spoken in a general way about facets of a community, and later will stress the significance of popular ideas about health and disease, we cannot overstress the variability in attitudes and needs of individuals in matters of illness. Our study leads us to agree with those who are concerned about the individual's needs amid Western health care systems where scientific medicine primarily views the body in terms of physical and chemical processes, and where community and social studies are concerned mostly with overall population and cultural patterns.[29]

CHAPTER 4

Self-Treatment in the Community:
A Cultural Force

Don't Take Calomel—Take Vega-Cal.

Just as Mr. Bass's community sets a stage of minor ailments interwoven at times with more serious complaints, it also provides a backdrop of self-treatment. A constant feature throughout Bass's lifetime has been discussion after discussion—experiences shared between him and his visitors—on the merits of countless medicines, purchased and homemade. Consideration of this promotes further understanding of the details and cultural background of his practice. It also provides some insights into the complex arena of self-treatment at a time of growing interest in patterns of self-care practices and the forces that shape them. The treatments described here—long commonplace among large sections of the population—highlight the constant search for new therapies and prompt questions both about patients' expectations and about quackery. Although generally Bass is revered as an honest herbalist, some people do consider him a quack.

CONTINUITY AND CHANGE IN SELF-TREATMENT

As one looks at twentieth-century self-treatment in the Mackey-Leesburg community, largely through the recollections of Bass and other informants, there is a temptation to see it as possessing a unique regional flavor.[1] Yet, while local testimonies and enthusiasms have dictated the popularity of certain items, many features are common to self-treatment everywhere. This universality and its roots in the past—contributing to self-treatment's long-standing cultural presence —helps us see why Mr. Bass views his activities ("always part of my life") as practices happening "ever since time."

It is customary to trace the story of self-treatment—where the patient chooses what medicines to take without the immediate advice of a regular practitioner—back to classical times, often with the presumption that it was necessary because doctors were scarce. Just as often, however, there were other reasons, including low cost, convenience, self-reliance, and distrust of doctors. Because numerous medicines used for self-treatment were also commonly prescribed or recommended by regular physicians, tracing the character of self-treatment is not easy, at least before the vernacular literature of the sixteenth and seventeenth centuries. This literature, with its frequent mention of such "irregular" practitioners as piss-prophets (who examined urine), itinerants, magical healers, ministers who treated bodies as well as souls, common herbalists, and herb women, reflects not only patient choices separate from regular medicine, but also belief that a basic knowledge of about sixty herbs was essential.[2]

The vernacular literature also gives a sense of eclecticism and, by references to herbs marketed by herb women (e.g., *Carduus benedictus* sold by the basket, red poppies by the peck, violets by the pint or measure, and scurvy grass by the basket, bushel, or peck)[3] and frequent mention of "ignorant" people, indicates a distinction between home and regular medicine. The distinction, at least until the eighteenth century, is nevertheless blurred, in part because few plants were exclusive to either practice and also because medical knowledge was not as professionally restricted then as it is today.

Much of the knowledge of the use of herbs for self-treatment was handed down from one generation to the next, orally and through collected notes. The formulas (or "recipes"), which range from simple teas to extracts, were eclectically acquired from renowned physicians, quack doctors, neighbors, "old wives," and newspapers.[4] Conspicuous in many notebooks, particularly until the nineteenth century, were magical or astrological remedies and directions for collecting, preparing, and administering the herbs linked with magic and astrology. While the recipe-book tradition petered out in the nineteenth century, later examples still contain a broad spectrum of recipes for foods, beer, soap, candles, and other miscellaneous items besides medicine.[5]

The same or similar formulas, though frequently with much less emphasis on magical associations, were also sustained by a variety of published works covering self-care, ranging from the majestic sixteenth- and seventeenth-century herbals of William Turner, John Gerard, and John Parkinson to cheaper, less cumbersome works like the long-lived *Herbal*, by Nicholas Culpeper (published in 1652 with an astrological focus and still in print), John Wesley's pointedly antiprofessional *Primitive Physick* (1747), William Buchan's more balanced *Domestic Medicine* (1769), and such publications as the *Gentleman's Magazine*, cookery and household recipe books, and the ephemeral almanacs commonplace from the eighteenth century to the present.[6] The vast home medical literature, which featured approaches and marketing strategies from easy-to-follow recipe-style books (often combination cookbooks) to works more concerned with educating the public about preserving health and medical care for routine problems and emergencies, catered to both the "educated and the uneducated."[7]

Differentiating the various readership levels of domestic medical literature is not always easy, though that written for the "uneducated" is generally less discursive and includes relatively simple recipes and, more often, astrological notions. Yet whatever the content of the variety of writings on domestic medicine, a core of treatment common to regular medicine is conspicuous. This, plus a fairly common lay possession of key medical textbooks, contributed to a widespread ethos of common understanding between regular practitioners and laypeople. While we will not explore this ethos here in any detail, some instances from seventeenth-century England of laypeople's searches for new remedies illuminate patients' relations with physicians and suggest the timelessness of situations found in Bass's practice.

Correspondence from the early 1600s between an English doctor, John Symcotts, and his patients is a rich source of information. The letters are full of talk of humors—"sharp humours," "offensive humours"—typical of the Galenic medicine of the time and understood by physicians and patients alike. Of special interest is the exchange of information about formulas. One patient wrote to Symcotts: "There is another tried medicine which as I am told, never fails, which is: let two leeches be laid to the plate of [your] foot where the gout is until they drop off themselves, then put your foot for a while into warm water, then take it out and lay on some what you will to stop the blood."[8]

Sometimes the free exchange of information created confusion. Symcotts wrote to a patient on 1 June 1633: "Whatever your neighbours ignorantly talk against physick your own judgement can inform you that for easing of so p[rincipal] a part, the voiding of the humour by blisters has been improper and remed[ies] applied for mitigation might easily rept that viscous humour into the noble parts." Symcotts's understanding of and insight into his patients and his general interest in self-medication is not unique.[9] A sense of understanding between physicians and patients is discernible down to the present time, although the physician often had an employeelike role until the nineteenth century, and the character of the relationship has not been constant.[10] By the nineteenth century quickening changes in medical practice—including concerns about physicans' behavior and the profession's status in society, new medical theories, changes in diagnosis and therapy, statutory changes toward the end of the century, and growing medical commercialism, all to some degree set in a framework of support for science—helped bring about a more dominant role for physicians.[11]

A number of consequences accompanied this trend. One was that the distinction between self-treatment and regular medicine sharpened. What physicians and those concerned with public health believed laypeople should and should not do medically became more clear-cut.[12] Medical commercialism—manufactured products such as medicine chests, small electrical machines, invalid foods, patent medicines, many types of baths, synthetic spa waters, and so on—as well as virulent debates over new medical sects also helped define the limits of self-treatment and undermined many long-standing practices of using herbs.

Some consequences were a deterioration in understanding between physician and patient amid growing communication difficulties and a sharpening disquiet among physicians about many facets of self-care. The disquiet ranged from worry that patients would turn into hypochondriacs to the view that self-treatment often led to delays in calling in a medical practitioner, who then found a disease so far advanced that little could be done.

Linked to this was the view that home or traditional medicine, which relied on locally gathered herbs, was often too mild and out-of-date compared with regular medicine. Items expunged from the regular medical literature during, say, the revision that took place in the eighteenth century often retained a place in domestic medicine, even though generally considered obsolete. Additionally, the incorporation of more and more chemical remedies into regular medicine in the last decades of the nineteenth century gave it a feeling of progress and separateness.

Criticisms of herbal remedies, particularly in the context of magical associations, were also incorporated into the harsh nineteenth-century attacks on quackery and medical sects such as homeopathy. Such attacks were strengthened by data from improvements in chemical and pharmaceutical analysis and the growing concern placed on protecting the public.[13]

Amid such concerns some physicians viewed self-treatment with a measure of ambivalence. After all, none could deny its value in many circumstances. This ambivalence, conspicuous in the twentieth century, has meant that physicians have paid little attention to everyday self-treatment unless adverse effects occurred. In turn, this has further strengthened the view of separateness between self-treatment and regular medicine that is felt keenly by Bass and is hardly softened by the current growing interest in self-care within the medical profession.

As facets of the voluminous story of self-treatment in the Mackey-Leesburg area are considered, sufficient detail from an overwhelming amount of data is given to show both the diversity of medicines used and why Bass feels that those who call him a quack do not appreciate the deep roots of his practice.

PACKAGED HERBS

Although botanical remedies are the main concern of this story, they have not always been the most conspicuous feature of self-care in the Appalachians or elsewhere in the United States. Indeed, by 1900 interest in botanicals had long been declining, though more so in regular than in home medicine. While interest was greater in rural Appalachia than in many other places as the twentieth century opened, sales of alternative, over-the-counter "patent" medicines, which were far more convenient to use, were expanding.[14] Nevertheless, up until the 1940s—and still today in parts of the country—pharmacies and other stores carried herbs conveniently packaged in one- to four-ounce cardboard boxes. This method of marketing, used by such well-known pharmaceutical companies as Parke-Davis, helped sustain interest not only in old favorites like boneset, catnip, sassafras, and yarrow after most people stopped collecting them, but also in less popular herbs such as fringe tree, five-finger grass, and chickweed.[15]

One of Bass's early commercial activities was supplying packages of dried herbs ready to be made into tea. Commercial precedents for this enterprise included Simmons's laxative, which, says Bass, "we kept in our home all the time—take a packet in a quart of water, make a tea, strain it, add sugar and take two tablespoons as a dose."

Despite the continued availability of herbs, most people born between the 1920s and 1940s never acquired an interest in them; in part the ready availability and reliance on "family" and over-the-counter medicines made it unnecessary, even apart from changing social attitudes.

FAMILY AND STORE-BOUGHT MEDICINES

"Family remedies"—medicines prepared in the home—included herbs, though a tendency existed by the nineteenth century for family remedies to refer primarily to such grocery and other household items as alum, borax, cream of tartar, honey, and unbranded medicines such as Epsom salts, Seidlitz powders, and castor oil. Their ready availability at low cost contributed to their significant role in self-care until around the 1940s. In fact, despite the extensive sale of patent remedies, home medicines have always been a powerful force in domestic care. While they rarely have been studied in terms of effectiveness, they, along with knowledge of how to remove stains from clothes and methods of cleaning silver, have been an integral part of the home economics of countless households and continue to be reported in surveys of "traditional" practices.[16]

The following recollections of some of the more popular medicines are from the memories of Bass and his visitors, and it is clear that they have contributed much to his knowledge of therapy. He vividly remembers purchasing ingredients from the old Mackey store ("Mackey would tell you how to use them") and still occasionally recommends a few—"they're easier to use than herbs"—thus keeping alive a generally safe popular tradition from which he learned a great deal.[17]

One of the best remembered and very popular ways of using family medicines was in poultices. These were employed particularly to "draw out sores" and to relieve cough and cold symptoms (sore throat and congestion of the chest). Poultices, especially mild ones for sores, were "made of almost anything," like flour and lard, Irish potato, light bread, onions, or such herbs as mullein. Pine tar, sulfur, turpentine, and coal oil (i.e., kerosene) were commonly added. The poultice mass was generally spread on a piece of cheese- or flour-cloth (muslin), which was then applied and kept in place overnight.

There is perhaps no end to personalized or family variations of the poultice, which often contained herbs. Bass recalls: "When they'd get something like the flu or the grippe, as they used to call it in the old days, why the mother would fry onions in vinegar and then she'd take and mix flour with that or meal and make a poultice and put it on a cloth on the chest and by the next morning they'd have no cold. It would have been sweated out."

Many accounts exist of overuse of such poultices: " 'Thank goodness you're here, Doc,' a man's hoarse whisper came to me from the bedroom whence came the whimpering, and the scent. 'Peggy's got the pneumonia for sure. She's been ailing a week and we done all we could for her. Her grandma even wrapped her in an onion jacket.' "[18]

Another popular poultice included kerosene, turpentine, camphor, and vinegar, to which was added "meal or flour so it wouldn't burn." It was then put on a flannel cloth (such as a piece of an old pair of pants) and applied to the chest. Occasionally a "mash" of boiled herbs was applied, a remnant of the once-popular application of fomentations, but Mr. Bass does not believe they were as effective as poultices.

If the ailment was deemed potentially serious (for instance, "side pleurisy"), plasters, or "harsh poultices" as they were sometimes called, were used. Made with a paper or leather backing, they were stickier than poultices and hence could be kept in position longer. A common plaster contained pine tar (to aid sticking) mixed with lard and perhaps opossum, raccoon, or skunk oil or fat. "Hunters, in particular," says Bass, "used these." All animal fats, he adds, were felt to be "good at healing," because "animals eat natural products" and hence "have herbs in their system."

Of all the plasters, Bass remembers best the strong ones made with mustard. One recollection he often shares with visitors runs: "I've had the headache so bad you know it run me crazy, but Mother would fix the mustard plaster and just blister my head; it would make it feel good while it was there." The excellent reputation of mustard plasters is derived, in part, from the confidence many physicians continued to have in them until at least the 1940s. Their continuing medical popularity is reflected in various explanations in early twentieth-century medical textbooks to account for the action of mustard, mostly on the basis of counterirritation. Hare, for instance, was characteristically speculative in saying that it acted by "reflex action or the conduction of a nervous impulse to a center which, when so stimulated, sends out an impulse to the part of the body which is diseased."[19]

In addition to poultices and plasters, treatments for coughs and colds included soaking the feet in hot water to which mustard or commercially made Vicks VapoRub had been added, and rubbing the chest with salves. Vicks was sometimes "diluted" by mixing with lard, especially for children, an example of the commonplace activity of modifying over-the-counter medicines into family preparations. Two other popular cough and cold remedies were turpentine and kerosene, generally taken orally with sugar, while camphor dissolved in whiskey was rubbed on the forehead for a headache or fever. Whiskey, undoubtedly the most common vehicle for all sorts of medicines, was also used in the Mackey-Leesburg area and throughout the South to dissolve rock candy, thereby forming one of the most popular cough and cold remedies until recent times.

It is hard to say which was the most popular family remedy for sore throats, astringent alum water (a teaspoonful of alum to a quart of water, sometimes with salt added), or the ever-available kerosene, which had a reputation as a panacea. Another popular throat remedy, often used if the above failed or because of personal preferences by lovers of molasses, was a mixture of baking soda and molasses.

Cuts, sores, and skin problems were commonplace and family medicines were frontline treatments. ("Lots of old people had old

sores that just wouldn't heal.") Apart from the poultices already mentioned, applications of kerosene were the first choice of many people
for sores and even cuts. However, for the latter alum was a favorite
styptic, as it was for poison ivy rashes and "breaking outs." Athlete's
foot was treated sometimes with baking or "table" soda, which also
was used for burns. Borax was employed on occasion, though more
often as a wash for sores. ("Lots of old doctors used it. A friend of
mine who used to drive an old doctor said, 'No matter what kind of
sore or breaking out—the doctor used it.' ")

The ready availability of family medicines helped make them popular for minor stomach ailments; for example, regular soda (for "sour
stomach": one-half teaspoonful in water), baking soda (for indigestion, sour stomach, and cleaning teeth), and hot black pepper or ginger tea (for stomach cramps). Many stomach conditions were treated
by laxatives, of which castor oil was possibly the all-time favorite.
Epsom salts, considered a "cooling laxative," were also popular, more
so than the occasionally used cream of tartar (sometimes mixed with
table soda).

Numerous other household remedies were employed for a broad
spectrum of problems: boric acid for an eyewash, for diaper rash,
or, mixed with powdered alum in Vaseline, as a salve, especially for
children's sores; saltpeter was often used as "a kidney medicine for
man or beast"; salt solutions were instilled into the nose for sinus
problems; and kerosene and turpentine were employed as a liniment
for rheumatism and muscle aches. Of special interest, because of its
reputation in the Mackey-Leesburg area, was a "dough" made from
mud daubers' nests and vinegar used for swollen joints. Bass often
found the nests for others to make the dough.

As much care and attention went into "getting over" an illness as
into "curing" it. Chicken broth was common for supportive care, as a
"strengthener"—a long-standing notion—but if that didn't work, says
Mr. Bass, "you killed a squirrel and gave them squirrel soup. I've
killed many a squirrel for a sick person. Some of them got well, some
didn't, but you see it's easily digested: just put a little meal or cornbread on it. Now oatmeal is also good. I lived on oatmeal since I had a
sick stomach. Sorghum molasses is also good. It's high in iron; that's
the reason it's so healthy for us." Bass might well also have said that a
mixture of sulfur and molasses has been extraordinarily popular as a

"strengthener" and blood purifier, while in his region the ubiquitous buttermilk was perhaps a close second.[20]

The wide range of family medicines, including countless others not described, is generally little known today among people under the age of forty; exceptions include sodium bicarbonate as an antacid, boric acid eyewashes, and poultices for boils. Their relatively rapid demise during the 1940s and 1950s in the face of the ever-growing popularity of new over-the-counter and prescription-only medicines —some more effective, some more convenient but not more effective, and all more expensive—raises a question. Did family medicines go out of fashion because they were largely ineffective, or were they just pushed aside by other treatments? The latter seems to be the primary reason, at least judging from the once-widespread acceptance of most of them within regular medicine and the strong testimonies from Mr. Bass and others of his generation that they provided symptomatic relief.[21]

PATENT MEDICINES

Patent or over-the-counter medicines were a popular and conspicuous part of self-treatment as Tommie Bass was growing up. It was said that a patent medicine bottle was commonly found in mountain cabins throughout the Appalachians.[22] This contributed to what was called the nostrum evil, but Bass views patent medicines otherwise and is upset by the opinion that they are "quack" remedies with the connotation of being fraudulent. They have shaped his thinking in many ways. He has a strong appreciation of the long history of many of them, an enthusiasm for the entrepreneurship by which they were marketed, and confidence in the effectiveness of the many plants used in them, plants he still employs and recommends.

The cultural presence of patent medicines is long-standing and pervasive. After slow growth in numbers in the eighteenth century —when imported British medicines were widely used—American patent medicines (with such evocative names as Ayer's Ague Cure, Chickener's Sugar Coated Pills, and Dr. Osgood's Indian Cholagogue) gained a conspicuous place in the nineteenth century. Types of medicines widely advertised included corn and bunion salves, depilatories, tonics, hair restoratives, preparations for whitening hands and beautifying the skin, purgatives, and cures for coughs, colds, asthma, consumption, deafness, eye troubles, fits, mad dogs, congestion, venereal disease, gout and rheumatism, hernias, impotency, bladder infections, fevers, and liver and kidney problems.[23]

Many nineteenth-century American medicines were marketed honestly and fairly, but out of fifty thousand different medicines made and sold in the United States around the turn of the century—no other product exceeded them in the amount of money spent for national advertising[24]—claims for many were undoubtedly excessive, and sometimes deliberately misleading. The 1906 Food and Drug Act was only partly successful in controlling abuses and reshaping attitudes. The act, by prohibiting interstate commerce in misbranded and adulterated foods, drinks, and drugs, curtailed some of the outrageous claims, but references to curing kidney and liver ailments lasted for many years, due largely to a Supreme Court ruling which held that the law did not prohibit false health claims. The tide of medicines continued to be enormous in the 1920s and 1930s, encouraged by intensive advertising in newspapers, on the radio, and by ephemera from book matches to fans, as well as by ready availability from general stores, drugstores, and door-to-door sales.[25] Bass has a sharp memory of the Watkins dealer, who then, as nowadays, traveled around and took orders for future delivery for "Watkins's brand of liniment, stomach medicine, machine oil and floor polish."[26]

Yet slowly the scene for proprietary medicines changed, leaving Bass and others feeling more and more that they were second-class medicaments. The 1938 Food, Drug, and Cosmetic Act, which replaced the Food and Drug Act of 1906, was most significant.[27] This new legislation enacted more stringent requirements that led to many drugs becoming "doctors' drugs" available on prescription only. Although the 1938 act did not specifically distinguish between over-the-counter and prescription drugs, the FDA's 1939 *Annual Report* reached the administrative conclusion that the 1938 statute allowed the FDA to limit such drugs as sulfanilamide to physicians' prescriptions to ensure adequate supervision. Bass certainly blames "consumer protection" (though he does not use that expression) by the FDA for downgrading and removing from the market some of the "old-time" medicines with their herbal ingredients. Yet also significant to their disappearance were the social upheavals of World War II, new types of medicines that came on the market in the 1940s and 1950s, and, as recognized by Bass, changing commercial practices.

Bass recollects clearly the names of countless proprietary medicine manufacturers, many of which survived a long time after they were founded in the nineteenth century; these included nationally known names such as Pierce, Thacher, Chattanooga Medicine Company, De Gear, St. Joseph, Simmons, Lydia Pinkham, Sloane, Watkins, and Vicks. Of all the medicines, Bass views Pierce's with the highest regard and (incorrectly) the proprietor, R. V. Pierce of Buffalo, New York, as "one of the first main doctors we had in the country." Pierce's national reputation rested on his home medicine book and such medicines as Dr. Pierce's Favorite Prescription, which Bass believes saved his mother's life "a couple of times." Just as he recollects the botanical ingredients of many medicines, he remembers that Dr. Pierce's ("a ladies' medicine, five bottles formed a course of treatment") contained squawvine, black cohosh, black-haw bark, and Solomon's seal. A reason for the popularity of Pierce's remedies in the Bass family household was that, unlike others, they did not contain alcohol but used glycerin, a reflection perhaps of contemporary efforts to improve the quality of medicines.[28]

Children's medicines are also remembered well by Mr. Bass, the result of growing up with three brothers and two sisters. Castoria was a favorite: "There was hardly a kid nowhere that was not brought up on that. I wanted to stay a baby a long time so I could take it, just like syrup." Other "favorites"—or at least widely used items— were Syrup of Figs, Santonin Worm Syrup, and Grove's Chill Tonic. Of only vague memory were the many preparations containing opium such as Mr. Winslow's Soothing Syrup, often used to quiet fractious children; they were not used in the Bass household.[29]

Another once-popular category of patent medicines were liver medicines: "liver regulators," "liver pills," "liver tonics," and so on. One example, Taylor's Vega-Cal, made by the W. D. Taylor Company of Bessemer, Alabama, is of special interest. Bass has, among his bric-a-brac, old bottles for the product and a tin advertising sign: DON'T TAKE CALOMEL—TAKE VEGA-CAL (VEGETABLE CALOMEL). GETS THE BILE. TASTES GOOD—ACTS BETTER. At least up to the 1930s this contained a high concentration of alcohol (12 percent) as well as cascara, senna, peppermint, and cassia in sugar syrup. As the name and advertisement indicate, this product illustrates an emphasis on using botanical remedies rather than the mercury preparation calomel. Bass still appreciates Vega-Cal, for he remembers that many of the old-time medicines contained calomel and "cramped the hound out of you," and affected the gums if used often.

Calomel—sometimes called the "Samson of the Materia Medica" —was commonly used in large quantities during the nineteenth century and often produced serious side effects.[30] Its use continued after heroic doses went out of fashion around mid-century. Bass remembers with graphic clarity taking calomel as a child, always followed some hours later by a dose of castor oil to aid its removal, a regimen long popular, though sometimes with the more drastic purgative jalap.[31]

The last category of patent medicines discussed here is liniments. Of the many remembered by Bass, two stand out: the best known, Sloan's Liniment, "the World's Liniment Recommended for Rheumatic Aches & Pains and Sprains & Strains," is still available. (Bass keeps calendars dating from the 1920s, supplied by the Coleman-Belcher drugstore in nearby Centre, that advertise Sloan's Liniment and other medicines.) The second, Dr. Brown's Magic Liniment, advertised its value as a "guaranteed specific for all manifestations of rheumatism including sciatica, muscular and inflammatory lumbago and backache; neuralgia of face, stomach, spleen and ovaries, also painful menstruation, cramps, etc." Nowadays, in promoting his own liniment, Bass continues to proclaim a panacea reputation for liniments, but his enthusiasm is backed by the testimony he has heard over the years.

Not surprisingly, Bass does not remember (he never knew in detail) the ingredients of most proprietary medicines. Nevertheless, he has an intuitive idea of the contents of a large number. For example, mayapple and senna in laxatives; corn silk and boneset in kidney remedies; wild cherry in cough medicines, cayenne pepper in liniments; sassafras and sumac in liver and blood medicines. Some laxative preparations, with tonics added, were also considered good for the liver; for example, C. F. Simmons's liver medicine contained angelica, mayapple, goldenseal, and gentian. Bass testifies to the effectiveness of many plants which were ingredients, "so we can go along one hundred percent when we remember the old-timers." Bass has also stressed that polypharmacy—the large number of ingredients in some compounded preparations—justifies his own approach to formulations.

MEDICINE BY MAIL

No discussion of self-treatment, especially in rural areas, can omit the impact of mail-order companies—large ones, such as Sears, Roebuck, and many smaller ones. Throughout his life Bass has purchased items from them, and he knows of many people who used home remedies from Sears catalogs until at least the 1930s. One 1930s catalog, still treasured by Bass, advertised not only a host of proprietary medicines, including St. Joseph's range of "family medicines," but also health foods and such popular nonbotanical tonics of the day as cod-liver oil, iron, liver extract, and glycerophosphates. These foreshadowed the present-day emphasis on vitamins, minerals, and health foods. Mail order companies were influential in many ways. A decade or so after the 1938 Food, Drug, and Cosmetic Act, promoters were still claiming that diseases like cancer and diabetes could be eradicated with recipes sent by mail. Busts could be built up and virility quickened. In the beckoning world of direct-mail promotion almost anything could be found, and stark examples of quackery existed that could never survive over-the-counter marketing.[32]

Efforts by the post office to control some of the most flagrant frauds have been partially successful, but innumerable doubtful products remain readily available today, especially in the areas of nutrition and improvement of sexual image. Even money-back guarantees, which provide much confidence for people like Bass, are no safeguard against misleading claims. A real difficulty exists in distinguishing fraudulent from genuine claims, especially in the area of herbs.[33]

SELF-TREATMENT TODAY

The 1940s and 1950s brought a period of decline in the popularity of family medicines and the disappearance or lowering in social standing of many "old-timer" patent medicines. Up to then Mr. Bass had learned how to treat symptoms economically using commonplace kitchen items, the use of many plants employed in patent medi-

cines, and to appreciate that entrepreneurship often brought success
to medicine makers. His sense of confidence in family and patent
medicines has been encouraged by the fact that, in his younger years,
many physicians prescribed them. He recalls that some local practitioners seemed to prescribe "nothing more than a mustard plaster"
for many complaints. Dr. Cross in his Gadsden drugstore commonly
recommended family medicines, even though much of his business
success depended on the sale of patent medicines advertised in Sears,
Roebuck's catalogs and elsewhere. Only a few of the more popular
medicines, such as Lydia Pinkham's Vegetable Compound for "hot
flashes" and Dr. Hitchcock's Laxative Powder, survived for long after
World War II. Advertisements for them continued to appear in local
newspapers, and slogans like "Stop taking harsh drugs for constipation" helped sustain the notion that botanical remedies were better
than those prepared from chemicals (see *Cherokee County Herald*,
24 October 1951, p. 7).

Other indexes of change are easy to recognize. For instance, while
over-the-counter remedies have remained a central feature in drugstores (an estimated 350,000 kinds were available in 1970), many new
types such as steroid creams, antihistamines, and vasoconstrictors
have appeared. Furthermore, medicines are now commonly marketed
on open shelves, supermarket-style, a reflection that the entire image
of pharmacy has altered from a cottage-level activity to a big-business
atmosphere.[34] Associated with this is the availability of antibiotics,
tranquilizers, and other "miracles" of modern medicine available only
on prescription but often prescribed with impunity. The postwar generation has undoubtedly grown up with the view that germs should
be killed with antibiotics.[35]

Although recent legislative changes allow some prescription-only
medicines to be sold over the counter, and new emphases on prevention have fostered some feeling of common ground between regular medicine and self-care, the general tenor of postwar changes has
sharpened the difference between self-treatment and regular medicine in the minds of Bass and many of his visitors. They often express
disquiet with "official" or establishment medical views, at least those
that argue that the public should be protected from anything that is
not demonstrably safe and effective. A common feeling exists that
"wolf" is cried too often by the FDA and medical scientists. Certain

paradoxes are also recognized that seem to underscore professional medicine's sense of ambivalence about self-treatment. For instance, despite concerns over safety, entrepreneurship and hard selling of medicines is dominant in drugstores and supermarkets, aided by television and other advertising. Instant medication for many ailments is promoted. Such medical entrepreneurship is comfortable to Mr. Bass, whose activities may be seen as part of it.

A further aspect of the present-day over-the-counter medicine scene that gives Bass heart is that at least a few of the old favorite medicines are still available, testimony for him of the power of herbs and reinforcing their cultural presence. Examples include some produced locally (e.g., cumarindine), and others from farther afield such as Dr. Pierce's Golden Medical Discovery, Black Draught, and Carter's Little Liver Pills.[36] The continuity contributes to the cultural ethos that exists between him and some older visitors, both white and black.[37]

Another heart-warming feature of self-treatment for Bass is the conspicuous recent development of health food stores which sell—among other things—crude drugs, often in capsule form. The nationwide impact of this development is conspicuous not only in urban settings, but also in such rural areas as Bass's. Around two hundred herbs are obtainable from local health food stores and drugstores and from distributors selling capsules of herbs from their homes or businesses.[38] In March 1983 Bass started helping a local business in capsulated herbs, generally promoted as "concentrated foods in capsulated form" (see chapter 6). Indeed, capsulated herbs have dramatically changed the style and scope of his practice.

His association with the health food movement has also exposed him to a new level of antiestablishment opinion toward medicine which only adds conviction to his faith in herbs. Further, when he hears that more and more chiropractics are using herbs, he believes that the overall reputation of herbal medicine will ultimately improve. In some ways Bass's attitudes and sympathies mirror an eclecticism toward self-treatment that is as marked today as in times past when legislation was freer. Certainly recent studies have demonstrated that very large numbers of patients undergoing regular treatment take alternative therapies.[39]

Noticeable features of self-treatment over time—such as uneasy relations with professional medicine and particular confidence in remedies stamped by local testimony, especially if they fit into prevailing concepts of disease and therapy—not only help us understand some of the background of Bass's attitudes, but also those of his visitors. Expectations among the latter often depend on and vary according to the illness, changing confidence in physicians, past experiences, and willingness to try a "safe" remedy, one without side effects.[40]

Another issue is that some people do call Bass a quack, particularly if they do not know him well. Yet such an attitude—in line with those who see the public as generally credulous and gullible about medicine—ignores the pervasiveness of many attitudes behind self-treatment, some dependent on class allegiances and a sense of separateness from the medical profession. All this makes it overly glib to label Bass gullible. Those who do are ignoring his patterns of thinking, which remain untouched by the analytical frameworks established by lengthy formal education.

CHAPTER 5

Acquiring Herbal Knowledge:
A Popular Tradition

I've known about the biggest part of plants since I was a little boy. I've helped people all my life. Just like a politician I've always had herbs in my system.

Our discussion of Mr. Bass's personality, life, and setting has shown that many experiences—for example, the influence of his parents, tending and treating animals, and observing countless minor ailments in a small community—provided him with opportunities to learn about herbs and medicines. As we look in more detail at how Bass acquired, piecemeal, a wide repertoire of knowledge, we consider first two factors that helped to create a framework for his learning: his place among traditional practitioners and some of his concepts about plants. In many ways these have substituted for his lack of formal education. A question surfaces, considered later in detail, about whether or not knowledge of herbs accounts for all of Bass's success.

A SPECTRUM OF PRACTITIONERS

While Mr. Bass is the only long-standing public herbalist in his area, he consciously draws upon the tradition of folk practitioners and reflects many of their characteristics such as authority and personal disinterest. His sense of tradition becomes especially noticeable when he feels defensive about his practice, as in the presence of doctors.

The number of traditional practitioners who play a significant role in health care in American communities today is far fewer than before the 1940s, when alternative health care was much less formalized. In those days herbalists (often called yarb doctors), faith healers, granny women, and such "specialists" as bonesetters, blood stoppers, and medicine-show doctors were most influential on Bass's development.[1]

Of particular influence were granny women, or granny midwives, such as Molly Kirby in Mackey-Leesburg, whose services went beyond midwifery and were often compensated by gifts of food or by gratitude alone.[2] The herbal knowledge of many granny women falls within the Anglo-Saxon tradition, which is characterized as primarily secular with reliance on experience. In America the tradition owes much to British and Irish immigrants, though undoubtedly it has been reinforced by those from other European countries as well.[3] Mr. Bass works within the same tradition and it is of special interest that Molly Kirby sent some of her patients to him for herbs. When she died, sometime around 1940, these people continued to go to him for herbs as well as advice.

White male herbalists known to Bass, such as "Doc" Nelson of Gadsden, fall within the same tradition. Mr. Bass recalls:

> Doc was not a doctor. He told people he was, but he just played with herbs. He took a course with the Meyer's herb people. One time Doc had me gather a bunch of pine tops. He used them in making his cough medicine. And then he wanted plantain. We gathered big sackfuls of that. And chickweed and sweet gum leaves to put in his cough remedy. He died some time ago, but I still see someone every once in a while that took his medicine. One of the men who used to deliver milk—said he had ulcers— went to old Doc for something in a mayonnaise jar that was yellow and tasted like mayonnaise in a way. I said, "Partner, that's mayonnaise with ground-up yellowroot and goldenseal." He said it sure did heal his ulcers.[4]

Herbal practitioners like Doc Nelson and Mr. Bass developed their practices slowly, first offering advice to neighbors and then gradually attaining a local or regional reputation. Practitioners elsewhere in the Appalachians also illustrate this and the secular-experiential approach to using herbs.[5] One is Kern Kiser, who in 1973 was selling herbal remedies from his home in southern Appalachia. Initially, his interest was aroused by being treated for a sting by an "old man—a thoroughbred Indian." Kiser built up his knowledge after trying many herbs and finding they "worked good."[6]

Neither faith doctors nor his father's ability to "blow out" burns apparently had much influence on Bass. He generally remains skeptical about white practitioners who employ nonnatural concepts, even in conjunction with herbs. His skepticism rests on the opinion that some practices are fraudulent. Bass is unappreciative of the many practitioners who have become part of the present-day wholistic movement without a clear lineage from the past.[7] On the other hand, he is enthusiastic about what he has heard of curanderos and other "native" practitioners, above all, American Indians.[8] He particularly admires the spiritual conviction of Indian medicine men and knows that many became practitioners through acquiring a "gift."

One example (unknown to Bass) is Vernon Cooper, a Lumbee Indian of Robeson County, North Carolina. He acquired the gift in 1917, and in 1980 he was still treating patients by means of prayer, massage, and herbal remedies.[9] Just how he acquired his detailed knowledge is unclear, but important influences were his grandmother, who was a midwife and herb doctor, and a homeopathic practitioner, Dr. Jesse Hair. As a child, Vernon Cooper helped gather herbs and prepare hair tonics. Later, like Mr. Bass, through a variety of jobs—"a little of everything but turpentining"—he assumed an authoritative role in his community.[10]

Mr. Bass is less certain, indeed less knowledgeable, about the bewildering array of black practitioners. These, often difficult to classify precisely, have been called healers, herb doctors, root workers, readers, granny advisers, spiritualists, and conjure men and women. Black practitioners are sometimes grouped according to how their skills were acquired—by "gift" or learning—or according to their mode of practice.[11] Diverse treatments reflect diverse approaches: use of herbs, rituals, having the patient wear special clothing, strings, or amulets, or merely providing reassurance. Time spent with clients is equally variable, as is the location of practices—from a chapel to an officelike setting.[12] Whatever the practice, an underlying religious conviction is commonplace, just as it is among many practitioners in other ethnic groups.[13]

Religion is not a conspicuous feature of Bass's practice, but as he recounts his belief that God provided the herbs of the field for a purpose, it is clear that religious faith is one of the many components of the herbal tradition in which he practices.

CONCEPTUALIZING PLANTS

A more subtle aspect of the traditions that shaped Bass's activities is the way he and herbalists before him perceived relationships among plants not as botanical families but as "families of useful herbs." After his early years of constantly observing and learning about plants and animals, mostly from his mother and father and neighbors, a framework emerged whereby he, perhaps unconsciously, classifies plants and looks for similarities and differences among them. This has not only helped him to retain and assimilate a vast store of information, and to "inventory plants" (his phrase) in collecting areas, but also to ask himself questions about plants new to him.

Bass first learned plant names and plant identifications from family and friends as well as from books, pamphlets, and flyers. His ready recognition of "substitutes" and "facsimiles" for plants he had heard or read about but could not find in his locale and his appreciation of "wild" and "tame" plants suggest that from experience he soon saw relationships and affinities in which to place new information acquired orally or from reading. Many vernacular plant names include the word "wild," like wild bergamot, wild carrot, wild cherry, and wild lettuce. He generally considers that wild plants provide "stronger medicines" than cultivated ones. In addition to "classifying" plants by their usefulness, he recognizes a few natural groups such as a "family of bonesets," or the many "hyssops." [14]

The way Mr. Bass uses vernacular names and groups some plants is analogous to that employed in cultures unaffected by the scientific study of botany. [15] The constant comparison of one plant with another apparently illustrates what has been called the "horizontal expansion" of names over time; that is, defining new plants or groups of taxa by the addition of a descriptive word to an existing name, like red oak and white oak, broad dock and yellow dock, broad-leaf plantain and narrow-leaf plantain, and so on.

Assuming that such comparisons reflect the development of knowledge of plant relationships, Bass's use of vernacular names underscores the idea that folk knowledge of plants is not always as far removed from "scientific" taxonomy as is sometimes supposed. "Man," it has been said, "is by nature a classifying animal," but while it is "one thing to describe typological regularities," it is not easy to understand how knowledge of them emerged.[16] A consideration of Bass's knowledge suggests that analogy and comparison serve as the basis for recognizing and remembering plant groups.

Particularly interesting is his accentuation of the adjective part of vernacular names, many of which reflect comparisons from everyday life, from religion to shirt buttons. Examples include bee balm, blazing star, boarhog root, butterfly weed, buttonbush, carpet weed, devil's shoestring, elephant's foot, lady's slipper, and shepherd's purse. Many vernacular names suggest medicinal properties; this serves as another authority behind such herbs as Indian physic, pleurisy root, ague root, ague weed, ague bark, alumroot, and feverwort. According to Mr. Bass, the reason why these medicinal plants possess additional names not indicative of therapeutic properties is because people view plants in different ways, or because some names do contain medical allusions, such as Indian sage and marsh sage for boneset.

It seems clear that the motivation behind Bass's mental classification of plants—pinpointing similarities and differences—is a utilitarian one; some consider utilitarian factors to be the basis of folk classification in general.[17] It is increasingly obvious that the origins of Western natural science owe much to the recording by classical authors of folk classifications and the subsequent sharpening of taxonomic criteria for distinguishing one organism from another. It has been pointed out, too, that during Renaissance times the tendency for herbals to focus on individual plants rather than, as hitherto, on a group of plants, was more for the sake of horticulturalists and notions of individualism than for strictly medical criteria.[18] Bass's practice rests on categorizing herbs, but it also suggests that continual first-hand observations of nature have been important in maintaining folk classifications.

If Bass's utilitarianism—with specific interest in medicinal properties of plants—encourages a lack of interest in the niceties of scientific distinctions (for instance, his "substitute" brooklimes are based solely on similarity of habit and habitat), he is at least part of a broad tradition. He can be seen to be both eclectic and conservative insofar as he places much confidence in his own experience. Partly because of this, he claims less of herbs than is generally found in modern advocacy herbals compiled primarily from secondary sources.

A MATRIX OF INFORMATION

So far we have noted the effects of both oral and printed sources of information on Bass's development. We now elaborate on these in looking at two periods in Bass's practice as an herbalist. The first, up to around 1960, was typified by a modest but growing level of activity ("it was more a hobby time"); the second is his more recent growing influence locally and regionally.

How usage of herbs and other medical knowledge is transmitted from one generation to the next, and how it and folk beliefs in general are sustained, are topics of great interest. While oral traditions have shaped Bass's life in many ways, especially because he has lived in a community in which oral talents are widely appreciated, they were probably no more important than printed sources. Mr. Bass has been reading since the age of six, and it is now often impossible to pinpoint which printed sources provided him with new information or merely reinforced—by his selective reading of information and ideas which fit into his existing framework of knowledge—that obtained from his parents or "other rural folk who learn from one another." Transmission of information brought together from oral and written sources —generally so closely intertwined that it is impossible to determine which has had the greatest influence—is commonly referred to as the "popular tradition."[19]

Much of our account illuminates the popular tradition and its diverse components and dynamic nature. It is often felt—erroneously —that traditional medicine is static. Yet as we observed Bass incorporating new ideas, two points became obvious. One is that new information often does not replace existing ideas; instead it is incorporated into an existing framework, which may then be modified. Second, much of the new information is derived from professional medicine, which has been an important factor in sustaining belief in certain herbs over time and contributes, like patent medicines, to creating channels of communication between visitors and herbalists.

The backcountry life of Bass's parents provided ready circumstances for young Tommie to start learning to identify medicinal plants. Although he feels that his mother had the greatest influence on his development, his father initiated at least two major activities in his life: trapping and fur dealing and gathering medicinal plants for the market.

Tommie Bass's father followed a long and continuing tradition of gathering herbs in Appalachia.[20] An occasional collector of "sang" (ginseng), he shipped it and a few other herbs to such wholesale companies as the St. Louis Commission Company, Funston Brothers of St. Louis, and Higgins and Waters of Baltimore, all of which sold medicinal plants for the collectors on a 10 percent commission. The companies helped collectors, including young Tommie, by supplying pamphlets containing pictures and descriptions of plants and by identifying plants sent to them. Particular interest was aroused in plants which brought the highest price per pound, and, on the basis of this "pedigree," Mr. Bass still considers these of special medical value. Aided by low shipping costs, Bass sent substantial amounts of herbs to the companies.

By the early 1920s, when Bass was a teenager, the aura of the Appalachians and its wealth of medicinal plants began to encompass him more and more. It is reported that approximately 75 percent of all crude drugs collected in the United States have come from western North Carolina, eastern Tennessee, and southwestern Virginia.[21] We estimate that of approximately 2,500 plant species in the area, 1,100 or so have been reported to have medicinal properties; some are still collected for national and international crude drug markets.[22] The Appalachians are well known, too, for the practice of traditional medicine among the scattered population in the hollows and valleys, a population mostly Anglo-Saxon in origin. Although the employment of traditional medical practices has declined during the past fifty years or so, a core group of about thirty medicinal plants is still widely employed, with another three hundred or so botanicals and store-bought items used on occasion.[23]

As a young man drawing on Appalachian lore, Tommie Bass became a self-taught field naturalist while honing skills with the broadax, bucksaw, mattock, sickle, hoe, carpenter saw, steel trap, and so on acquired as a backwoodsman and through many jobs. Much of his domestic knowledge, such as handling the butter churn and gathering a wide range of greens, has also contributed to his practical knowledge of nature. He knows dozens of ways of making pocket money. For instance, he often tells boys how to collect worms for fishing by spraying a one-to-one dilution of bleach onto an area of soil to bring them to the surface. These interests and skills were not pursued by his younger brothers and sisters. "They don't know a thing about nature or natural things. In fact, they was more of a city people." Aside from his character, his role as first son and principal help to his father was significant. Perhaps, too, by the time he was in his twenties he recognized that his knowledge of herbs was appreciated and allowed him to contribute to people's welfare.

When Bass was first learning about medicinal plants, those sold through the commercial market—often for regular medicine—were called "official" medicines. This pedigree still serves him as testimony to their effectiveness. Equally compelling testimony is the presence of plants in a large number of over-the-counter medicines or patent medicines (considered in chapter 4), as well as his father's distribution of a homemade rheumatism medicine along with products put out by the American Remedy Company.[24] It was in connection with his father's activities with this company that Bass developed a lifelong wariness of doctors' attitudes. It is not outright suspicion, but an inherent worry about what they think about his activities: "The doctors got in after Dad; they never did arrest him. He went out and got a bunch of the people to come in to one of the doctor's offices and said, 'Doc, you ask them what I told them.' One said, 'Bass didn't tell us it'd do anything.' All stood behind him."

Apart from recommending and selling herbs, Bass has always been attracted to the convenience of patent medicines and the entrepreneurship of selling them. He has sold them almost continuously since he acquired unsold stock from the local general store in 1926. Much of this business, as with herbs, has been carried out through mail order, a noticeable feature of rural life. One of Bass's early advertisements in the *Alabama Farmers' Bulletin* (1 March 1945) is typical of those he used for the next thirty years: "Wanted: Star of Grub root, Star grass root, Lady Slipper, Snake root, Black Haw bark or root, Calamus and Blood root, etc. Write for prices—A. L. Bass, Leesburg (Cherokee Co.)." Correspondence generated by these ads added to his knowledge.

The 1920s and 1930s were a "haphazard time" for the herb market, Bass remembers, because of the "lopsided nature of the business." A writer on Appalachia indicated in 1924 that "only a few medicinal roots can be sold at the store where a (company) buyer comes perhaps once a year. Going 'sanging' (to dig wild ginseng) used to be a common and profitable recreation which brought one a bit of money as well as a pleasant ramble in the woods."[25] Regardless of the slow market, Mr. Bass's knowledge continued to expand. "About 1925, when I was 17, I didn't use medicinal plants myself at that time, but there's hardly a main plant out here, that is, mayapple, yellow dock, alumroot, poke-root, dandelion, boneset, wild cherry bark, and those things, I didn't know about." This was the time, too, when local people started to ask Mr. Bass for advice about herbs and to share their own knowledge. For instance, he remembers a neighbor querying whether redshank, recommended by granny midwife Molly Kirby for a child's colitis, was good for diarrhea.[26]

Bass's growing reputation from this time, through the 1940s and 1950s and then into his more active period from 1960 to the present, was fostered by his unquenchable thirst for knowledge, best described as eclectic abandon. His sources included almanacs, herb buyers' lists, information sheets and calendars furnished by local drugstores, the radio, and domestic medicine manuals. Comments on some of these help to illustrate the pervasiveness of ephemeral items in contributing to or sustaining popular traditions.

Produced in the tens of thousands since around the mid-nineteenth century, almanacs have been a significant source of information on botanicals and home medicines in general. Some almanacs, such as those from the Illinois Herb Company, focus specifically on herbs and herbal products: "Herbs are Nature's Way to Health."[27] Bass recalls that some herb company almanacs were like medical books, with long lists of herbs and their uses.[28] The bulk of "medical" almanacs, however, were issued by patent medicine companies and "were always available in the local drugstore." These almanacs, simply written, found their way into most of the homes of Bass's visitors. Apart from advertising medicines, they gave a lot of general information on health matters. Almanacs for Morse's Indian Root Pills, for instance, included notes, still remembered by Mr. Bass, on liver disorders.[29] While it is difficult to assess the precise influence of almanacs, many of Mr. Bass's visitors have much detailed knowledge of their contents, and, as they say, the almanacs are always lying around.

Apart from health-oriented almanacs, such general almanacs as Grier's—widely circulated in Bass's community—have commonly carried advertisements for long-standing popular medicines like Black Draught, sss Tonic, Vicks's products, Lydia Pinkham's, and Grove's Tasteless Chill Tonic.

The same products were frequently advertised in newspapers and on the radio. Bass loves to talk about early radio, and it is clear that it quickly became a cultural force in his life. He recalls listening to the radio in Leesburg in 1927 and attributes much social change to radio's role in education and in helping to "bring the country together." He remembers wholesome, "clean shows," and much advertising of proprietary medicines such as Vicks, Black Draught, Dr. Miles's medicines, Pinex (a cough medicine "you mix yourself" and "add lemon and sugar"), and especially Hadacol. The latter perhaps had the biggest impact in the South around 1950: "You could hardly turn any radio station on at that time in the day or night that didn't have it on"—"it really straightened out people." In Hadacol's heyday the advertising bill ran to $1 million a month, including about 700 daily papers, 4,700 weeklies, and 528 radio stations.[30]

Apart from almanacs and radio and newspaper advertising, a main resource of information in the Bass family home was R. V. Pierce's *The People's Common Sense Medical Advisor*, one of the most popular home medicine books of the late nineteenth and early twentieth centuries, and described by Bass as a book "uneducated persons could understand if they could read." However, it was not one of the more elementary home medicine books and it, like many others, promoted an ideology of maintaining health through education about the body.[31] It is difficult to estimate how much this ideology affected individuals in rural areas like Mackey-Leesburg. It seems, though, that for Mr. Bass, the Pierce volume provided two areas of information: (1) descriptions (with diagrams) that encouraged a mechanical view of the body; namely, that it "works like a motor-car engine," in which special attention should be paid to such "filters" as the liver and the kidney (see chapter 7); and (2) specific information on individual remedies: family remedies, medicinal plants, and R. V. Pierce's proprietary medicines. Another late-nineteenth-century work in young Tommie Bass's home, used to supplement Pierce, was H. B. Allen's

Useful Companion and Artificer's Assistant, which provided general information on diseases and various family remedies.

Although Bass still possesses and uses these two volumes, J. E. Meyer's *The Herbalist* has had the greatest influence. It was first published in 1918 (the same era as Pierce's and Allen's books), when botanical remedies were still widely used. Not only does it contain precise information on many plants but it also reflects the influence of Eclectic botanic medicine. Bass sells a 1975 edition (essentially unrevised from the first edition) in which herbs continue to be described in terms of such general medicinal properties as bitter, diaphoretic, expectorant, pectoral, astringent, alterative, febrifuge, and diuretic.

Another herbal used and sold by Bass is Jethro Kloss's *Back to Eden*, first published in 1939. The 1975 edition—"704 pages of old-fashioned, time-tested good health advice"—has a more evangelical tone than Meyer's work. It underscores a "natural" approach to health, a concept with which Mr. Bass has much sympathy. This concept is reinforced time and time again by such phrases as "God's original plant for restoring health" and the "fundamental principle of healing consists of a return of natural habits of living." Apart from succinct if somewhat hyperbolic accounts of herbs, Kloss includes much general information on diseases, water-cure treatment, diet, cooking, aluminum poisoning, and so on. (Bass, like so many other advocates of herbal teas, emphasizes the dangers of using aluminum vessels.)

The natural approach to treatment is reinforced in countless advocacy books published in recent years. Two booklets, well thumbed by Bass, are Claudia V. James's *Herbs and the Fountain of Youth* and H. E. Kirschner's *Nature's Healing Grasses*. James's book in particular stresses the importance of "natural medicine and healthful living." As is commonplace in much advocatory literature, it is a mix of religion, history, science, and references to the dangers of regular medicine and treatment. For example: "Many patients have succumbed to the effect of radium and X-ray treatments in the hands of inexpert manipulators of the deadly machines."[32]

Popular magazines, particularly *Prevention*, also have had much influence on Bass and many of his visitors. Founded in 1948 (and reaching a circulation of over one million in the 1960s and 1970s),

Prevention has been a major plank in the teaching of health promoter Jerome Irving Rodale (1891–1971) and his sons. It stresses that natural or organically grown foods are the foundation of good health—a view that reinforces the writings of Kloss, James, and others. The restoration of a natural diet was the primary objective of the elder Rodale's "prevention system for better health."[33] Bass has probably derived more knowledge of and enthusiasm for minerals and vitamins from *Prevention* than from any other source, as well as the widely held view that natural vitamin C is superior to synthetic. Articles mentioning the value of herbs reinforce his existing knowledge, while references to minerals remind him of the healthful properties of mineral springs.[34]

Bass has gained little scientific understanding about vitamins from this reading, for, like many others, he has integrated vitamins into older conceptual frameworks of tonics and stimulants, perhaps part of the reason why vitamins are widely believed to give "pep and energy."[35] In fact, it is not easy to acquire a good understanding from such advocacy literature as *Prevention* because, while scientific papers are often referred to, much of the information—given out of context or misinterpreted—has the character of pseudoscience.

Bass has undoubtedly acquired much of his conceptual framework via the spoken rather than the written word, as reflected by the countless things he has "known all my life" and the remarkable number of sayings and beliefs from Alabama and southern Appalachia that he knows.[36] He says that the reason he has heard so many sayings is because of his contacts with many people through his innumerable jobs and his life as an herbalist. He reckons he has learned of only a few "new things" through reading; it seems clear that oral information has had the greatest effect on him. Specific examples are given in the monographs in volume 2, where Bass remembers learning about a medicinal plant from a neighbor (for instance, devil's shoestring and New Jersey tea), although he knows his reading about them has reinforced his convictions.

Bass believes that he has learned much from the Indians, particularly the Cherokees, who have been a key feature in Appalachian history—even apart from reading an authoritative small booklet by Hamel and Chiltoskey entitled *Cherokee Plants*. Although the extent of specific Indian influence on white medicine is often overestimated, the ethos of Cherokee medicine, at least the widespread use of herbs, has been very significant to Bass. Although some rather scornful views of Cherokee medicine were published in the nineteenth century, many writers have stressed the "hundreds of years" of Indian experience in using indigenous plants. This not only reinforces confidence in much Anglo-Saxon knowledge, but also influences Bass and many of his visitors. The "authority" of Indian knowledge is easy to find in Appalachia today, for instance with such vernacular plant names as Indian chickweed, Indian hemp, Indian pennyroyal, Indian pink, Indian plantain, Indian sage, squawroot, squawvine, and wahoo.[37]

A COMMERCIAL EDGE

The 1960s saw a considerable expansion of Mr. Bass's activities, in part following the increasingly widespread interest in natural foods and herbs. A good deal of the expansion came about from his commercial activities, which amplified his network of sources of information considerably. Undoubtedly entrepreneurship has been a significant force in the part he plays in the popular herbal tradition, even apart from promoting patent medicines.

During his early fifties, wanting to devote more attention to herbs, he expanded his mail-order activities. Another significant development was the opportunity to collect plants for a wholesale herb dealer, Doc Sanders, who "lived in Pickens County, Alabama, but his post office was in Prairie Point, Mississippi." "We got to writing back and forth. He had me send him herbs. I shipped him queen-of-the-meadow and horsemint and watercress plants, and, oh, just quite a lot of wild plants—wild ginger, ratsvein. He wanted me to ship him bugleweed, but I didn't know what it was then. He just used the hound out of that. You see he shipped herbs all over the country. I sold him ground-ivy by the hundred pounds and chickweed." Much of the business with Sanders was on a contract basis, and it is the only time that Mr. Bass felt he made any money out of herbs.[38] He also learned a great deal. "Doc Sanders was the one that teached me about the goosegrass and wild yam. If I was doubtful of what he wanted, he would send me samples." The employment of samples was, in fact, not foolproof (see "Skullcap", vol. 2).

Bass's local visibility also increased in the 1960s through gathering more and more herbs for local people—including Doc Nelson of Gadsden—operating a trade barn (1963–67) where he had an herb rack, and his friendship with George Butler, a reporter for the *Gadsden Times*. For many years the herbalist and journalist, an enthusiastic student of herbs, went on Sunday rambles in search of plants. Butler wrote occasional articles on herbs for his newspaper: "It's Time Again for Those Spring-Tonic Poke Greens" (28 April 1968); "Yellow Root, Popular Herb" (11 April 1971); "It's Chickweed Time Again" (1 April 1973), and so on.[39] Bass says the effect of newspaper publicity —which has increased immeasurably in recent years—made him a "pretty famous guy in the way of herbs after 1962."

So far we have indicated eclectic sources of information, oral and printed. Mr. Bass is somewhat like an indiscriminate magpie in the way he gathers information, but clearly the information best retained is that which reinforces existing ideas. Even so, he correctly emphasizes that much of the knowledge he puts into practice rests on his own experience in trying out remedies and observing the results through visitors' testimonies: "I've got a lot of my learning from actual experience." The results, as seen in later chapters in this volume and in volume 2, are strikingly in line with historical usages, except, he says, where he has used recent information without subjecting it to experience.

While we have focused on Bass's developing knowledge of herbs and the factors sustaining a popular tradition, it is appropriate to ask here whether other factors have strengthened the tradition in his hands by giving it authority. Bass certainly believes that most visitors have faith in his knowledge about herbs—an index of the respect for his integrity. "A lot of people who come have knowed me all their lives. I wouldn't tell them anything I cannot back up. Do not think I am a soothsayer, I am not putting a spell on them." However, despite his views, he recognizes the possibility that a number of visitors see him as a healer, perhaps as a shaman rather than a medicine man. "Some people who come to talk to me seem to go away feeling better, but I don't have any power."[40] Even those who do not see him as a healer recognize him as a special individual.

The symbiotic relationship that exists between Mr. Bass and the community in which he lives merits further comment. Tommie Bass is widely respected even among many who have little or no sympathy for his herbal practice. This respect rests not only on his community service but also on his personal characteristics: his mild manner, self-deprecation, fatalism, self-reliance, teetotalism, and firmly stated views, which he shares willingly with friends and neighbors. Mr. Bass's apparent good health and simple existence are thought-provoking in an age of widespread materialism and acquisitiveness. In many ways he acts as an integrative force in the community, both by encouraging open communication and by virtue of his integrity. His integrating role is furthered because, while he is religious, he has not developed strong loyalties to any one church, and because his many jobs have mitigated against carrying over comraderies from the workplace to his everyday life. Further, his age, his bachelor status, his quiet demeanor, and his graphic turn of phrase allow him to interact with various social groups in the area (rural elites, town elites, small farmers). These groups have expanded and become more diffuse in recent years.

Mr. Bass, then, is part of a number of social networks, and through them he is able to pass along advice about health matters (sometimes "practical common sense" as much as about herbs). It is appropriate to speculate that this may have more significance than merely contributing to the corporate sense of community, since more and more medical sociologists are arguing that the presence or absence of social networks are important factors in recovery from many illnesses, including asthma, heart attacks, cancer, stress (depression and anxiety), and schizophrenia.[41] While no studies have been undertaken in Bass's region to see if extended social networks have a measurable effect on the health of individuals, it is clear, on a subjective basis, that Bass improves the well-being of many local people apart from suggesting or dispensing herbs or offering advice.

CHAPTER 6

The Practice: Setting and Visitors

I'm a hurting and sickly woman.

This account of Bass's activities, witnessed between 1980 and 1987, describes two phases of his practice. The first, up to 1983, followed a pattern essentially unchanged for forty years, although since the 1970s there have been growing numbers of visitors, all helping to make these later years a golden age in distilling a lifetime's experience. The second phase, beginning in 1983, is characterized by an enthusiastic promotion of commercially prepared capsules of herbs that has reduced many of Bass's long-standing practices to a minimum. As we consider various features of his practice, some commonplace to traditional medicine, a question already raised is underscored: Is his success in treatment due solely to herbal medicines?

PRACTICING FROM THE YARD, SHACK, OR WOODS

First-time visitors to Mr. Bass are generally fascinated by the haphazard scene of hand-painted notices, rickety sheds—some full of sacks of herbs—a shack serving as home and office, and all manner of secondhand items, empty bottles, and bric-a-brac for sale and giveaway. All this is situated on an acre lot with a sizable, somewhat run-down, 1920s-era porched frame house bequeathed to him in 1979. Mr. Bass prefers the shack to the house, which he uses only for its kitchen and bathroom, and for storage.

The chaos in what Bass calls his junkyard is deceptive, however, because whether he is looking for herbs or an old newspaper, he can generally find anything. The profusion of items is a measure of salvaging, recycling, and self-sufficiency. Nothing is thrown away; sooner or later someone will come along for the old bottles or hubcaps.[1]

A visit with Bass generally takes place in the yard, on the porch, or inside his shack, depending on the weather. In the winter a coffeepot of warm sassafras tea on top of a laundry stove greets the visitor to the cluttered shack, with its walls lined with old calendars and photographs of friends and relatives. Pictures of President and Mrs. Reagan and Senator Jesse Helms, also on the walls, are testimony to a spirit of republican independence. Often a visit is brief, but time is always available for cordial conversation, which ranges over local events, reminiscences, and references to mutual acquaintances, births, marriages, and deaths, all laced with Bass's stories, jokes, and testimonials about the effectiveness of herbs. When people leave, the last comment from Mr. Bass is often, "I'm sure glad you came."

During many a conversation in the heyday of his practice, following an initial exchange of pleasantries, a visitor mentions an ailment or worry. Bass usually responds, at least for such common problems as ulcers and rheumatism, by indicating that he might be able to provide relief ("ease") rather than a cure, and that the visitor may be a "guinea pig to see if the medicine works." He often assures the visitor that the medicine is safe. Usually no charge is made for the "trial" of medicine. ("I'm going to make a present of that. Don't tell on me.") If the medicine "works" the visitor is told to return for more and then the cost is commonly in the range of one to two dollars.

Visitors, except for many regulars who want further supplies of, say, yellowroot for ulcers or a tea for diabetes, often arrive in groups of two, three, or more. Initially only one person may admit to a medical problem (e.g., rheumatism), but eventually everyone leaves with herbs (enough in a plastic bag to make a gallon of tea) or advice, perhaps for obesity, nerves, or stomach ulcers.

Others arrive solely to talk about herbs, to get help with the identification of such plants as heal-all, chickweed, or queen-of-the-meadow, or to obtain advice for friends or relatives. On some occasions visitors leave with turnip greens or other vegetables from Bass's garden.

Much advice is given over the telephone; in fact, the telephone, as it has in medical practice in general, has become a central feature of his practice and has contributed much to his mail-order business.[2]

Bass has long had a general-store license to sell not only his locally collected herbs, salves, and other medicines he prepares, but also a range of commercially prepared products such as tablets or capsules of alfalfa, comfrey root, gotu kola, and senna. He appreciates that some people find tablets or capsules more convenient than making teas. After all, he says, a tea can be made from a tablet. His sale of herb books such as Meyer's, usually without markup and with Bass's autograph on the title page, encourages good turnover and relationships.

The number of visitors calling each day varies; sometimes when the weather is bad no one appears, but usually two to five people come by. Not all want help on medical or herbal matters. Some may be solicitous friends who try to ensure that Mr. Bass looks after himself properly. Others come for nonmedical services such as sharpening saws (from pruning to chain saws) or skinning animals for furs. Neighbors' children might ask about where to get straight fishing poles. On some days, most frequently fine-weather Saturdays or Sundays, up to twenty-five visitors arrive, even more if there has been recent newspaper publicity about Bass.[3]

Bass's practice, or at least the sale of herbs and prepared medicines, extends beyond people who visit, write, or telephone him directly. Some "dealers," who at one time or another have benefited from taking Bass's remedies, sell or have sold considerable quantities of Tommie Bass's herbs and medicines for a relatively small commission (which nevertheless exceeds Bass's own return). One outlet from 1976 to 1984—proclaiming "We have Tommy Bass Herb Medicines" —was a small, two-room frame store, overflowing with secondhand clothing, china oddments, and knickknacks, which ran a permanent "garage sale" on the outskirts of Centre. Bass's herbs and medicines attracted many customers. Favorite sellers were chickweed, yellowroot, and blueberry leaves, the latter for "high blood" and sugar, and Bass Salve and Bass Rub.[4]

A tape recording of Bass's firsthand advice was available for customers to listen to. A transcript of some of the tape, appended to this chapter, provides both a sense of his entrepreneurship and the power of testimonials. The latter have been significant in encouraging people to visit him. It is not easy for those who have not listened to Bass to appreciate the rhythm of his spoken word, reminiscent perhaps of the flow of words from a pitchman of an old-time medicine show. He regrets that he never saw such a show, nor took part in one, but is ever ready to mimic the pitchman.[5]

Another dealer in Bass's herbs and preparations is the local "rabbit man" who, since 1980, has been selling—along with rabbits and slingshots—Bass Rub, Bass Salve, and a few herbs such as sassafras and bloodroot at local trade days, generally four a week at local towns. People from all walks of life try out the herbs and preparations.

Visitors often join Bass on walks in nearby woods and fields because it is well known that he entertains everyone with his detailed knowledge of nature. Clearly his authority, his reputation as an herbalist, and his influence on people rest not only on his knowledge of herbs and how he employs them, but also on his general understanding of nature.

Bass's role as a backwoodsman provides him with more than a reputation as one skilled in the ways of nature. He is often viewed, unconsciously as well as consciously, as a typical pioneer from times past. He enjoys being called a backwoodsman and often points out that early American pioneers were, like him, basically fur trappers. Some attitudes toward him reflect tenets, sometimes called myths, of American culture: the promised land, the earthly paradise, and pioneers with the innocence of Adam.[6]

Religious beliefs shared by Bass and many of his visitors encourage these views. He holds that God's hand is readily seen throughout nature, and that God's creation of animals and plants is totally good: "All natural things, like herbs, are good, even the weeds of the field." Nature and God, for Bass, are virtually synonymous. He often remarks that "when the good Lord made the world everything was perfect, until he found out he did not have anyone to operate it. So he took some of the herbs and made Adam."[7] Bass believes that an ever-present God is similar to Indian concepts of plant spirits.[8]

Bass's intimate feeling for nature, reflected in his many metaphors and his beliefs about weather lore and planting, is, like that of many visitors, more practical than poetic. Nature serves mankind: "God put things here for us. If we put them to use, God's gonna bless the world; he didn't mean for things to be wasted." Nature, too, is to be husbanded. "Like our bodies," he stresses, "nature is not to be abused."

VISITORS: PROFILES AND ATTITUDES

The informal nature of Bass's practice makes it difficult to determine accurately the number of people calling for help, their backgrounds, the nature of their health problems, and their reasons for choosing Bass. In addition to participant observations and structured interviews (employing a set pattern of questions and accepted problem-solving techniques), tape-recorded diaries were prepared by Bass at the end of a day or, at most, after two or three days during a nine-month period. Only a limited number of questionnaires were employed and independent clinical assessments made because requesting each visitor to fill out a questionnaire tended to hinder, even destroy, the informal nature of their associations with Mr. Bass. Many visitors do not even tell him their names.[9]

Visitors, especially those who have never tried to analyze their reasons for visiting Bass, found questions about their attitudes toward herbal practice difficult to answer. Specific questions, too, often elicited answers clearly shaped by politeness and efforts to be helpful. Some visitors are defensive about visiting an herbalist and perhaps overstress their disquiet about side effects of prescription medicines and over-the-counter items such as aspirin, as well as their frustrations with physicians' behavior. In many cases one feels that comments on reasons for taking herbs merely rationalize the real reason, which relates to a sense of personal failure in an illness and the attendant psychological need to do something.[10] Efforts were made to overcome uneasiness through extensive casual (albeit structured) conversations. We tried to minimize educational differences by recognizing outlooks based more on experiences and relationships rather than those oriented toward aims and goals.

Mr. Bass says that the social composition of visitors has altered within the past ten years. As he talked about changes and his visitors, the shortcomings of stereotyping people were underscored. Possibly because of location, and possibly because we did not meet a random sample of the entire populace, the negative aspects so often attributed to Appalachian people were rarely observed.[11] Although attitudes such as individualism and the feeling of man being in the hands of God and nature were often discerned, a recent observer of Appalachia is surely correct in saying that it is difficult to categorize its people.[12]

The annual number of visitors, letters, and telephone conversations reached about two thousand in 1980–83. Each year he received about six hundred first-time visitors.[13] Dealers' sales of Mr. Bass's salve, liniment, and dried herbs exceeded about five thousand separate transactions a year. Senior citizens (about twice as many women as men) predominated among visitors, as they always have. Since 1980, however, there have been more younger men and women, aged between thirty and sixty (plus a few in their twenties). In 1983 about 30 percent of his visitors were between thirty and sixty, while younger people, perhaps the most noticeable recent shift in clientele, numbered about 10 percent.

By 1983 the least-educated members of the community were no longer so dominant in Bass's practice as they had been, nor did they all fall within E. L. Koos's class III, described in his influential study of an American rural community (*The Health of Regionville*) as characterized by low incomes, rented homes, the constant anticipation of unemployment, little insurance or credit, and a tendency to seek medical attention for only a small range of symptoms.[14]

Our study of visitors shows that most (about 70 percent) fall into Koos's class II; namely, wage earners with steady employment in skilled to relatively unskilled jobs. Younger people (under thirty) in this class have often finished twelve years of school. Older citizens have generally acquired more spendable income in recent years, much of which is used for health-related items.[15]

Class I of Koos's social stratification comprises a mixed group of "the successful people" in the area: "the town banker, a successful businessman, the resident manager of a local manufacturing plant, the doctor, the minister." Some have college educations, many do not. Although only a small number in this class visit Bass, their regard for him adds prestige to his activities.

Another conspicuous recent shift in Bass's practice is the growing number of whites. In 1983 they accounted for about 60 percent of his visitors, replacing blacks as the predominant group.

Visitors arrive at various stages of an ailment or severity of a symptom; some just hope to "nip" an ailment "in the bud," and it is clear that a spectrum of concerns and worries over symptoms are at play.[16] The precise reasons for the visit and the choice of Mr. Bass are frequently difficult to determine because many people, often with multiple problems, have not tried to analyze their motivation for seeking his help. Just as a wide range of obvious and less-obvious reasons explain visits to professional medical personnel, so a singularly complex array lies behind visits to Bass. It is clear, too, that many visitors have multiple reasons for a visit, so that singling out particular factors can cause oversimplification. Recent discussions suggest that a trend toward more self-reliance in American society, toward more self-management—and invoking "basic" American ideas of individualism—is especially significant. This is a persuasive interpretation with some validity, but in the context of Bass's practice (as with much self-care in general), it serves primarily as fertile soil to nurture more specific reasons.[17] Lengthy discussions with ninety visitors, plus additional help from Mr. Bass and access to his correspondence, have shown that both obvious and well-known as well as somewhat more subtle factors are commonly at play.

One conspicuous reason for a visit, especially among senior citizens, both black and white, is financial hardship, not only from low incomes but also among those comfortably off until hit by multiple medical problems not covered entirely by insurance or Medicare. Economic difficulties are recorded in many letters written to Bass. The following (original spelling) is dated January 1983:

> I'm writing concerning the herbs, roots, weeds, etc. I read about you in the Anniston Starr. I'm real interested about finding out about these. My mother has a weight problem which she can't loose weight no way she tries, she also had tyroid problems which now they've got them under control. But she still can't loose weight. I would very much appreciate you writing me back and giving me a list of what these are, how to identify these. How to fix them and your price list. I need information on: Red clover, Devils shoe string, Rabbit tobacco, Ground Ivy, Goose Grass, peach tree leaves, Calamus Root, Squawvine, Sumac berries, what tree bark is it you can chew to stop the tooth ache,

which plant to use to cure a stomach ache & what can you use to cure a ear infection in a small child. The reason I'm writing to you for these is we don't have money to go to the doctor. In this one year about a month apart my mother & sister-in-law have had operations and my brother had an ear operation cause he couldn't hardly hear out of it. And we just can't afford to see the doctor they don't get to work but once or twice a week. Oh could you please send something to help my Daddy he stomach is pretty big. I think he's got prostrate gland trouble and send something good for indigestion please help us out and write us back we need your help desperately.

That an overwhelming burden of multiple medical problems lies behind many who approach Mr. Bass is often clear: "I am a Black woman age 70 and a Hurting and sickly woman, I get monthly income of my Dead Husband, I want you to send me some medicine, I will pay you for it after I get my check if you can Help my complant my nerve is real bad. I have gas and Bloated Stomach. Body won't Stay up womb hang low and the doctor say womb full of little tumors please help me."

About 50 percent of Bass's visitors—most without economic difficulties—concurrently visit their own physicians for such problems as rheumatism and urinary tract infections. Sometimes this reflects uncertainty about visiting herbalists,[18] yet, resting on a fatalism sometimes sharpened by bouts of illness, many—especially the elderly—have an open and empirical mind toward health care. As one said, "Did you ever see a cocky old person? As you get older you back away and look more." Even some who regard herbal medicines with doubt keep Bass's tonic in a refrigerator and take a glassful on occasion, possibly three times a day, in case it might be helpful. Many elderly persons have a feeling that their doctor has given them up, that regular medicine has failed, and invariably they remember the employment of herbs in the past, especially by parents and grandparents.[19]

Some open-minded visitors, mostly those with time on their hands, have developed a policy of shopping around for medical advice, not restricting themselves to their own physician and Mr. Bass. One visitor, a seventy-five-year-old retired schoolteacher suffering from shingles, visited in turn on a single day a chiropractor, Mr. Bass, and her regular physician.[20] Others clearly shop around looking for relief for a long-standing problem. A retired steelworker, aged seventy-five, had a hiatal hernia and an ulcer. A physician gave him a medicine that "didn't work," a chiropractor admitted he could not help, another physician said he would not operate, and yellowroot from the local health food store did not help with pain which came after eating and at night. Bass suggested a formula with goldenseal. A few of Bass's visitors have tried other herbalists, like the one who runs a practice with set office hours in the Appalachian town of Flintstone, Georgia.

Cultural and ethnic characteristics bring many visitors to Bass. Numerous blacks purchase just one or two herbs which they believe have "special" powers and which they cannot get elsewhere, like ginseng, angelico, bloodroot, Solomon's seal ("a lot of the colored folk call it John-the-conqueror-root") and five-finger grass.[21] The roots of the last two, like the better-known buckeyes, are often carried as good-luck tokens. Bass tells many stories about the association of good luck with buckeyes, which, over the years, he has sold and given away by the sackful. He says that it is best for them to be given away, for buying a buckeye does not bring the purchaser luck. "My doctor's a buckeye" is a punchline in at least one of his stories about blacks.

The precise role of popular or folk beliefs and superstitions in bringing visitors to Mr. Bass—at least for herbs—is difficult to determine. While Bass openly denies believing in medical superstitions (or "witchery"), he seems to only really doubt beliefs involving animal products, which, he says, are held mostly by blacks. He remembers many that refer to the use of fresh blood of animals—obviously felt to possess special powers—and he recently heard about a child being held over the smoke of burning chicken feathers to treat convulsions.[22] However, he is reluctant to dismiss even these outright, and certainly he would never question the astrological or "superstitious" beliefs of a visitor, not only because they were an integral part of his upbringing, but also because of his innate feeling for the unity of nature.[23]

He says that most whites are as superstitious as blacks. Like many of his visitors, he accepts readily the fact that inexplicable things happen. Fate, he believes, has sometimes brought people to him before they visited a doctor or had surgery; he considers that occasionally the visit has changed the course of management, even to avoiding surgery.

While some of his views about blacks, in line with nineteenth-century attitudes considering them a race inferior to whites, contribute to racism today, these thoughts never intrude into the relationships between him as an herbalist and his visitors.

Bass appreciates that not all blacks' interest in herbs is linked with a belief in their superstitious qualities, but he considers that he has learned less about herbs from them than from Indians, a view that mirrors the overall small contribution of blacks to white medicine.[24] Bass is delighted that Indian ancestry has become more conspicuous among his visitors in recent years. More and more visitors acknowledge that they possess Indian blood and tell him this is the reason for their interest in herbs; this, because of his great respect for Indians, is a considerable encouragement to him. "We just love the Indians. If we'd only made love to them instead of driving them out, we'd be in a whole lot different situation." He believes, with a touch of romanticism, that Indians have used every herb of value. Recent meetings with a Cherokee medicine man have reinforced Bass's confidence in Indian medicine, including reverence for the spiritual component of plants.[25]

Whatever the age and economic and ethnic background of each visitor, two attitudes stand out and merit particular comment: all have strong opinions about regular medicine and all have faith in natural products. Popular beliefs about the body and disease are considered in later chapters.

A few visitors, particularly those with a college education, are especially critical of many features of regular medicine; in frequently citing "bad experiences," they illustrate "priority gaps" between medical and consumer viewpoints.[26] One visitor who had recently suffered a heart attack admitted considerable anxiety over his condition and showed real frustration with the impersonal side of medicine: "I'm not down on doctors, but I'm down on some of their attitudes. Patients go through their offices fast enough that they [the doctors] are going to make a killing and retire early. Next! Next! Next! I've tried to ask the doctor about my condition when he'd be pushing me out the door. I ain't going to stay with that guy. You don't have no confidence in a guy like that. We've lost that feeling my grandmother had—a neighbor."

The physicians used by Bass's visitors provoke a spectrum of negative attitudes; for instance, one is called a dope man, since it is felt he prescribes too much "strong" medicine, and another is viewed as "too easy and does not give enough information." Patients who are less explicit in their criticism often show a wistfulness for something better. The following account as told by Bass reflects a refrain observed time and time again among visitors, one of puzzlement about a course of treatment:

> A man came here from Centre. He drives a gas truck that sells the bottled and tank gas. I was out in the garden plowing; it was just as hot as a firecracker one afternoon, a Friday. He said something was the matter with his stomach. He had talked to somebody that had got some yellowroot and it didn't do him no good. Course, he didn't have an ulcer. He said he was fifty-two years old. He looked well. I told him, "Neighbor, how does your stomach do?"
>
> "Well, it just hurts and gives me troubles. I can't eat nothing. My doctor gave me a prescription and I got the capsules and when I take 'em, it makes me so sleepy I have to pull off on the side of the road. I've got to drive my truck; if I don't, I'll lose my job."
>
> I said, "Have you ever quit driving that truck? And see what happens?"
>
> "Yes sir, I quit three weeks and my stomach didn't bother me."
>
> And I said, "That's about what's the trouble; your nervous stomach and that shaking. I make a tonic. If you want to try it, I'll give you a bottle. It won't cost you nothing and you can see what it'll do."
>
> He says, "Well, I can't be hurt."
>
> So I let him have an eight-ounce bottle of this tonic I make out of herbs. He took it with him, that was on Friday. He come back on the next Friday and said he felt good and had eat everything except onions and his stomach hadn't bothered him. The last time he was here, he told me to fix him up a real large bottle. I fixed him a forty-eight-ounce Coca-Cola bottle and he took it with him. He said, "When this is gone, I'll be back after more."
>
> It was amazing that Dr. Miller would have prescribed those sleeping capsules when just all he needed was something to sterilize his stomach or help the gas on his stomach.

In a small rural community unfortunate or unhappy episodes with physicians become widely discussed and, perhaps, sometimes overly embroidered in critical terms. Such views are undoubtedly fed by criticism of the medical profession in newspapers, popular magazines, and talk shows, especially if it comes from a doctor about the practices of colleagues.[27] Criticisms of the medical profession rarely, if ever, lead to total rejection, but more a feeling—sometimes fed by a sense of republican independence—of wishing to "try out" alternative treatments and "Tommie Bass's common sense."[28]

The second attitude, most conspicuous among visitors under the age of fifty, though by no means restricted to them, is faith in "natural products" and deep concerns over side effects of "chemical" drugs and polluted environments. Some have a religious fervor, an almost blind faith in herbs. The intensity of enthusiasm sometimes generated is reflected in the following excerpts from a letter dated 31 January 1982:

> Just a few lines to say [we] enjoyed ourselves, talking and listening about the herbs of the Indians, Pioneers and of herbs of now—today. Tommy, we are sincere about learning about the Herbs and how Mother Nature protects her own. We are looking forward to our field trip with you to learn even more.
>
> Our neighbors . . . Mr. Smith & Mrs. Smith, when they found out that we are wanting to learn about Herbs, they told us that they would go with us and show us where to find yellow root and how to spot it. Boy was it fun. We gathered grocery sacks of yellow root and I've gathered some samples of what I believe to be red maple, Elderberry, Poplar, Sweet gum, black gum but we didn't find any black [haw] or squaw vine. . . .
>
> Our son, David, was running a fever the night we were there, visiting with you. Anyway when we got back to my sister-in-laws house, I fixed up a tea of Blood root—Mullen & boneset and by the next morning being Sunday his fever broke. I'm still giving him the tea and the Gensing has made me feel ever so much more energy that I had lost. Now if I can only get the other things took care of. Oh yeah I tried the Rabbit tobacco the way you told me too and do you know I got rid of the head ache. . . . Sunday morning I woke up with a migrain, but the rabbit tobacco did the trick again. It took my headache away. . . .
>
> I went today and bought a Composition Notebook so as I can keep notes while on our field trip. I can hardly wait. I'm really

excited about the trip and learning from "the Medicine Man." That's you. All I can so I too can pass on what you have taught me and will teach me about Herbs. I really want to learn how to fix up tonics and cough syrups that will help the body and sustain against having so many dr. bills, hosp. bills.

At least two young people in close contact with Mr. Bass have a similar fervor. One, a construction worker, began learning from him as an "apprentice" in 1980. Another, a housewife, in 1983 became a salesperson for a national company producing capsules of dried herbs. Indeed, people under thirty provide some of the staunchest testimonials supporting Mr. Bass's practice. Like others of the same generation everywhere who have an enthusiasm for herbal medicine and "natural food supplements," they are particularly concerned about the dangers of side effects of synthetic drugs and believe in the value of "granny's natural remedies." Steroids, aspirin, and sleeping pills produce particular worry. "My daughter has had eczema all of her 22 years and can no longer take the cortisone cream," wrote one correspondent requesting Bass's help. Such concerns are fed in part by memories of past tragedies with chemical medicines. One example of the latter, still remembered in Bass's area, is the many deaths that resulted from taking a contaminated sulfanilamide preparation produced by a southern pharmaceutical company, J. E. Massengill of Bristol, Tennessee, in 1937. Even more indelibly printed in people's memories are thalidomide abnormalities from the early 1960s.[29] Such episodes have become or are becoming a part of environmental folklore and serve as a constant warning about the dangers of synthetic drugs. For some people such concerns are reinforced by a general fear of change, which, as we discussed, is an element of nostalgia for the past.

Bass's views on environmental hazards summarize those shared by many visitors:

> Now all these vegetables we buy nowadays, they all have insecticide on them and it gets into the system and does harm. Now they also use chemicals to take the leaves off the beans and the cotton. I've never figured it out: medical people are trying to take it. The way I feel about it, if you smoke or take snuff or something like that, it gets into the stomach and lungs and it seems like the

biggest part of cancers are there in the stomach and do the damage there. In my years of watching people, I think women must stop smoking and you wouldn't get all these birth defects.

Reasons behind visits to Mr. Bass are made especially complex by factors rarely expressed and sometimes not consciously recognized by visitors. One factor is an attitude toward herbal remedies that allows failures to be accepted without loss of confidence and alternatives to be eagerly tried, unlike when medicines prescribed by physicians fail.[30] Of course, flexibility is easier because many problems brought to Bass are those for which the drugstore rather than the physician is often the first port of call. Such problems, sometimes self-limiting, sometimes merely a feeling of general unwellness, often elicit the response: "I don't want to bother the doctor," or "it's not bad enough for the doctor," or "the doctor couldn't do anything last time." Above all, reassurance is wanted—some would say informal counseling—and Bass's open door, like the drugstore, encourages many visitors.[31] Everyone is put at ease by Bass's nonthreatening, nonjudgmental atmosphere. His is a place to shop around to find new medicines, or to take and receive the "practical common sense" of a charismatic individual—common sense communicated via shared concepts. Many such concepts and lay health beliefs differ markedly from notions of modern medicine. This attitude and the nonjudgmental atmosphere contrast with that of many doctors, and it helps those who are afraid to consult physicians about their health. Whatever the precipitating reasons for visiting Bass, time spent with him can produce a sense of well-being, as borne out by countless testimonials.

Regular visitors have high praise for his medicines. Typically, one informant told us his wife would take only Bass's cough medicine: "She'd tell anybody it helped her. She's still taking it. She wants to be sure she can get some more." Mr. Bass's recent enthusiastic support for capsulated herbs, considered below, has contributed to more and more public testimonials for herbs. At local meetings of distributors and salespeople, testimonials are given before the group about the effectiveness of the capsules for numerous chronic problems ranging from Crohn's disease to rheumatoid arthritis. Such testimonials are sometimes delivered in an impressive aura of religious conviction reminiscent of many aspects of life surrounding Bass.

It is difficult to overemphasize the power of testimonials in encouraging the use of particular medical advice and herbs. The influence of friends and relatives on laypeople is unquestioned—it is a vast network of health advice.[32] Likewise, testimonials have shaped many a physician's practice. The accounts of herbs in volume 2 illustrate the fact that regular practitioners have commonly placed confidence in a plant if its efficacy was supported by just an occasional testimonial from other physicians. On the other hand, one of the most conspicuous features of regular medicine, especially during recent decades, is skepticism of testimonials, of any evidence of successful treatment other than that derived from double-blind clinical trials. This perplexes Bass and most of his visitors because their personal experiences—their firsthand observations–are being questioned. In this they are part of a long tradition of debate about the relationships between folk and scientific knowledge, and about the failure of most laypeople to understand scientific methods.[33]

Curiosity is yet another factor behind visits to Bass, one which seemingly lies behind many visitors not returning. Mr. Bass says this is not necessarily because they found his remedies ineffective, but because it was too much bother to make teas from uninviting-looking herbs. Some also fail to return because they do not hold the same popular beliefs as Mr. Bass; while numerous visitors become increasingly caught up with his charisma, others see him as merely old-fashioned.

This account of the diversity of responses to the question "Why do you visit Mr. Bass?" mentions many that have been discussed by other commentators on traditional practices worldwide. What is significant is the complex matrix of factors at play, some of which can be more important for one individual than another. The vagueness of many responses may reflect the confusing intermingling of various factors or even the inconsequential nature of some people's feelings. Often it is merely that a visit provides an uplift in the sense of well-being ("it makes me feel good") or the feeling that herbs are "good" or "helpful." The expression "helpful" is apt because it recognizes that relief is often temporary; at the same time it allows people to retain a sense of self-responsibility, of being in control of looking after their symptoms.

THE HEALTH FOOD DIMENSION

The key features of Bass's practice as it is described above are the employment of crude drugs collected locally, the employment of concepts once part of professional medicine, and the preparation of teas and other medicines made either by him or by visitors. Yet by the summer of 1984 this practice had dwindled conspicuously, surviving only for some long-standing visitors. Beginning in 1983, Bass has increasingly become an advocate and promoter of manufactured products, herbs sold in gelatin capsules as "health foods," "nutrients," or "food supplements." Thus, he became part of a social movement mushrooming nationwide in rural and urban areas. This herbal movement is a complex of many alternative medical practices, but with common themes—particularly the emphasis on preserving health rather than curing disease. Creating an optimum state of health is promoted in various ways, but frequently in the context of restoring balance through such factors as food, exercise, and cosmic influences. Western concepts are sometimes bolstered by non-Western ideas, especially concepts of balance (yin and yang), as well as a sense that exotic remedies have much to offer.

As the transition in Mr. Bass's practice is briefly considered—in many respects it is another instance of the dynamic character of traditional practice and the changing patterns in self-care—the question can be asked whether herbal medicine everywhere is likely to follow the same trend.

When Bass first heard from a local housewife of her opportunity to become a distributor of capsulated herbs for a national company, he was immediately enthusiastic and gratified that the herbs that he had been using and recommending for a lifetime were becoming widely available, even though promoted as "concentrated food in capsulated form." At the age of seventy-five he was finding the gathering of herbs increasingly irksome. Furthermore, he was disillusioned by so many visitors relying on him to make the medicines because they were "too lazy" to make their own teas.

Many other factors, each reinforcing the other, contributed to Bass's rapid transition. Especially significant was the promotion of capsulated herbs using concepts already familiar to him—in particular, four concepts of health and disease with strong cultural overtones. One is the mechanical-chemical view of human physiology, which gives the analogy of the body to an automobile engine and the need to remove "waste products" ("toxins") to prevent clogging of the vessels, concepts discussed in chapter 7.[34] A second concept deals with ideas about balance, that balance is health (some see this as wholism, or holism), an idea that is particularly congenial to him. Third is religious support for the efficacy of herbs. Not only do biblical texts encourage the promotion of herbs (e.g., "He causes the grass to grow for cattle and herbs for the men" [Psalms 104:14], and "the leaves of the tree were for the healing of nations" [Revelation 22:27]), but also at play is Bass's sensitivity toward the integrity of the Mormons, who manufacture the capsules he sells. He has even heard—perhaps as a result of a misguided promotion—that this is linked to the healthiness of the Mormons because of their way of life.[35] The fourth concept is that dangerous poisons exist in the environment, including nonprescription drugs ("you do not catch a disease, you eat it"), an idea which has bolstered the long-standing, almost intuitively held belief that "nature and natural products are pure."[36]

Notions of balance and the purity of nature—like many cosmic and philosophical notions embraced by irregular medical practices—have deep cultural roots, roots eclectically combined, which accounts for much of their pervasiveness. Influences and beliefs include the healing power of nature; that America is a garden with fertile fields offering pure food, rather like the original Garden of Eden; legacies of such entrepreneurs as Sylvester Graham (of Graham Cracker fame);[37] fifty years or so of belief in the health-giving value of vitamins; increasingly widespread acceptance of many onetime "counterculture" health movements;[38] and the overt symbolism in the promotion of remedies when associating the "goodness and safety" of herbs with the "goodness" of the family, rural life, God, patriotism, and freedom of choice.

Also important in Bass's transition has been the opportunity to help the proprietors of a new health food store and other distributors, thus allowing him opportunities to exploit his love of entrepreneurship—which has carried him through many occupations and activities—with advertising in newspapers, on the radio, and in talks at local meetings and trade days. Recent newspaper advertisements that have focused on herb history not only echo the style of some advertisements (c. 1920) for Dr. Pierce's remedies, well remembered by Bass, but also underscore his own long experience. For example: "The export of ginseng did much to save the infant United States from economic collapse after the Revolutionary War. This is true not only with ginseng but with numerous herbs. Tommie Bass recalls the days when he and his father gathered and sold herbs to companies and individuals which Tommie still does to this day, not just for economic reasons but for the benefit of mankind. Herbs serving man yesterday, serving man today." By 1985 the considerable local success in the sale of capsules was itself considered testimony to their value.

The sale of capsulated herbs has led Bass to advocate uses of herbs (e.g., for hypoglycemia) beyond the knowledge and experience he has gathered over the years.[39] The commercial success of capsulated herbs has given him confidence in the "truthfulness" behind their promotion, including recommendations new to him. Though he sometimes points out to visitors his lack of experience with some of the new products, we are both intrigued and a little disquieted to see how commercial forces have blunted the edge of reliance on experience, not only with Mr. Bass but also with many of his visitors.

Other trends are noticeable. One is the tendency among new sellers of capsulated herbs to make diagnoses of ailments beyond anything attempted by Mr. Bass. Diagnostic practices include iridology (a "television into the body" as Bass describes it) and other techniques not accepted by regular medicine. Conversations between health food store employees and customers often reveal popular concepts. These, as seen in the following exchange—encouraged by the nonthreatening store atmosphere—can lead to taking multiple herbal medicines.

> SALESPERSON: This [herb] is real good to work on the upper tract of the intestines. And this one is good for the lower bowel.
> CUSTOMER: Well, [my mother] had gall bladder trouble and. . . .
> SALESPERSON: Well, now, this is good for her liver and her gall bladder. Get a cleanse for her to do with olive oil and lemon juice. Then if she has any stones, she'll pass them.
> CUSTOMER: This right here?
> SALESPERSON: Well, no, she can take this daily, this'll help strengthen and get the toxin out of the liver and the gall bladder.

And we'll give you instructions how for her to do this gall bladder cleanse which is just olive oil and lemon juice, and she can
do that in her spare time. I have one man in Georgia that passed
half a dozen gallstones, doing this, and his doctor said. . . .
CUSTOMER: Well, we'll try, I'll try that and let's see. She's really
nervous, she's had the shingles but they are cleared up. However,
it's left her in a nervous condition and this severe pain where the
shingles were. Do you have anything that might could help that?
SALESPERSON: Yeah. One thing would be this salve. We have a
lot of people use this for shingles, and she can rub this, use this
externally, and then we can put her on the A or the calcium for
her nerves. How's her circulation?
CUSTOMER: Well her circulation seems to be pretty good.
SALESPERSON: How old is she?
CUSTOMER: Eighty-six.
SALESPERSON: Let's put her on calcium 'cause this'll help her with
her circulation.[40]

Many readers of this dialogue will undoubtedly view it as quackery, and others, even if they see no deliberate fraud, will consider it
misleading to the public. We discuss this later, and it is merely noted
here that while some alternative practices are totally unacceptable
scientifically, there is much testimony from patients that they provide
social and, hence, in a broad sense, medical roles through offering
circumstances that, if nothing more, encourage placebo responses.

Recent changes in Bass's practice extend to promoting "new" botanicals such as gotu kola and show a new emphasis on the importance of "all-around" sound nutrition. During most of his years as an
herbalist he has given visitors little specific information about food in
relation to health, although he is fully cognizant of the importance of
nutrition. The limited advice he has given parallels the general trend
in regular medicine during the twentieth century of paying relatively
little attention to nutrition.

Mr. Bass, at least up to 1986, had some reservations about the new
health food movement, such as the tendency to use excessive quantities. Some reducing formulas, for instance, are recommended in such
doses that they produce bowel movements three times a day. Bass is
ambivalent, too, about the marketing of "medicinal" herbs as foods,

though he accepts that many have tonic actions and contain vitamins and minerals. On the other hand, while he believes that taking
some herbs over a long period of time is valuable, like many people
he primarily sees the herbs as maintaining health more by specific
medicinal actions. In fact, he says it is all because the FDA won't recognize herbs as medicines that they are sold as foods. This is certainly
the case, and, as discussed later, we believe that it produces some
unfortunate social consequences.

In many ways Bass does not recognize just how much his practice has changed. By early 1986 there had been a further change in
emphasis. For many reasons, especially religious ones, he now sees
herbs as "vegetables," with both medical and nutritious qualities.
Arguments he once used for cabbage (see Cabbage, volume 2) are
extended to many herbs. It is clear that some local preachers have
played a significant role in countenancing natural remedies.[41] In one
sense an increasing spirituality is at play, a trend observed in other
social movements embracing healing and religion.[42]

Although Bass appreciates that some visitors prefer to make their
own teas rather than buying capsules (since that ensures obtaining
the "genuine article"), he does not think that, generally, personal involvement by visitors in their own treatment is important. We have
seen that for many people visits have become more perfunctory, with
much less time spent discussing herbs and how they should be prepared. Furthermore, Bass is less often available in his shack for casual
callers as he spends more time in the local health food store or in
another community speaking about herbal remedies and advocating
capsulated products.

The changes focus sharply on the issue raised at the beginning of
this chapter, whether factors other than herbs lie behind his success
and reputation. Bass does not believe the help he has given over the
years is diminished by spending less time with visitors, by not using
herbs from local fields and woods, by not expecting visitors to make
their own teas, and so on. His conviction in the physiological value
of herbs is strong. Our observations suggest that most visitors agree
with him, especially those who accept the notion that capsules, compared with teas and other herbal remedies, provide accurate doses
and "that the whole, not just extracted goodness is present." Innumerable testimonies on the value of capsulated herbs are striking and

need consideration by the severest critic. Bass, in fact, always down-plays the idea that herbal medicine works because herbalists spend more time with patients than do regular physicians. Just how many visitors want the personal touch, are skeptical about the quality of commercially prepared products, or object to and cannot afford the higher prices, is not clear, though few have been identified in four years of observing the transition in Bass's practice.

It is clear that the milieu of Mr. Bass's practice has been a sig-nificant feature behind his success in the past. If it is now less so for many visitors, the new dimension to his practice is in keeping with a cardinal characteristic of his service to the community, that he accommodates a variety of individuals, concerns, and worries. He believes unquestionably that his new activities make him more generally useful.

APPENDIX:
Excerpts from Tommie Bass Tape in General Store

Hello, friends, this is Tommie Bass down in Leesburg and we thought we'd make Mrs. Woodall a tape and kind of tell you how to use some of these products that she has on sale, I mean, in the store here. And she hasn't had the opportunity to have the experience that I have. She got more brains in five seconds than I'd have in my whole lifetime, but trouble of it is you know you got to kind of have a little experi-ence, especially in this herb line. Course I'm not a doctor, I'm not no son of a doctor, I'm not anything but a hillbilly without a guitar. But anyway, we're going to talk some right now about what the most people is interested in—the reducing herbs.

Well, we have three different ones and right now at the present time [about the ninth of April 1982] we have what we call the goosegrass. Some of you may have read about it, or seen the picture of me having it in my hand in the *Gadsden Times* two weeks ago. It's a weed; it don't look like grass, but it runs along the ground. But anyway I won't try to explain that cause most people can't understand what it looks like until they actually see it.

And if she doesn't have the goosegrass, why she has what we call the chickweed. And if she doesn't have the chickweed, why she's got what we call wild carrot—or some people knows it as Queen Annie's lace.

It all comes in gallon bags—makes one gallon of tea—boil it in a gallon of water for about twenty or twenty-five minutes and then you strain it into jars. If you have a gallon jar, of course, you use it, and if you have to use two half gallons, why, of course, you use that. And if you don't, you can use four quarts. But anyway, after you boil it and strain it, if you don't have a jarful, why you just fill it up with clear water. And I recommend that you drink at least three six-ounce glasses a day, that's three times a day. But if you're having a snack between meals, why, be sure you drink a glass of tea. And now you sweeten it any way you wish, don't worry about the fat; that's what the tea's there for. It kills the calories in your food. It also kills the fatty substance.

One lady said her and her husband ate lots of eggs and things like that and she called got what you get in your veins. Well, I said, this tea is a purifier; drink it; sweeten it any way you want it, just like you do iced tea. And if you want to lose weight faster, well drink an iced-tea-glass full three times a day, or four times if you wish to, cause there's no harm in it whatsoever. It's not a narcotic, it's not a dope, and it's got no caffeine in it. It'll make you sleep like a baby, and by the way most people, they tells me, that they don't take it because they want to reduce, they take it cause it makes them feel good. . . .

Now the goosegrass, it don't last long. It's like the Irishman was who went in to buy him a watch, and he told the fellow in the jewelry store, he wanted a good watch. Well, the fellow says, "Pat, here's one that'll last you a lifetime." So Pat carried it home with him and by the way it run two weeks and stopped. So he got so mad he could eat a banana and he wasn't even hungry, and he went back to the man and he just teared him up. He said, "You said this thing would run a lifetime." And the fellow said, "I didn't think you'd live two weeks." Well, now, that's the way this here goosegrass is.

You can use the chickweed. One of them is going out of season now, but another one's coming in. Chickweed's kind of like a family, there's another one coming on all the time, so that's the way the chickweed is. But goosegrass is not that way. It don't stay here long.

But now there's Queen Annie's lace, it's actually a carrot, why, it will be here 'til next fall. And if you're going to gather it yourself, why you just gather the herb, you don't use the root. You gather the herb and make the tea just like you do out of the goosegrass or the chickweed. We had it put up there, but it's better to buy the two-dollar bag on the counter, it generally takes at least two gallons to cause you to get to where you're losing weight like you want to. Because the first gallon just kind of cleans up your blood and purifies it and when you first start to drinking it, it may act as a kind of a laxative. But after you drink it a few days, why, it won't bother you at all. And it works on the same system that water tablets does that the doctor gives you but it works it through your pores. . . .

And now we're going to talk about the cough medicine. As far as it's concerned, it's complete, made ready-to-go. You don't have anything to do with it, but just take it according to directions, and there's not anything in it that'll harm you. It's made of wild cherry, mullein, and yellowroot, and redshank (or New Jersey tea root, if you want to call it that), and sweet gum bark, and rabbit-tobacco, and sumac berries. And of course then the sweetening part of it is honey and sugar and some of it I put up a kind of a oil in it, I can't say it'll work, but it's the one they put in these here popular cough drops. . . .

There was one lady come to me and her husband—I didn't see the woman—but her husband said the doctor told her that she had arthritis of the spine. But I never seen the doctor and I don't know whether he said that or not, but I do know that after the woman used the Bass Rub; why one of her granddaughters told me that, by Ned, she didn't have no arthritis any more. Well, now, if she didn't actually have arthritis, she was strained or sprained or something—it'd ease that. And bursitis, it'll just ease that right quick. And bee stings and frostbite and all that kind of thing, and poison ivy—it'll do away with it. . . .

Mrs. Woodall's got nothing here in her place that will harm you. It's all the same thing that you'd get in the drugstore. Now we're not a doctor, we're not knocking no doctors, not knocking no druggists, if you want to go down to the drugstore and buy the same thing, why you do that. You can't buy what we have here, because it's made out of the natural ingredients, right out of the woods.

Of course the goosegrass and the chickweed and the wild carrot, it needs washing. We clean it just as clean as we possibly can, but it's just like when we buy beans, or peas, or rice, or anything like that out of the store, we always wash it, or I always do. And my womenfolks and everybody I was ever around did because you can't keep it clean, you see. . . .

We're going to quit now and say thanks to everybody for listening at us. But we're gonna play the rest of the tape out on the harp and, of course, it'll punish you, but you won't have to listen to it if you don't want to. . . .

CHAPTER 7

The Practice: Treating Ailments
and Symptoms

Sometimes it's all colds and rheumatism. I
don't say I cure them. Most people come back
over the years.

A SPECTRUM OF SYMPTOMS AND AILMENTS

Herbal medicine offers an overwhelming number of alternative remedies (sometimes called resources) for treating a host of ailments. Unfortunately, comparatively little discussion is available on the choice of regimens, the relative popularity of each herb, and how their uses are justified.[1] Through the years, a practitioner's or layperson's choice of herbs has generally depended on such considerations as cost and availability in addition to reputation. In turn, the latter often depended on changing theories about disease. Whether or not a condition was considered inflammatory, a blood poison, or due to germs often shaped (and still shapes) treatment. Changing classifications of diseases also are relevant, and regimens can still be found that seemingly are legacies of a time when dyspepsia was classified as a nervous rather than a gastrointestinal disorder.

In this chapter Bass's herbal therapies for a variety of ailments are considered. Some well-established concepts are noted additional to those already mentioned, and the interplay of rationalism and empiricism is further illustrated. Most of Bass's concepts are rooted firmly in past centuries, but sufficient historical background is given for each ailment only to demonstrate a continuity of ideas once widely held. Comments and assessments of the practices are generally conventional, that is, based on concepts derived from current medicine and science, rather than from herbalists. Nevertheless, as discussed later, we feel that such approaches as removing herbs from the market unless they contain constituents proven to be effective in the same manner as prescription drugs—reflected in the regulatory philosophy of the U.S. Food and Drug Administration—is sometimes overly rigid.

Bass's visitors and correspondents ask about countless ailments from which they or their relatives suffer. Listed below are those he encountered during the nine months between November 1982 and July 1983. They are given in alphabetical order, but many were seen over and over again among about fifteen hundred people. The "diagnoses" are in Bass's own words or those of visitors, who frequently relayed a diagnosis obtained from a physician. The wide range of ailments— often symptoms rather than precise diagnoses—is of special interest since it illustrates a broad spectrum of needs and concerns, many of a minor or self-limiting nature. Not only is it a mix of types of problems commonly taken to a family practitioner and those self-treated (sometimes with the advice of a health professional), but also it includes what have been described as "folk" or ethnomedical ailments.

allergy	need straightening out
asthma	nerve anemia
asthma and sinus trouble	nerves
bad spells	nose bleeding
bad throat	obesity
blood condition	pinched nerve
breaking out on skin	prostate gland trouble
bursitis	relative on kidney machine
constipation	relative with cancer on bone
cough and cold	rheumatism
Crohn's disease	rundown feeling
diarrhea	shingles
dizziness	sinus trouble
earache	smoking too much
emphysema	something for lady friend
erysipelas	sore mouth
excess body fluid	sprained ankle
female problem	stomach

foot almost rotting off	sugar
gall bladder trouble	swelling in leg muscle
herniary	swollen feet
high blood	teething (baby)
high blood and sugar	tired blood
high blood pressure	trouble with knee
hives	tumor in lower part of stomach
improve hair growth	ulcers in the stomach
kidney complaint	wanting to build up nature
migraine	worms

"Over the years," says Mr. Bass, "the commonest problem has been coughs and colds, but other big things are poison ivy, sinus and allergy, obesity, rheumatism, ulcers and hernias, nerves, sugar diabetes, high blood pressure, and gall-bladder trouble." Another conspicuous problem, a "general feeling of unwellness," he says, is rarely mentioned specifically.

Anthropologists commonly distinguish two types of complaints in the above list: ethnomedical and biomedical. Ethnomedical ailments are defined as those based on beliefs and practices which arise from "indigenous developments" and, unlike biomedical ailments, are not explicitly derived from or understood through modern medical concepts. The distinction has arisen from growing interest in lay notions of disease, responses to illness, and attitudes to treatment and to the regular medical profession.[2]

Ethnomedical ailments in Bass's list include "high blood" and "sugar." Yet contrary to what might be expected from other studies, including some in the Appalachians, Mr. Bass says "high blood" is high blood pressure, and "sugar" is diabetes.[3] However, when it is suggested to him that "high blood" might mean blood out of balance (e.g., too thick, or "low blood" if too thin), he responds that this is the cause of the high pressure, and adds that it is the reason why a blood purifier or tonic is always helpful in treatments. In other words, like many of his visitors, he employs modernized ethnomedical concepts, just as physicians sometimes interpret patients' complaints into current medical ideas. By using blood purifiers for high blood pressure, for instance, Bass's practice contains elements of transition, of revision and compromise. In fact, while he and many visitors link symptoms with modern diagnostic terms, their explanations for the symptoms often rest on such notions (no longer acceptable in regular medicine) as toxins and mechanical blockage of tubes.

Given the trend toward modernizing terms, as well as a close association of many ethnomedical ideas with regular medicine of the recent past (plus a tendency for certain physicians to explain concepts to patients in what can be called ethnomedical language), distinctions between ethnomedical and biomedical explanations are sometimes hazy.[4] Certainly the accounts of Bass's treatments, which illustrate how he and many visitors join and synthesize past and modern ideas about symptoms and disease (a process called syncretism by anthropologists), serve as reminders of a dynamic relationship between lay and professional medicine, as well as how misunderstandings over diagnoses can arise between physicians and patients.

Bass generally accepts diagnoses presented by visitors at face value. Usually he does not take into account a possibly incorrect self-diagnosis, that the patient may have misunderstood a doctor, or that a complaint may be a visitor's way of drawing attention to other, more worrisome, problems. Assessments of Bass's practice also have relied heavily on visitors' diagnoses, although tempered with many independent clinical observations made at Bass's "office." Clearly, self-diagnosis and self-assessment of health problems are often unreliable, but careful observation and questioning suggests that complaints by visitors generally reflect physical problems rather than questions of morale and self-image.

Little evidence was found that the physical expression of anxieties, bad moods, and worries (somatization) is widespread among Bass's visitors. At least, on close questioning, only a few visitors felt they were or had been under stress, which itself is a reminder of the difficulty of assessing minor stress and that there are some who believe that it may be evoked too readily as a causative agent in disease.[5] Little difficulty exists in clinically diagnosing some ailments (e.g., shingles and poison ivy rash) in the setting of Bass's practice, while for many others (for instance, cough and burning urine) there is little reason not to accept the visitors' own accounts. By the same token, since Bass treats mostly symptoms and self-limiting problems, independent clinical assessments would, in many cases (though not, for instance, for hypertension, cirrhosis, etc.), be of limited help in assessing a visitor's opinion of whether or not *relief* or ease (not cure) resulted from treatment. Some objectivity emerges in assessing Bass's practice when visitors say, as they often do, that Tommie Bass helped them continue at work, rather than taking time off, and when forty-three out of a series of seventy visitors who had complained of tiredness and "rheumaticky" pains testified to some relief persisting at least two months after treatment. In addition, a few visitors were followed for three years or so, which provided some longer-term data for interpretation and helped with making generalizations.

To appreciate the circumstances of Bass's practice, one must remember that he sees himself as an "outback druggist" as much as an "herbist." He knows that medicinal plants are (or have been) the basis of many drugstore medicines: "A lot of people go down to the drugstore and they're just like an old sow under a hickory nut or acorn tree just eating the acorns and never looking and seeing what's coming. And so that's the way people is with medicine. They don't realize they have it right around them."[6] This analogy is apt in many ways. Traditionally pharmacists have provided much over-the-counter advice on relieving symptoms diagnosed by customers, just as Mr. Bass does.[7] Many problems brought to Bass—such as coughs, colds, sore throats, poison ivy rashes, insect bites, earache, headache, indigestion, sprains, and muscle aches—are widely self-treated with over-the-counter medicines. Even his popular "slimming aids" are little different from certain commercially prepared regimens.

Bass stresses that because he does not make diagnoses he is not practicing like a doctor. This is only partly correct. Occasionally he "translates" some vague symptoms into, say, liver or kidney problems or a stomach ulcer for which he can recommend herbal remedies, while he often differentiates rheumatism from arthritis. If his long experience and intuition tell him that a problem is serious, he recommends a visit to a doctor.

Viewing the practice as one that largely treats symptoms places it apart—at least conceptually—from the cornerstone of modern medicine, the determination of the causes of diseases and their cure through specific drugs. On the other hand, everyday traditional practice like Bass's, which commonly relieves symptoms, can be invaluable for the patient by improving function and easing stress.[8]

A very important question is whether dangers to health exist in Mr. Bass's practice. The possible toxic effects of herbs are considered later, but here other issues are noted. Herbal treatment for high blood pressure and for diabetes undoubtedly worries physicians. Several patients with adult-onset diabetes, some on insulin therapy, who take Bass's tea for their "sugar" say laboratory tests confirm that it reduces their blood-sugar levels (see "Blueberry", volume 2). Most visitors do not tell their physicians about the treatment, generally because they are not asked. Clearly a physician's efforts to maintain constant blood-sugar levels are complicated under such conditions. One sixty-five-year-old man on fifty units of insulin a day had a blood-sugar level of around two hundred milligrams percent. When he added Bass's huckleberry tea (while still continuing the insulin), he reported the sugar level dropped to around one hundred milligrams.

Even greater concern is expressed over Bass's recommendations for cancer, despite his cautious approach. Advice is generally given to relatives worried about a patient, and in every case Bass emphasizes that herbs are not alternatives to regular medical treatment but they might help and will do no harm. The incidence of relatives providing supplementary treatment for patients is probably common everywhere, and Bass may not contribute much to increasing the incidence in his area. Nevertheless, his reputation may encourage some laxity toward follow-up examinations and, on occasion, delays in regular medical treatment. Certainly delay is not uncommon with the "prostate trouble" frequently brought to Bass. Sometimes, too, he advises a delay in elective surgery until herbs have been tried. Such recommendations are often nonspecific: squawvine ("good for all female complaints"), for instance, is given to help cancer in female organs.

Yet another issue that has occasioned criticism of Bass is his treatment of protracted cases of shingles. However, he has had much experience and, so far as we ascertained, all visitors had first been evaluated by a physician. Bass's treatment calls for frequent application of an astringent wash (e.g., prepared from redroot); he has received much testimony that it alleviates the problem. Perhaps concern should be raised over Mr. Bass's management, which includes a sympathetic ear and time, only if a physician has not first ruled out underlying pathology and tried conventional medical treatment.

LAY BELIEFS: SOME RATIONALES FOR TREATMENT REGIMENS

The interplay of empiricism and theory noted earlier is conspicuous when we look at how medicinal plants have been used in practice. At first glance Mr. Bass's approach to treatment—shared by many visitors—has few theoretical underpinnings, yet a closer look shows an intriguing coherence based on the employment of concepts, now often called folk, popular, or ethnomedical, which at one time or another have generally been part of regular medicine. In considering some key features of lay beliefs about health and disease—some of which have become especially conspicuous amid the current promotion of herbs as nutrition products—it must be appreciated that the attitude of a particular individual toward the cause of illness commonly may involve multiple factors, some of which are linked, somewhat irrationally, to specific events in their lives.[9]

The legacies of humoral theory and its role in therapy described in chapter 1 have filtered into Bass's recommendations of "hot" blood purifiers and the application of "cool" astringents in the treatment of ulcers and "external cancers." Much of his approach, however, reflects a mechanical view of the body and its disorders. For instance, "the damp goes right through you," and "the cold has run to my chest." Indeed, Bass's key view of the body is that it works like an engine. Similar views are held by many of his visitors, and this popular model of illness—sometimes described as the "plumbing model"—unquestionably serves as a significant basis of communication and rapport between patient and herbalist.

The concept of "cleaning the engine" is implicit in much of Bass's treatment; it reflects, too, the age-old idea (given little attention today) of approaching the disease in a general (constitutional) manner as well as specifically treating the lesion. The general approach is to "get everything working well," to help the body fight the disease. "One of the main problems today with people is bad blood," says Bass. "Why doctors do not give something to clean out the system I do not know; for instance, give blood purifiers or laxatives [depending on the condition]; further, a tonic is always helpful. Even if the carburetor works well you need a good fuel line."

The mechanical view, or engine analogy, often embraces the notion that poor health is due to chemicals, "poisons" or "toxins" introduced into the body. Indeed the notion has been widely underscored in recent years by many promoters of health food products. Overlying the mechanical and chemical notions of the body is the belief that everything should be in balance. It is easy to suggest that this notion is a legacy of ideas that health is a balance of four humors, but among Bass's visitors and others the concept of balance is best seen as an intrinsic, almost intuitive one bound with many cultural and religious notions that reinforce it.[10] The deep historical roots—creating a cultural presence—of the concept of balance and of mechanical and chemical approaches help us appreciate this.

Mechanical notions have been conspicuous since belief in humoral theories began to decline in the second half of the seventeenth century. "That the animal body is a pure machine," as one author wrote in 1709, is just one of many early succinct expressions of the concept.[11]

Although alternative explanations for the origins and courses of diseases often exist concurrently, a clear thread of mechanical views, particularly among laypeople, can be easily traced up to the present. Innumerable writings have continuously reinforced the idea. A 1770 British almanac remarked that since a clockmaker should know the make and machinery of a clock or watch before attempting a repair, "how much more important is it that a physician should know the make and machinery of the body, which is an infinitely more curious machine or piece of clockwork than anything contriv'd by man."[12] Nineteenth-century popular medical literature commonly fostered the idea of the animal machine with both direct and indirect allusions. For instance, George Beard, in his popular *Our Home Physician* (1875), opened a brief review of anatomy and physiology with comments about the "nice and tender machinery." Statements throughout the work reinforce this idea; for instance, arteries are called "elastic tubes" and the kidney is said to "drain the system of its redundant water."[13]

Mechanical analogies have remained commonplace in this century and are found in a range of popular writings, from Arthur Keith's *The Engines of the Human Body*, first published in 1919, to modern works that compare the body to electronic circuits and computers.[14] The advertising of patent medicines, much of which reaches Mr. Bass via almanacs, also reinforces the concept with such descriptions as lubricating, flushing, and cleansing the intestinal tract, and "if your radiator leaks and your motor stands still, 'A-give her Hadacol & watch her Boogie up the hill.' " [15]

It is clear from listening to Bass that the engine metaphor provides a consistency, an internal logic, to much of his thinking. For instance, he often says that medicines acting on the liver do so by "cleaning" it and thereby aid the liver's role of "sieving blood" to remove bile. The mechanical notions are reinforced by the concept of cleansing the body of chemical toxins, which first reached Bass through his interest in internal intoxication (or "autointoxication"), an idea popularized in the early decades of the present century.[16] In part associated with the idea of visceroptosis—kinking in the intestines producing stasis—autointoxication was the alleged absorption of toxins, leading to chronic poisoning. The concept was early promoted and disseminated not only by such establishment medical personalities as London surgeon Sir William Arbuthnot Lane, but also in novels, plays, and popular medical books.

Whether popular medical works such as Charles M. Campbell's *The Lazy Colon* (1924), with its explicit diagrams, encouraged needless worry among readers is debatable; but this type of publication unquestionably reinforced, indeed helped to cement, the concept of toxins in the public mind. The concept, particularly in terms of focal sources of infection, was also widely disseminated at the time by countless appendectomies, tonsillectomies, and tooth extractions on the grounds of removing alleged sites of infection. Thus, when criticisms were expressed in the 1930s in such popular works as Jerome W. Ephraim's *Take Care of Yourself*, it is doubtful they had much immediate public impact. While the concept of autointoxication was certainly disappearing from regular medicine at that time, it only went fallow in the public mind; recent interest in toxins in general has brought the concept back to the forefront in the minds of many.

Clearly, as has been indicated, mechanical-chemical concepts serve as a logical framework for much of Bass's practice by readily rationalizing the use of blood purifiers, diaphoretics, and purgatives as a means of maintaining an efficiently running machine. Furthermore, they are open-ended concepts that readily embrace other popular ideas and thereby contribute to the persistence of ethnomedical explanations, and of much of alternative practice today.[17] It needs to be said that mechanical/chemical-balance explanations are most noticeably used in relatively minor complaints. In contrast, in life-threatening (e.g., cancer) or incapacitating (chronic rheumatism) problems, patients initially raise the question—implicitly if not explicitly—"Why do I have it? Why me?" In such cases spiritual and metaphysical questions and explanations come to the fore, but an overlapping of ideas exists; if "cleaning" the engine (body) brings it to a normal or balanced state, then, in a spiritual sense, the notion of balance seeks to clean badness with goodness.

TYPES OF MEDICINES

In addition to the concepts discussed above, many treatment regimens that were once popular in regular medicine but now are considered redundant are still conspicuous in herbal medicine today. Some are faint reflections of the past because of changed incidences of certain diseases (the "itch" and "fevers" are less prevalent) or changing concepts and classifications of disease. The liver, for instance, is no longer implicated in many general illnesses, and such therapeutic approaches as errhines to produce sneezing have disappeared as a valid part of many treatment regimens. Of the categories of medicines no longer generally accepted or recognized by regular physicians, we comment here only on alteratives and blood purifiers (including diaphoretics). Such medicines as tonics, errhines, and expectorants are considered later, under the ailment for which they are principally used.

Classifying medicines has always occasioned vigorous discussion and disagreement.[18] Of the various types, alteratives and blood purifiers, once widely used in both regular and home medicine, have been the most difficult to classify. In many ways they are catchall or "rag-bag" groups. Alteratives have always been defined somewhat vaguely, and definitions have changed little from the early eighteenth century to the beginning of this century. In 1708 they were said to be "medicines that change the humors, and restore them to their former state, either by diluting, thickning or, by little and little separating the pure from the impure by opening obstructions and strengthening the parts; whence they are called aperient, astringent, incrassating and specifick."[19]

Later definitions sometimes mentioned blood impurities, or merely stated that alteratives produce beneficial actions which defy physiological explanation.[20] Nineteenth-century writers listed large numbers of plants possessing alterative properties, though by mid-century many—such as white oak, plantain, daffodil, and stonecrop—had fallen from favor.[21] Some of the best-known alteratives still listed at the end of the century in a standard textbook were the botanicals colchicum, dandelion, and mezereon, and such inorganic substances as mercury, potassium, sodium iodides, iodine, and arsenic.[22]

Alteratives faded further from regular medicine or were reclassified into other pharmacological groups during the early decades of the present century, reflecting both an uneasiness about the lack of knowledge of their pharmacological properties and the appearance of new synthetic medicines. Though alteratives persist today in herbal medicine, and in fact have been given something of a rebirth by new scientific concepts, Mr. Bass does not use the term, instead calling many of the old alteratives "blood purifiers." [23]

Confusion between alteratives and blood purifiers can be discerned as far back as the eighteenth century. Interest in "disease poisons" in the blood was fostered by William Harvey's celebrated studies in 1628 showing that blood circulated in the body. Regular medical textbooks included more and more references to putrid blood, especially in fevers, for which alteratives, diaphoretics, and vulneraries were recommended for "purifying" or to sweeten humors.[24] Blood purifiers, a term established in the nineteenth-century popular (but not professional) medical literature, included a seeming rag-bag of substances, mostly diaphoretics and diuretics, some alteratives, and such "diluents" as water and whey.[25] Bitter substances were also included, partly on the grounds of analogy to cinchona bark (containing quinine), which "cured" fevers considered to have an underlying etiology of putrid blood.[26] Many purifiers were bitter, astringent medicines with a high tannin content.

Mr. Bass has a firm conviction in blood purifiers. Part of his working knowledge rests on the once-ubiquitous practice of giving blood purifiers as "spring tonics." "Up to the 1920s or so, all rural folk drank sassafras tea in the spring, and if they didn't have that, sarsaparilla. Another popular one in the South was pine-tops tea. A few people would drink boneset or peppermint. For children catnip was used.[27]

Generally speaking, the herbs were gathered in March and the teas drunk through that month and perhaps April. Sometimes the teas—at least sassafras—were drunk not so much as a spring tonic but because the cows were dry, a common happening in the spring." Present-day pharmacological knowledge offers no justification for blood purifiers. Clinically, however, some users find that the bitter taste provides an immediate sense of improved well-being. Further, blood purifiers that are diaphoretics (i.e., substances producing sweat and once believed thereby to remove impurities from the blood) have a physiological effect, thus suggesting that they "work."

Numerous diaphoretic plants had the added reputation of being valuable irrespective of alleged blood-purifying properties. Diaphoretics like the famed boneset were specifically regarded for fevers, but Bass comments that they are no longer used much since fevers are not as common as in the old days. He adds that some of the old fever remedies were not nearly so good as antibiotics, and he considers that, sometimes, drinking large quantities of warm water promotes perspiration independent of botanical ingredients, just as whey and tea (when assisted by external warmth, fires, or blankets) have long been well-known home diaphoretics. Bass believes that all diaphoretic plant remedies are best taken as warm teas; such observations deserve to be kept in mind during modern investigations on fever remedies, even those with a specific reputation for malaria.[28]

SPECIFIC AILMENTS

We now consider the most common ailments brought to Bass ("colds and rheumatism seem the biggest things") as well as those, albeit commonplace, which illustrate further how historical usage is part of the aura of Bass's practice and help with understanding much of his logic.

Colds, Coughs, Sore Throats, "Bad Chests," Sinus Problems, Allergies, and Flu

Like drugstores, with their myriad over-the-counter cough medicines, herbal practice offers innumerable remedies for the treatment of symptoms. Many of Bass's approaches can be discerned in regu-

lar and botanic/domestic medical textbooks of the nineteenth century and earlier, though with less emphasis on constitutional treatment and omitting almost all nonbotanical remedies.[29]

The inordinate attention given to respiratory complaints in the
nineteenth-century regular medical literature centered mostly on
diagnosis and the use of new instruments like the stethoscope, introduced in 1819. Common symptoms were generally discussed only if
they suggested serious illness or were the particular concern of the
public, such as indicators of "falling into consumption."[30] Ailments
like the common cold attracted little formal attention, partly because
treatment regimens were well known and established. Depending on
the state of a patient, treatment included gentle laxatives (perhaps
more vigorous if the case was complicated), diaphoretics to produce
sweating for the relief of inflamed membranes or to "break" a cold, expectorants and inhalations to render mucous and catarrh less viscid
and thus aid its removal, and, perhaps, counterirritants, such as plasters on the chest, to relieve congestion. If the general state of health
was poor, or if the illness was protracted, tonics also were given.[31]
Of the various approaches, particular attention was commonly given
to diaphoresis because many doctors attributed colds to obstructed
perspiration.[32]

A variety of remedies were popular, the most common falling into
the categories of diaphoretics, expectorants, and inhalants. Of these,
diaphoretics like boneset and sage are little known nowadays because
they were replaced during the latter part of the nineteenth century
by such chemicals as phenacetin, antipyrin, and salicylates (aspirin
from around 1900).

The innumerable and diverse expectorants and inhalants, a few still
in general use, illustrate the many choices once available to practitioners, and still open to the modern herbalist, for tailoring treatment
to the condition and wishes of the patient. Expectorants have been
divided into those acting topically (i.e., directly on the respiratory
tract like the popular inhalants) and those acting systemically (via the
bloodstream). By 1900 inhalants included the chemicals iodine, carbolic acid, chloroform, and ammonium chloride, though such botanical products as balsam of Peru, balsam of Tolu, horehound, and
turpentine remained popular. Systemic expectorants included such
"sedatives" as ipecacuanha (also a "nauseant") and bloodroot; "stimu-

lants" like squill and creosote; and "demulcents" like mucilage of acacia and licorice. Anodynes (e.g., hydrocyanic acid) also were employed with expectorants.[33]

The literature and classification of expectorants is confusing, partly because ideas resting on analogy (for instance, the mucilaginous nature of certain drugs) led to the employment of substances for which seemingly little clinical justification existed. Because theory also has provided professionally needed underpinnings to physicians' empirical practices—especially at times when much disagreement exists in therapy—debatable theoretical concepts often were uncritically assimilated. This helped cement into practice some drugs of doubtful or slight efficacy, though these were usually employed only when first-line treatments failed.

In contrast to other cold remedies, errhines—remedies used to excite secretions in the nasal mucous membranes and to promote sneezing—are almost totally forgotten. Bass can recall one or two, like wild ginger and such commercial preparations as Dr. Marshall's Aromatic Snuff for Cold in the Head. The latter, said to be introduced in 1835, lasted well into the twentieth century, long after errhines became generally unfashionable within regular medicine.[34]

The modern treatment of colds still rests on relieving symptoms, and Bass's botanicals are perhaps less dated than those used for many other ailments. Certainly, many people ask for advice about the vast number of remedies they have read about, especially aromatic plants. Many questions are asked about inhalants, for which Mr. Bass generally recommends rabbit-tobacco in steaming water.[35]

Bass's most popular diaphoretic (to break a cold, treat flu, or cool fever) is boneset. This, one of the most common home remedies in the nineteenth century, is, he stresses, free from the side effects of aspirin. Many accounts of boneset describe it as valuable for treating intermittent and remittent fevers. Intermittent fevers were generally considered malarial, and a wide range of remedies, many proprietary, were prescribed or marketed. While it is doubtful that any had specific antimalarial properties, the possibility exists of an antipyretic effect that complemented the body's immune reaction to an attack of malaria.

Mr. Bass considers boneset superior to chicken soup, which produces a sweat "if taken hot." Other favorites include onion and hot ginger tea, but "any hot tea may be good." Just as popular with Mr. Bass is wild cherry bark, which had untold popularity among physicians and laypeople throughout the nineteenth century and into the twentieth as a cough medicine ingredient. It was viewed as having both tonic and sedative properties and, by some, as an expectorant.[36]

Both boneset and wild cherry are widely recommended by Mr. Bass in the form of single-ingredient teas, especially when he gives advice over the telephone. Yet, despite confidence in these teas, like many herbalists he generally prefers compounded medicines for coughs. ("In my opinion when three, four, or five remedies are added together, they work like a team.") A formula for one gallon of "herb mixture for coughs and colds" (with Mr. Bass's own explanations) is as follows:

> One teacup wild cherry bark ("it's a wonderful medicine for everything")
> One teacup sweet gum bark or leaves ("it's kinda like turpentine")
> One teacup boneset ("good for fever")
> Half teacup redroot (redshank or Jersey tea; "it's a wonderful tonic")
> One teacup mullein ("good for catarrh")
> One teacup rabbit-tobacco (also called life-everlasting; "good for asthma and sinus problems")
> Two bundles red sumac ("good for flavor and for vitamin C")
>
> All to be simmered in one gallon of water for fifteen or twenty minutes. Then four pounds of sugar or honey are added, or six pounds to make a cough syrup. (Corn syrup can be used.) The dose is two tablespoonfuls as often as needed.

Mr. Bass varies the formula of this palatable medicine at times by substituting a herb he has available, perhaps comfrey or wild ginger—which also have reputations for easing coughs and colds—or bugleweed. Furthermore, he is always ready to try out new suggestions. Recently he heard that calamus was helpful and added it to the mixture. Testimony from visitors that this "improved" the medicine confirms, in his mind, its usefulness, though he admits perhaps more as a flavoring than for its physiological effectiveness.

One characteristic of Bass's practice is that he adapts formulas to suit an individual's confidence in a particular herb. Anyone who values slippery elm bark to soothe coughs and throat irritations might receive the following, a formula especially recommended for "dry coughs":[37]

> Half cup slippery elm bark
> Half cup wild cherry bark
> Half cup sweet gum bark
> Half cup mullein leaves

> All to be boiled in one gallon of water and then four pounds of sugar or honey added.

Generally, Mr. Bass does not differentiate between dry and productive coughs; however, if a visitor has catarrh with the cough, he may suggest an additional inhalation, probably a bowl of hot water containing rabbit-tobacco or peppermint. Bass might well add a tonic, too, or even a laxative on the basis that the body is a machine and needs to be kept running well during an illness.[38] For a bad cold on the chest Bass recommends applying a plaster made with onion or mustard to the chest. For people who do not have the time to prepare such a plaster, he may suggest hot flannel sprinkled with turpentine.

Frequently a sufferer from a cold complains not so much of the cough but of a sore throat, catarrh, sinus problems, and general malaise. Bass frequently is asked about sore throats. These, he says, were generally called "raspy throats, but now we call them laryngitis," (another example of the "updating" of medical terms discussed earlier). He has heard of a range of sore throats in the past, such as relaxed throat (a sensation of a "lump in the throat" and pain on swallowing) and catarrhal sore throat, but, he says, "folks call them all the same now."

He has many suggestions for sore throats, all employing astringent substances like persimmon and redroot. He remembers that putrid sore throat was another name for diphtheria. This, he says, was difficult to treat "before shots came along." It required "strong medicine," and he has in mind such astringent recipes as the following from the nineteenth-century family papers of North Carolina resident James Woodard: "Take the bark of runing brier root, sassafras root and shoemake [sumac] root, the kind that bear berrys, persimmon bark, an equal quantity of each. Add sage, honey, hyssop, alum, appletree moss. Simmer them together." [39]

For persistent catarrh, about which he is commonly asked, Bass has a number of suggestions: "My old remedy was to smoke sumac berries, fig leaves, or jimsonweed leaves. And some people would smoke rabbit-tobacco. Mullein is another good one, it's real good. Now my daddy, one of his main things for catarrh was pine dust. Sweet gum is also good, it's like turpentine though it don't taste like it."

Sinus problems are also commonly brought to him: "I tell them about rabbit-tobacco and horsemint. Some don't know the plants. I tell them to ask some old person—a neighbor." Bass adds that, "a lot of sinus trouble is allergy." In recent years the number of queries about allergies has increased. "I tell them if they know what they're allergic to (sneezing and stuffed-up head) to avoid it and to get some horsemint, and make a tea and drink it." This is to "relieve" the head. Additionally, he suggests drinking a tea made from ragweed or goldenrod in bloom, which "acts like a shot." Though he says they don't cure all the time, he relates many testimonials: "A man from West Virginia told me he had four shots and it didn't help him like ragweed tea." Many other suggestions are made if the above recommendations fail, like a tea made from "ivy." However, he says, these are "folk cures and I haven't tried them." [40]

Mr. Bass recognizes a link between allergy and asthma. He doesn't like making recommendations for asthma because it is difficult to treat, but says the "old" treatment of smoking jimsonweed can be helpful. He considers that its value is increased by adding fig leaves. Alternatively, the latter can be smoked alone, as can mullein or lobelia leaves. Smoke from pine sawdust is also "a favorite with old-timers." Other specific recommendations for asthma are chewing a comfrey leaf during an attack and taking a tea made from wild plum bark. Additional suggestions include "general" ones for chest complaints, like rabbit-tobacco and red sumac, either smoking them or using as teas, as well as inhaling herbal medicated steam.

With all his caution and his use of botanicals, Bass's practice reflects a mild, noninterventionist tradition of care rather than the type of interventionist care noticeable, for instance, during much of the nineteenth century. In fact, the cautious approach has been typical for much of the long history of self-treatment and is meshed with preventive measures such as avoidance of sudden changes in temperature or getting the feet and head wet. Another popular, well-entrenched belief, "feed a cold and starve a fever," is often mentioned by Bass, and it is clear that new medical ideas have been incorporated into the notion without changing a belief once sustained not so much on sensory perceptions of cold and hot but more on theoretical ideas.[41]

Among popular beliefs in general, relatively few superstitious and magical concepts apply to colds, at least in comparison to other ailments. In fact, the only one known to Mr. Bass is "when you first take off your shoes to go barefoot in the spring, wash your feet in cold water and you won't catch a cold all summer." This, he says, was part of "spring cleaning" and accompanies the drinking of sassafras tea. Nowadays, all such beliefs are commonly dismissed, especially by physicians and scientists, who argue that germs (or viruses) cause colds. On the other hand, some evidence exists that climatic factors may sometimes have a role in initiating a disease.[42]

Bass treats colds and attendant symptoms by providing relief. No sense exists of trying to cure, but, equally, modern medicine has yet to develop a weapon to destroy cold viruses. Since most plant remedies are no longer used in regular medicine, and have not, for the most part, been chemically studied or clinically investigated under controlled conditions, it is difficult to comment on their value. Furthermore, although testimony to their efficacy is considerable, this is based on use under a variety of circumstances, often in conjunction with other medicines (including antibiotics from a physician). Nevertheless, we venture here and elsewhere some remarks on efficacy. The comments cover the likelihood of some positive response apart from a placebo action (discussed later). Our remarks are sometimes based on evidence from medical textbooks published when the plants were commonly used and sometimes from more recent chemical, pharmacological, and clinical studies.

Undoubtedly Mr. Bass's "mainline" product is his compounded cough medicine. Like many such medicines still available, it contains one or more "expectorants" to aid removal of phlegm. In his formula the sweet gum and mullein are considered to serve this purpose, as are, to a lesser extent, the wild cherry and rabbit-tobacco.

Even if these are effective expectorants at appropriate doses, doubts arise about their value in Bass's preparation. The expectorant reputation of sweet gum, for instance, seems only to apply to the dried exudate known as "American storax"; we found no record of sweet gum bark or leaves having expectorant properties. Mullein's reputation, while firmer in the literature, is also problematical. Although the soothing, demulcent property has been widely considered helpful, doses recommended in the nineteenth century (e.g., four ounces of fresh leaves to a pint of milk three times a day) are far greater than those provided by Bass's medicine and his recommended doses.[43] The expectorant property of wild cherry bark—perhaps in reality sedative rather than expectorant—has long been attributed to hydrocyanic acid formed as a decomposition product of the glycoside prunasin. However, boiling is considered to destroy the enzyme responsible for the breakdown of the glycoside and it is unclear what concentration of hydrocyanic acid, if any, is present in the cough medicine. Rabbit-tobacco has perhaps the best reputation for chest diseases but it never became popular in regular medicine.

The whole issue of the effectiveness of expectorants is an open one. The tenor of medical thinking in recent years is that most traditional expectorants are ineffective, though some medical authorities keep an open mind.[44] Unfortunately, controlled studies are few, and most that have been undertaken deserve repetition, if for no other reason than that they suggest positive results. Examples include turpentine oil, pine oil, anise oil, and eucalyptus oil.

Other ingredients in the Bass cough medicine (boneset as a tonic and to bring down any temperature, and redroot) are present in doses smaller than those recommended in the past. It has been said, too, that neither plant is effective anyway, though this ignores the particularly strong testimonies to the value of boneset in colds and fevers, and recent suggestions that an immune stimulant action may be present separate from the diaphoretic property.

The lemon taste of sumac serves as flavoring, although it is hardly detectable amid the considerable amount of added syrup. While the medicine is palatable, it cannot be said to be enticing, unlike some well-known cough remedies; in addition, the doses are small compared with those recommended during the nineteenth century.

Bass's cough medicine thus clearly has ingredients which may well produce symptomatic relief, but only if used in doses greater than he recommends. Although many doubts have been raised recently over cough medicines analogous to Bass's, particularly over the expectorants, H. K. Beecher has argued that many patients with coughs due to diseases of the respiratory tract derive great psychological satisfaction from cough remedies, even when it has been objectively demonstrated that the remedies fail to reduce either the frequency or the intensity of the cough. This seems to be providing ease rather than provoking a placebo response.

Bass's treatment of asthma is of particular interest because of the wide range of plants recommended. Only jimsonweed has been generally accepted within regular medicine, and no evidence exists that the others have any specific effect on bronchial constriction. Yet in wondering about the recommendations (all of which have long pedigrees), possible confusion because of the many misconceptions about asthma needs to be borne in mind, along with the fact that, initially, asthma is often misdiagnosed as a common cold.

One respiratory symptom rarely brought to Mr. Bass nowadays is internal bleeding. Until the 1950s his advice was sought frequently about sputum flecked with blood, rather than the frank spitting of blood associated popularly with consumption (pulmonary tuberculosis). Mr. Bass's suggested treatments for bleeding from the lungs— the same as those employed for any "internal" bleeding—are readily found in the medical literature (regular and botanic/domestic) of the past; they include alumroot, blackberry, oak, redroot, and liverwort.

He considers the internal action of hemostatic botanicals to be the same as when applied to external wounds, a view held by physicians in the past. Concepts about the mode of action of astringents illustrate not only how theoretical notions can change without any consequent alteration in clinical practice, but also how theory can justify the use of medicines with little pharmacological action. One of numerous rationalizations with apparently little impact on everyday practice appeared in Paine's *Materia Medica and Therapeutics* (1847). Paine believed that ultimately it would be conceded that astringents operate internally like all other positive remedial agents by modifying the living properties and actions of the secerning vessels, and by arresting the redundant secretions of blood or other fluids.[45] In part, this was based on the view that opium possessed the properties of an internal astringent, though it did not contain an astringent principle. It was not until this century that belief in the efficacy of internal hemostatic agents like tannins was discarded.

Rheumatism and Arthritis

Over the years a wide range of complaints of muscle and joint aches and pains have been brought to Mr. Bass. Some, like swollen muscles, have been described as ethnomedical illnesses, since the ill-defined symptomatology does not fit a biomedical diagnosis. Bass offers such explanations as "too much fluid," "muscular" rheumatism, or some form of "charley horse" (in the calves or elsewhere).[46] If the problem seems to be excess fluid (suggested by relatively little ache) he recommends the use of a kidney medicine (e.g., Queen Anne's lace) and a blood purifier.

Bass has seen many visitors with "some type" of paralysis, most often the result of a stroke. He generally recommends as the main medicine the regular use of his salve or liniment. Many testimonials to their effectiveness—at least in the short term—have been given. On one occasion, a visitor, his wife, and a friend all said that there had been improvement after using the salve three times daily for two weeks on a hand that had been paralyzed by a stroke twelve years earlier. So far as we can tell, the seemingly beneficial result rested more on faith in the salve and the physiotherapy attendant on applying it than on any known pharmacological effect of the medicine.

Most cases of "rheumatism" and "arthritis" reaching Bass are self-diagnosed or diagnosed by a physician. Some misdiagnoses exist, if only because a wide variety of diseases may produce joint pain, and the pain does not necessarily imply joint disease. Self-diagnosis generally describes muscle aches as "rheumatic" or rheumatism, and joint problems as arthritis (sometimes called bursitis), irrespective of a wide diversity of beliefs on causes (see below). Bass says that stronger remedies are required for arthritis than for rheumatism. For both complaints he is familiar with innumerable widely known magical and nonplant treatments, but he encourages only the use of plant remedies. Table 1 lists those well known to him, though he personally recommends only a few. Also listed are concepts, still employed by Bass, which were current in nineteenth-century textbooks.

Mr. Bass's treatment of rheumatism, like that of coughs and colds, embraces nineteenth-century ideas and approaches to management.[47] Although varied and complex, these commonly rested on seeing the disease as an inflammatory disorder linked to ailments of the ner-

Table 1. Mr. Bass's Principal Remedies for "Rheumatism." These remedies, used internally, are based on nineteenth-century concepts still appreciated by Bass.

Plant	Use
Angelico (root or leaves)	Tonic. Almost all tonics (see others below), especially bitter ones, are considered helpful for rheumatism. Sometimes the reputation is strengthened by analogy to cinchona bark, regarded for its febrifuge and diaphoretic properties, also viewed as beneficial in rheumatism
Apple (bark or fresh leaves)	Tonic
Bay (bark or leaves)	All magnolias are recognized as bitter tonics
Beech (bark or leaves)	Astringent; tonic
Black cohosh (roots)	Tonic
Boneset (leaves)	Diaphoretic; tonic
Bowman's root (bark)	Astringent; tonic
Button snakeroot (root)	Tonic; diuretic ("kidney medicine") considered valuable for rheumatism and gout (see others below)
Cucumber tree (bark)	Another magnolia (cf. bay above)
Devil's shoestring (root)	Bitter tonic
Gentian (root)	Bitter tonic
Hydrangea (bark, leaves, androot)	"Kidney" medicine
Indian hemp (root)	Diuretic; diaphoretic
Joe-Pye-weed (root)	*Eupatorium* sp. (cf. boneset above)
Poke (root, berries)	Well-established, almost specific, reputation for rheumatism
Prickly ash (bark or berries)	Bitter tonic. Well-established reputation for rheumatism
Queen Anne's lace (tops and roots)	Diuretic

Table 1 *continued*

Plant	Use
Ratsvein (leaves)	Diuretic; tonic; diaphoretic
Sampson snakeroot (root)	Tonic
Sassafras (root and root bark)	Diaphoretic; diuretic; blood purifier (blood purifiers helpful for rheumatism)
Skullcap (leaves and stem)	Tonic; diaphoretic
Wild yam (tuber)	Diaphoretic
Yellow poplar (bark)	Diuretic; tonic; diaphoretic

vous system or "poisons" in the blood. Poisons originated either "internally" (e.g., lactic acid) or "externally" from miasmas and damp weather. Treatment regimens, commonly rationalized by these concepts, called for "standard" antiphlogistic or cooling approaches (involving purgation, diaphoresis, and low diet), and sometimes diuretics, liver medicines, purgatives, and direct applications to the affected parts.

Of these practices, diaphoresis received much attention because it was often thought that rheumatism was linked with suppression of perspiration, which had to be restored to normal.[48] Although the concept of antiphlogistic treatment for inflammation has not survived as an entity, encouraging sweating is still widespread; for this Bass suggests the use of boneset tea, or, alternatively, almost any hot tea and aromatic stimulant, like angelico. Diaphoresis has also been (and still is) rationalized as removing "poisons," that is, acting as a blood purifier, a concept very popular with Bass. Additional features of his regimen may include the use of liver and kidney medicines to remove impurities and ways to generally "improve the system," such as with tonics.

One aspect of Bass's thinking on rheumatism, the genesis of which remains uncertain, is the value placed on plants containing what he calls "tannic acid." Perhaps this stems from analogy with the presence of tannins in such astringent medicines as bay and cucumber tree bark, which have well-established reputations in treating rheumatism. Another untraced concept holds that rheumatism is a kind of nervous condition. Bass explained this when talking about skullcap: "There's not anything better for the nerves. It is highly recommended for rheumatism, 'cause rheumatism is a kind of nervous condition, especially the kind that pains you awful bad. The old sore type may not be the nerves, but the pain would make you nervous if you're not. I don't know how many formulas that calls for skullcap in rheumatism, but it's a fine nerve medicine."

His favorite remedies are cucumber tree ("if I can get it"), bay tree, magnolia, prickly ash, and skullcap. Some ambivalence exists over another well-known plant, devil's shoestring: "It takes the place of cucumber tree bark and magnolia, but people who use cucumber bark can't be convinced." Pokeroot has an impressive reputation in the Appalachians, but Mr. Bass feels it is generally too strong a remedy and only recommends it occasionally for arthritis if other plants have been ineffective.

All the plants suggested can be used to make single-ingredient teas. He does not agree with those who say that making rheumatism medicines in whiskey makes them stronger, but he prefers compounded preparations. A good illustration is the following unusually complex recipe, custom-prescribed for a woman visitor. Mr. Bass's explanations of the purpose of each ingredient are included in parentheses.

> Boil the following in a gallon of water for thirty-five to forty minutes:
>
> one-fourth teacup sarsaparilla (blood purifier)
> one teacup clover bloom (blood purifier)
> one-fourth teacup wild cherry bark (strengthens liver)
> one-fourth teacup skullcap (for nerves, since rheumatism is a
>   nervous condition in "one sense of the word")
> two tablespoons mayapple (good tonic)
> one-fourth teacup dogwood bark (because rheumatism is
>   "crampy")
> one-half teacup yellow dock (to put iron in the system)
> one-fourth teacup squawvine (a lady's medicine)
> one tablespoon black snakeroot
> one-fourth teacup prickly ash (for rheumatism)
> one-half teacup goldenrod (blood purifier and flavor)
> one-fourth teacup ratsvein (for rheumatism)

one tablespoon goldenseal
one ounce Solomon's seal (another lady's medicine)

After boiling, four pounds of honey or four pounds of sugar are to be added and the whole is reboiled. The medicine is then refrigerated. A dose is two tablespoonfuls three times a day and night.

This grand example of polypharmacy is too complex for everyday use; most of his compounded preparations (like the following) are simpler but still embrace the concept of "working like a team."

one tablespoon each of:

powdered blue cohosh
prickly ash bark
powdered yarrow bark
sliced sassafras
black-haw bark

Simmer for twenty-five minutes in one quart water; strain; and take a wineglassful daily before a meal.

Following long-established patterns in self-care and regular medicine, Bass does not rely solely on internal treatments for rheumatism but believes also in the efficacy of external liniments. Faith in his "rub" is encouraged since it offers a chance of keeping medicines "out of the stomach."

The rub, reflecting family and patent medicines rather than botanicals, is well known locally not only through its widespread sales, but also through distribution of typed copies of the formula. The preparation contains no plant materials (apart from commercially prepared turpentine and camphor), and Mr. Bass stresses that it is easy to make since items can be purchased readily:

How to Make Bass Quick Rub
You use one pint of green rubbing alcohol, one pint of vinegar, one pint of household ammonia and two blocks of camphor gum and two tablespoonsful of turpentine. Mix all in a jar, the alcohol, vinegar, and ammonia, camphor, and turpentine. Let set overnight and you have a rub that will ease all pain. This [is] my own

recipe and I have sold this rub for many years. But I am past 74 years old so want to pass it on to other folks, it will kill the bite of bees etc.; also poison oak, ivy etc.; good luck.

This rub produces a rubefacient response typical of large numbers of commercial liniments available from drug and general stores that provide symptomatic relief for many if not all patients.[49] Mr. Bass sees it as analogous to the "old favorite and one of the biggest sellers, Sloane's Liniment."

While plants are not included in the rub, Mr. Bass recognizes that pine, mullein, and beech, for instance, possess rubefacient properties and have been widely employed in "rubs" for rheumatism and neuralgia.

When specifically questioned on rheumatism remedies, he comes up with a longer list of botanicals than in table 1. Many are found in collections of popular sayings and beliefs recorded in Alabama and elsewhere. Most of these are for external applications (e.g., turpentine, liniments, or washes like red oak ooze). Popular recommendations for the internal use of botanicals include some very well known to Mr. Bass, such as pokeweed, "poplar" (presumably yellow poplar), bloodroot, and ratsvein, and others less commonly employed, like oil of wintergreen, parsley, sassafras (as a blood purifier), holly, mullein, and wild cherry (this last more as a tonic).[50]

It is noteworthy that some readily available plants with similar sensory characteristics and properties to plants used by Mr. Bass, and recorded in accounts of folk beliefs and nineteenth-century writings on rheumatism, are omitted from the table of rheumatism medicines. Dogwood, one example, was once widely recommended as a tonic and substitute for cinchona bark; however Bass knows of only one person "trying it out," apparently because of sensory properties analogous to other rheumatism medicines.

The fact that the concepts behind Mr. Bass's use of rheumatism medicines are essentially those of the nineteenth century and earlier raises the question of whether or not the remedies have specific effects on rheumatism, such as an anti-inflammatory action. After all, reputations in the past were explained on the basis of diaphoretic action and removing poisons from the blood. Unfortunately, it is generally difficult to decide when theory merely rationalized successful empirical treatment and when it was employed to suggest new remedies in the absence of effective treatments. We believe, however, that many of Bass's internal remedies emerged on the basis of sensory properties and analogy with other rheumatism remedies. Certainly only a few plants such as pokeweed and cucumber bark stand out as having been consistently and strongly recommended for rheumatism. The force of the testimony for these, more than slavish copying from one source to another, may suggest a possible physiological action in rheumatism rather than a placebo effect. Plants that perhaps merit closer examination because of past levels of interest include prickly ash and those with steroidal saponins like wild yam. If specific activity exists, current speculations on how this may occur include anti-inflammatory activity linked with enhancement of the immune system or effects on prostaglandin metabolism.

Bass, as noted, prefers external treatments. Liniments like Bass Rub often bring relief through rubefacient properties, which are used not only for "rheumatism" or minor aches but also for sprains. The "medicated" odor of rubefacient preparations and the feeling of warmth and visible reddening of the skin on application encourage a sense of effectiveness. Testimony on the value of this type of preparation remains positive. However, the clinical significance of reddening or vasodilation, more conspicuous in preparations containing vasodilators like methyl nicotinate, is not altogether clear, even though it may lead to greater absorption, for example, of accompanying salicylates.[51]

Bass never recommends practices such as tying strings around a limb, carrying a buckeye or an Irish potato, or wearing copper bangles.[52] However, he accepts the power of suggestion, saying that "if people believe in those things they often work." He also indicates a sense of confidence when he remarks that some people are like rabbits, which start to eat green beans in the spring and continue to do so throughout the year. Patient idiosyncrasies, he says, help explain why there are so many alternative treatments for rheumatism and other ailments.

We met thirty-three visitors over sixty years of age with "rheumatism" who provided strong testimony for these views. They have generally taken teas of bark from the cucumber tree, bay tree, or prickly ash, and have used Bass Rub. Without exception they said they had been helped. None, however, had a severe disability, and only three had difficulty in getting about their homes, climbing stairs, getting in and out of bed, and dressing. Their views agree with Mr. Bass's that rheumatism and arthritis are linked with wear and tear and toxins, and underscore the importance of the common understanding about therapy. Unfortunately, the number of visitors who have not obtained relief from Mr. Bass is unknown, as is the incidence of periodic remissions which might account for the apparent efficacy of various herbal remedies.

Skin Conditions

General principles. Recommendations for skin problems ("I guess people ask me about one every other day") generally reflect dermatological care as it existed within regular medicine until recently— namely, constitutional treatment and the application of salves and washes developed on the basis of empirical knowledge. While the management of skin diseases has slowly evolved into the specialty of dermatology during the past two centuries, until the last two decades or so advances have been mostly in pathology and diagnosis rather than in therapy.[53] Many new treatments were introduced over the years, but relatively few remained well established. An exception, sometimes recommended by Bass, is Vaseline, a refined petroleum product introduced in the nineteenth century which has become one of the most widely used household remedies of all time.[54] Its introduction reflected a trend toward using blander remedies, or at least avoiding practices of deliberately irritating the skin.

Until the early years of the present century, a key feature in the treatment of all skin diseases was administering blood purifiers. Skin ailments were generally linked with blood impurities, or "vicarious secretions" deposited on the surface of skin eruptions.[55] Bass holds this view ("a sore is a poison") and is his own living testimony for blood purifiers. When asked why he has such smooth skin, he replies that he takes blood purifiers like teas made from sarsaparilla, boneset, wild cherry bark, or clover bloom. For those "with no time to prepare a tea," he suggests "old-time brewer's yeast" or the proprietary SSS tonic.[56] On the other hand, blood purifiers that are primarily diaphoretic have been specifically advocated for skin problems with underlying inflammation; for this reason Bass recommends boneset for erysipelas.

If a visitor has a shingles rash, a different underlying problem, "nerves," has to be dealt with. Additionally, as with all skin problems, the general constitution is considered. Bass believes that any tonic (including the new "tonics," like vitamins) can be helpful. Buttermilk is often mentioned both as an internal nutrient and an external wash for skin ailments.

Salves, according to Mr. Bass, are another "general" treatment, since they can be employed for all skin ailments. "Each family used to have its own," he says, such as Bass Salve, which his family brought from England generations ago. He believes that it started out as a preparation of hog lard, pine tar, yellow sulfur, jimsonweed, tobacco, honey, and powdered alum. Though it was a good salve, Mr. Bass modified it, largely because customers didn't like the greasiness and odor. His revised formula, which may vary according to what he has available, generally contains pokeweed, bloodroot, mayapple, yellow dock, boric acid, and powdered alum in hog lard, or occasionally in beef tallow.[57] Bass Salve has been used as first-line treatment for almost any sore, burn, "skin cancer," eczema, "what we used to call erysipelas," and one of "two kinds of psoriasis." Bass's rationale behind the multiple uses, apart from his experience, is his belief in the "unity" of sores, a concept that he extends to internal ulcers: "Anything that will heal one sore will heal another."[58]

The salve cools the "heat" of sores, says Bass, but, alternatively, "cooling" may be induced by astringent washes recommended for a variety of skin problems—from prickly heat rashes to varicose veins —an approach discussed widely in all levels of the medical literature of the past.[59] His favorite wash is an "ooze" (or tea) made from red or white oak, but he recognizes that some astringents have acquired local reputations for specific problems. In one instance, "An old dreyer and old logger, had a black feller who couldn't work and wouldn't say what it was. The fellow's brother told him his tool was all festered up, the inflammation was falling out of it. A Jersey tea wash was made and the tool bathed in it and three to four cups drunk a day. He was back at work in two weeks, but he wouldn't look at a woman. You could put sarsaparilla with it."

One general treatment commonplace within regular medicine, though less so in self-treatment and only dimly remembered by Bass, is the use of powders like powdered orrisroot or lycopodium for "drying up" cutaneous diseases. Nor does he use irritant substances like pepper, mustard, or stinging nettle, although he appreciates that the latter is a good Indian remedy. Not surprisingly, in view of his enthusiasm for salves and washes, he has little interest in the practice of counterirritation (discussed later).

Apart from the general approach of using blood purifiers, tonics, salves, and astringent washes, additional or supplementary treatments are suggested for many problems.

Sores, ulcers, and boils. For discrete sores and ulcers, Bass recommends the topical application of teas made from yellowroot or goldenseal, as well as taking them internally.[60] At the outset of treatment yellowroot is preferred as being milder; if it does not work, goldenseal is substituted, especially for stomach ulcers or for "herniary" ("the feeling in the stomach that makes it difficult to swallow").[61] Barberry, also well known to Bass, is considered by him to be of "intermediate" strength between yellowroot and goldenseal.

For people who have difficulty taking these very bitter roots, Bass suggests mixing them with mayonnaise or honey ("now honey is a healer within itself"). Specifically for sore mouths he recommends chewing on a root. Alternatively, particularly for a scalded roof of a mouth, he might recommend the demulcent slippery elm bark.[62]

Sores, especially boils or carbuncles (often called "risings" or "risens"), are commonly treated with poultices, one of the most widely used forms of "traditional" treatment everywhere (see chapter 4).[63] Of the countless poultices Bass knows, he most frequently recommends plantain beaten together with buttermilk, since it is easy to prepare: "If you bind it on at night, the core of a boil will come out by next morning." This may be optimistic, but certainly poultices to bring pus "to a head" are well established as providing relief, if not a cure.

Poison ivy. Mr. Bass has probably been asked about poison ivy rash more than any other skin ailment. He recognizes that "hundreds of suggestions" have been made to "give relief," many of which, he says, "are not favored." This includes the fairly well-known jewelweed. His own suggestions tend to be tailored to the amount of time a person has to prepare the remedy. In an emergency, vinegar or Octagon soap is recommended. Other soaps can be used, "but most are not strong enough."

If time is available, gathering and making a wash (a weak tea) from leaves of various plants is suggested. Plantain, made into a tea or boiled in milk, is "highly recommended" and considered more effective than soap. Alternative plants with astringent properties include white oak, Jersey tea, and rabbit-tobacco.[64] Bass believes that liberally applied washes are better than plant juices, which generally cannot be obtained in sufficiently large quantities.

Many people ask Bass about eating poison ivy leaves to build up resistance. He knows of three people who have tried it, but is wary of the idea and does not recommend it (see "Poison Ivy", volume 2).[65]

Occasionally Bass is faced with thunderwood poisoning (from *Rhus vernix* L., commonly known as poison sumac). As "one of the worst things you can get," he does not believe most of the poison ivy remedies work, and has recently concluded that aloe vera juice is best.

Ringworm and other infections. Ringworm, superficial skin lesions caused by a fungus, is viewed by Bass as similar to psoriasis, "but it's not so serious. I don't get asked about it like I used to." The best-known remedy, he says, is walnut leaf juice, "though I generally give yellowroot or goldenseal as well; the plants that will cure all sores." [66]

It is clear from personal observations that Bass is asked about many superficial infections, including impetigo. In addition to astringent washes, he recommends applications of iodine and potassium permanganate wash, and, "if it does not get better," going to the doctor.

Bites and stings. "There are so many remedies for bites," says Bass, "that people use almost anything." Plant remedies are, in fact, not commonly reported, apart from tobacco (juice or snuff). Bass usually suggests his salve, the type of greasy ointment often recommended in the past,[67] or for those who do not like the greasy preparations, a plantain wash.

Despite Bass's dismissal of practices he considers to be superstitious, he has often recommended a long-established regimen of rubbing three different leaves in turn on the sting—"any three leaves, such as sourwood, dogwood, and plantain." Testimony over the years has convinced him that this is helpful.

"Itch" (scabies) and lice. Scabies, a highly contagious disease

caused by the parasitic mite *Acarus* burrowing into the skin, was commonplace when Tommie Bass was growing up. "It lasted so long it was called the seven-year itch."[68] He is still asked for advice on occasion, although he recognizes that the complaint "I've got an itch" is no longer usually due to scabies. Treatment with poke, well known to Bass ("the oldest remedy in the world"), is well established in the popular tradition. It is used as a tea or wash, or by applying the sap directly.[69] Numerous alternative remedies, indicative of the once widespread nature of itch, are well known and include teas made from tobacco, plantain, red oak, white oak, or Jersey tea. ("Wash the skin like using soap and water, using a sponge. It will need to be done several times.")

"Lice," remarks Bass, "like herbs, are on the way back." Certainly the head louse can be found in many populations, rural and urban. Nit picking and combing are well remembered, but Bass says washing the hair with fleabane tea worked as well. He remembers that DDT began to be used for lice not long after it was introduced. Nowadays, he tells anyone requesting help to get a special shampoo from the doctor or druggist: "It's quicker and easier."

Burns. First aid for burns is usually requested by telephone. Bass knows a host of remedies, but says he has little experience to back them up. They mostly fall into the categories of applying butter and salves (emollients) and/or leaves such as plantain. In the last few years aloe vera gel has become his first choice, but he still commonly suggests applying ice for half an hour or so. Interestingly, this is a relatively recent idea: "When I was a boy it was not used for fear of running the fire in."[70] If the area remains sore after ice treatment, an application of sweet milk, bicarbonate of soda, and plantain is recommended. This, he says, is "cooling," but he argues that the plantain is valuable for its astringent activity. Other astringents, like Jersey tea, are almost as good and are used when readily available.

Yet another treatment Bass has occasionally recommended—apparently an example of treating like with like—involves warming grease and red pepper together and smearing the "salve" over the burn. Mr. Bass considers it a better remedy than applying butter, but he recognizes that butter is easier to use and that most people will not prepare compounded remedies. He does not believe other fatty remedies, of which countless numbers have been recorded, are as good.

Psoriasis. Mr. Bass has had as little success with treating psoriasis as doctors in the past. "Two types of psoriasis exist," he says, "the scaly type and the brown type. The salve helps the scaly, but not the brown." His general approach is trial and error. If the salve fails, Jersey tea might help. He adds, "A man on the mountain came down with it. I gave him a bag of Jersey tea root. It done him so much good he comes back all the time, if he can't find his own."

Jersey tea root has helped on other occasions, as related in another testimony:

> A woman with beautiful hair had psoriasis on it. I gave her a bag of Jersey tea (we call it redroot or redshank) and told her to make you a gallon of tea and wash her hair like it was a shampoo and let it stay on about an hour, and rinse it out with any kind of shampoo. Do it every day until it's used up. Her sister tried to stop her, but after three or four applications, the split ends went away. The pain stopped. Her sister run her fingers through her hair and said, "You tell that feller to send me some of that." It healed her scalp. Got it plumb out.

Warts. Warts, the product of epidermal cells infected with a virus, are commonly viewed as an enigma and a nuisance by physicians and sufferers alike. The diversity of treatments, almost as varied in regular as in traditional medicine,[71] have constantly aroused fascination. This is especially so for magical treatments, of which there may be more for warts than for any other ailment.[72] "Contagious magic" is still current in Bass's neighborhood: touching the wart with a piece of wood, a rag, and so on, and placing the item near another person, who, by coming into contact with it, may have the wart transferred to him.

Bass says the best-known magical cure directs the sufferer to "cut an Irish potato in nine slices, rub each slice over the wart nine times, throw each slice over the shoulder and 'don't look back.' "[73] He remembers, too, that in the past some people had the "gift" to remove warts without applying anything to them, merely "telling them to go"; many such practitioners, like a Mr. Alexander who lived in Leesburg during the 1920s, were faith doctors who cured a wide range of conditions.

The commonest treatment recommended by Bass, and long known

in domestic medicine, is daily application of the milky juice (latex) from many plants such as the fig tree, dandelion, milkweed, or wild lettuce.[74] "It takes two weeks to a month, just keep the juice on." Other well-known though less-popular alternatives are the application of astringent lotions such as plantain tea. Bass says even the regular application of castor oil has led to satisfied visitors. Occasionally he has recommended a caustic like lye, an approach in line with some modern therapies.

A more "modern" treatment is a combination of the old concept of getting the blood in good order and modern ideas of nutrition: "A good way to get rid of warts is to eat food high in iodine and vitamins like A, B-complex, D, E, and calcium, zinc, etc., to get the blood in order." Bass has received much positive testimony about this regime.

Of all the wart treatments known to Bass, only mayapple is still well known in regular medicine. He rarely recommends it, however, either in a salve or wash, since he considers it too strong.

Corns. Like many podiatrists, Mr. Bass indicates that the best treatment is to "treat the shoe." ("There are no foot problems, only shoe problems.")[75] But when asked for advice on softening corns, he suggests repeated applications of castor oil, soaking the feet in hot water, applying turpentine or kerosene, and then scraping.[76] Bass's favorite treatment is salicylic acid, and he sometimes suggests softening a corn in warm water and applying an aspirin tablet. Bass, like others, does not appreciate the difference between salicylic acid and acetylsalicylic acid (aspirin), but he reports that the regimen has been successful for many people.[77]

Piles. In recent years Bass has had fewer requests for remedies for itching associated with this common ailment, which is due to varicose veins rather than a skin problem. The decline, he considers, is due to the popularity of such widely advertised, over-the-counter, easy-to-use medicines as Preparation H.

His long-standing suggestions follow the line that "anything that is astringent will take the swelling out." Red oak bark ooze (tea) is a typical recommendation, although redroot is considered just as helpful.[78] Additionally, he is always ready to suggest that Bass Salve will help. ("All sores can be treated the same.") Testimony supporting the all-purpose effectiveness of the salve is in line with many old-time greasy remedies such as axle grease and lard. Well-known botanical remedies recommended by many herbalists today include hydrastis (see "Goldenseal", volume 2) and *Collinsonia canadensis* L., neither of which are known to Mr. Bass for treating hemorrhoids, nor do they have a strong historical pedigree for such usage.

"Cancer," including skin cancers and lumps. A conspicuous feature of the story of "cancer" is the vast number of remedies that have been tried over the years, so often with high hopes that are ultimately dashed. "It would be very tedious, and, at the same time, an unprofitable task, to attempt to offer a detailed account of the various articles of the materia medica that have been given internally with a view to the cure of cancer."[79] Aside from threads of optimism, most opinions over time have questioned the effectiveness of medical treatment for malignant diseases. A long history of comments from physicians and laypeople alike match the views of herb dealer C. J. Cowle, who in a letter to a friend on 7 January 1859 noted the "common notion that [cancers] are incurable"; interestingly, however, he went on to share an undisclosed cancer "cure." This perhaps reflects a view, often found in the past, that proposed treatments were not expected to be effective on every occasion. An implicit sense of trial and error is often discernible in medical writings on cancer. For instance, it lies behind the remark of B. Banister (1622) that "every cancer is uncurable or hardly cured."[80] Others perhaps appreciated a placebo action at play, a notion discussed explicitly by the early nineteenth century.[81]

Bass is cautious about making recommendations for "cancer" and suggests that any worried visitor see a doctor. However, he has supplementary treatments to offer. He knows of many of the "cooling" applications used in the past for external cancers (e.g., plantain and violet leaves) but generally recommends his Bass Salve or a tea prepared from red oak or bloodroot. Like many people, he has misunderstood recent developments in the employment of Madagascar periwinkle and he believes that an ointment prepared from any periwinkle would be useful.

Apart from external applications, Bass recommends tonics to build up the system. One which he also believes has a specific effect on cancer is clover—red or white, but preferably red. This has received little recent attention compared to such botanical remedies as chaparral, "Jason Winter's tea," and mistletoe.[82] Bass is much more circumspect than many herbalists, who not only recommend tonics, but also various "cleansing" regimens.

General comments on skin treatments. Commenting on the pharmacological effectiveness of diverse skin remedies is not easy. Until relatively recently the regular practice of dermatology employed demulcents, emollients, protectives, absorbents, irritants, and astringents largely on an empirical basis. Mr. Bass's practice, with its considerable usage of emollient and astringent medicines, is similar. It may be that he achieves a comparable level of success to that obtained by many physicians in the past. It is certainly impossible at present to determine the relative importance, in the results obtained, of physiological action versus such factors as his "authority" and local reputation in promoting a placebo response.

Bass's favorable experiences with greasy salve may be primarily the result of its role as a protective agent. On the other hand, with burns it is generally agreed that a significant cause of accompanying pain is the drying-out effect; this is felt to be minimized by the application of butter, oils, and salves, though they are no longer recommended by regular physicians. Modern discussions on traditional treatments of wounds often consider the possibility of antiseptic or antibiotic action (and occasionally wound-stimulating effects). Many suggestions have been published; for instance, the milky juice of a fig and certain essential oils are reported to have antibacterial properties, as do *Agave* species, honey, and sugar.[83] On the other hand, we have found no reports of antibiotic activity relevant to Bass's preparations.

Studies on the anti-inflammatory or immunostimulant activity of plant extracts are presently at an elementary stage and it is not easy to say whether or not, or how often, these concepts are at play. Nevertheless, many suggestions indicate that such properties may have a role in the reputations of some plant remedies.[84] Compounds such as coumarins, for instance, may be significant in melilotus (see "Clover", volume 2).

Basically, Bass's principal overall recommendation for most skin ailments is the application of astringent substances (mostly tannins). While these, with their precipitant action on proteins, have a long history of use on abraded tissues (the resulting mechanical barrier is considered to be valuable in encouraging wound repair), their anti-inflammatory action may be relevant. Astringent preparations, at least tannic acid, have been a popular treatment for burns during this century, as Mr. Bass recognizes. His confidence in this ("because doctors use tannic acid") lies behind his enthusiasm for plantain and New Jersey tea. Tannic acid, however, disappeared from the regular treatment regimens for burns around the 1950s. Another well-known past use of astringents is followed by Bass: the treatment of hemorrhoids, for which much supporting testimony exists. Notwithstanding the pedigree of astringents, it must not be assumed—as it sometimes is—that this covers merely applying a fresh leaf to a wound or sore, a favorite recommendation of many herbalists.

It is not easy to comment constructively on the various recommendations for poison ivy, though most are recognized as mildly palliative at best. Interestingly, Mr. Bass has little faith in jewelweed, which, of all the botanical remedies, has probably received the most recent positive testimony. Nevertheless, other testimony supports the value of his principal approach of liberal washing, either with soap (preferably Octagon) or with astringent lotions. It is fairly widely held that washing with soap degrades the causative chemical constituent, urushiol.[85]

Bass's knowledge of the use of irritant substances on the skin merits comment. Irritants like mustard have been widely employed over time as counterirritants (often producing vesication) to treat internal complaints such as "inflammation of the lungs and pleura, in gastric disorders accompanied by much pain, in colic, in neuralgias and neuritis, and for inflammations of the kidney."[86] Counterirritation was still widely discussed in regular medical books up to the 1940s. Bass's formula for mustard plaster, however, is much milder than plasters commonly used up to the 1930s, and it seems likely that it has relatively little physiological effect on most patients.

Despite the long-standing pessimism over the medical treatment of cancer, many modern researchers believe that folklore is a valuable tool for predicting plant constituents with antitumor activity, especially as so much disappointment has arisen over the enormous effort expended in an indiscriminate search of the plant kingdom for such agents. Encouragement for studies on folk medicine is provided by the long history of employing *Podophyllum peltatum* for cancerous tumors, polyps, and unhealthy granulations. Also, while the value of the Madagascar periwinkle alkaloids for some cancerous conditions was found by chance, at least one instance has been reported of an herbalist using it to treat Hodgkin's disease.[87]

Yet, frequently, positive laboratory results on plant activity have proved clinically disappointing. While many physiologically active compounds have been found in plants once recommended for tumorous conditions, cytotoxic activity is often too low (for instance, among tannins, phytosterols, or saponins), or there is an unacceptable general toxic effect. This, along with negative views about successful treatment in the past, suggests that clues garnered from history and folklore about potential new cancer drugs are likely to lead to blind alleys, at least without very careful assessment of the data. A particular problem is the difficulty in giving a modern diagnosis to the many lumps and bumps described in the past. Many were undoubtedly glands enlarged as a result of diseases like tuberculosis, known as king's evil or scrofula. Whether inflammatory, benign, or malignant, until the nineteenth century swellings were thought to be due to local aggregates of more or less abnormal "humors" or fluids. In fact, a clear line of demarcation between inflammatory and neoplastic tumors was not drawn until the second half of the century, and "cooling" astringent washes were generally used for all.[88] In other words, theoretical concepts have probably been a major factor behind the use of many "cancer" remedies; thus those employed in the past on the basis of their tannin content (e.g., redroot, as noted by Bass) probably merit low priority in modern laboratory investigations of plant products for antitumor activity.[89]

Other remedies, such as blood purifiers, must be treated just as circumspectly. It is very difficult to make laboratory or clinical assessments of these, as it is with tonics and eliminatives often recommended by herbalists for constitutional treatment. In the light of current knowledge, the historical record does not seem to offer much additional help in finding new chemotherapeutic agents, beyond a general empirical approach of studying physiologically active constituents. On the other hand, it may be that the effectiveness of a plant may be due to a general immunostimulant action rather than direct action on a tumor.

Cosmetics (including treatment for dandruff, brown spots, and more general depigmentation). No discussion on skin conditions is complete without some reference to cosmetics. Indeed, it is relevant to appreciate that the employment of cosmetic and perfumery materials has often embraced a distinctly medical component, particularly prior to the eighteenth century, when fumigating pestilential matter changed from using sweet, aromatic substances to employing vinegary preparations. In recent years, as part of the growing interest in herbs, Bass has been asked more frequently than ever before about herbal cosmetics. Some queries probably reflect the high cost of many commercial preparations or a fear of allergic responses to nonnatural substances. Certain suggestions from him are well established in the popular tradition and have long been recorded in countless books on household recipes and cooking.

Bass is especially knowledgeable on products for the hair, and for a number of years he has sold an herbal shampoo commercially prepared for him. It contains such hair "tonics" as sage and "other good herbs like peppergrass, peach leaves and chickweed." If the hair needs a conditioner, rubbing cottonseed or olive oil into the hair along with the shampoo is recommended.[90] By virtue of their "tonic" action, hair tonics are considered to have a beneficial effect on thinning hair; however, he gives "no guarantee" and does not believe that they help baldness.

If he is specifically asked for treatment of dandruff which does not clear up with a tonic shampoo, he recommends a wash: "Mayapple makes a good tonic to wash your hair; it helps get rid of dandruff. If I'd put it in a dandruff medicine, I'd get rich in thirty days. I'd take red and garden sage, redroot, walnut or pecan leaves, mullein, and mayapple. If you just love the redroot, you can use that."

To acquire a clear skin, Bass also recommends blood purifiers and good skin hygiene. A good tonic, he adds, is lemon juice, which has long been recommended for a variety of skin conditions. However, if skin remains "unhealthy," the "best treatment, nowadays, is aloe vera; in the old days, to keep the skin soft, a lotion of peach or sassafras leaves was often used. Beef tallow could be added to make a salve."

There are many suggestions for specific blemishes like brown or "age" spots. He has always known about age spots, but in the old days, he says, people did not worry so much. His first recommendation is generally lemon juice, but "the sap of any milkweed or fig tree can be tried." A tea of white oak bark used every day, especially at night, for many weeks is also suggested at times, but with "no guarantee" that it works.

One long-standing query—in many respects a similar issue—is from blacks who wish to lighten their skin color. While Bass recommends lemon juice, he recognizes this is not necessarily suitable for large areas and says that slippery elm bark made into a thick "stew" and applied regularly is well known. On the other hand, the use of a white powder (e.g., corn starch) is commonly employed. Depigmenting practices are fairly widespread among black populations worldwide, and many commercial preparations are marketed; many contain hydroquinone, which interferes with the formation of melanin pigment.[91]

"Nerves," Tonics, and Sedative Medicines

"I have that run-down feeling," "My spirits are low," "I have a fit of blues," or "I have trouble with the nerves" are frequent complaints heard by physicians, pharmacists, and Mr. Bass. These complaints, as they are brought to him, are generally relatively minor cases of depression or anxiety. No evidence was observed that the complaint of "nerves" fits a relatively unique clinical syndrome described by other authors (though some common features exist), nor have we found many visitors who believe that their "nerves" is a physical disorder of the nerves. On the other hand, most other studies have been undertaken in a medical setting where there is a strong tendency to describe problems in biological terms.[92] We have found that "nerves" is generally used as another term for "my spirits are low," or for mild depression or anxiety.

Bass has no dealings with severe mental disturbances, but does say that strong doses of the nerve medicines he generally recommends would be helpful. He appreciates that recognizing the seriousness of a mental problem is not easy.

Anxiety and worry are viewed by Bass and many of his visitors as largely a female problem: "They fly off the handle and cannot stand their husbands"; or "Some of the ladies who they work to death in the chicken plant keeping up with the machines, their nerves just go to pieces if they are young or old." Men, on the other hand, are not immune: "I wish the wife would leave home, and the children are running me crazy." Depression, like anxiety, he believes, is more common among women than men, and affects all ages.[93]

Bass has a tendency to see a nervous component in many complaints, and it is difficult to determine whether this reflects the current debate on the role of stress in disease or attitudes he acquired as a young man. Certainly it is necessary to appreciate that nervous disorders were viewed in the past as possessing a very protean character, and this has seemingly influenced Bass and other herbalists of his generation.

Expressions like "my spirits are low" have a long history in lay and professional medicine. It is part of the title of George Cheyne's influential work, *The English Malady* (1733), which contributed to the eighteenth-century trend to see more and more problems as medical or nervous disorders.[94] In fact, it has been said that in the eighteenth century almost every disease might be called nervous.[95] A prime exponent of this view was the influential Edinburgh physician William Cullen (1710–90). His writings, which were still being published in America in the early decades of the nineteenth century, described "neuroses, or nervous diseases" as "all those preternatural affections of sense and motion which are without pyrexia." The wide range of neuroses included apoplexy, paralysis, fainting, indigestion, epilepsy, hypochondriasis (or "vapors" or "low spirits"), tetanus, palpitation of the heart, hysteria, mania, and melancholia.[96]

Some of these categories disappeared from regular medicine in the nineteenth century as new theories of the causes of nervous diseases emerged. This affected self-care less than professional medicine, partly because changes in therapy were, in fact, commonly changes in regimen, and the use of many long-standing drugs persisted to a greater or lesser extent alongside new ones. That—plus, for instance, continued concern with paying attention to the constitution —helped sustain many lay beliefs (e.g., concepts of vapors), despite the growing influence of new medical theories that tended to distinguish more sharply between neurological and psychiatric disorders. Depending on the condition and constitution of the patient, treatment regimens might include light diet, exercise, laxatives, bloodletting, blisters, and opium. Additionally, tonics and stimulants were given on the basis of "strengthening" fibers or nerves, or, more generally (such as with aromatic, saline, acid, or bitter substances), to act on the vascular as much as the nervous system. Implicit in the writings of Cullen and others is a combination of whole, or constitutional, and more localized treatments, on the basis that regimens should be tailored carefully to a particular patient and condition. In practice this was obscured for a number of reasons; one was that some drugs in the categories of narcotics, sedatives, and stimulants were so often employed that usage tended to become rote.

Nineteenth-century discussions on these categories of drugs are somewhat confusing because of different definitions and classifications. Narcotics, such as opium, belladonna, hyoscyamine, nicotine, laurocerasus, and sweet almond were commonly understood to be substances that reduced the irritability of the whole body through acting on the brain and the nervous system. Sedatives, on the other hand, were usually felt to have more localized actions and anti-inflammatory effects. While they often were incorporated into regimens involving bloodletting and purging, some sedatives considered as antispasmodics with specific actions on the gastrointestinal tract were employed, particularly for nervous disorders. The sedative antispasmodics were a diverse, physiologically active group of substances, which included heavily scented products like musk and civet and the plant product asafetida. All had the common characteristic of a disagreeable odor, however, hence the name fetids.[97]

Cullen's account of nervous disorders, like many others, suggests that theory was employed not only to rationalize empirical data but also to suggest potential new drug uses and regimens. For instance, Cullen's explanation for the action of fetid medicines apparently opened the door to the use of any plant with a harsh smell: "Since all disagreeable sensations are sedative, or means of weakening the energy of the brain, so I conceive that our foetid medicines, by obviating or moderating the increased excitement which begins spasmodic affection, may be the remedies of these." Similarly, he argued that all stimulants—generally more sharply aromatic products like lavender, marjoram, camphor, mint, and vinegar—had a common action of "increasing the mobility" of fluid contained in the nerves. Stimulants were sometimes referred to as nervines, but this term came to be widely used for all substances acting on the nerves.[98]

William Buchan and other writers of popular medical texts appreciated the sedative/stimulant regimes described in Cullen's writings but were cautious about the use of medicines and tended to emphasize, more than Cullen, non-drug treatment. For instance, an 1805 edition of Buchan's *Domestic Medicine* said about neuroses that "it would be an easy matter to enumerate many medicines which have been extolled for relieving nervous disorders. However we shall omit mentioning more medicines and again, recommend the strictest attention to DIET, AIR, EXERCISE AND AMUSEMENT."[99] Buchan, like Cullen and other physicians of that time, was concerned with the "equilibrium" or constitution of the body as a whole: attention to diet, fresh air, exercise, and amusement was in keeping with regulation according to nature. The same factors, once called nonnaturals, are still recognized today as helpful ways to cope with depression, despite the medical emphasis on drug treatment. They include activities like seeing a friend, going for a walk, eating properly, traveling to a different climate, and trying to work out the reasons for feeling depressed.[100] One way to complement such factors was medical treatment with tonics, and these were frequently used by nineteenth-century physicians and laypeople alike.

Many explanations were put forward to justify the variety of substances employed as "tonics" and "stimulants." Although medical books often separated these on the basis of tonics having a general restorative action and stimulants augmenting the action of particular organs, in practice much overlap existed. The alleged pharmacological effects ranged from acting on the body's fibers, acting on the stomach, and promoting secretions, to merely some "inherent" action.[101] While disagreement about the nature of the actions persisted throughout the nineteenth century, a web of closely interwoven factors encouraged the growing popularity of tonics. A particularly important one was the commercial promotion of patent medicines in general, many of which were described as tonics (see chapter 4). At the same time the use of tonics was fostered by changing concepts which suggested that certain ailments were becoming less "vigorous" than hitherto. Patients who showed diminished excitement along with a low temperature and weak pulse were sometimes supported with alcohol or tonics. Similar ideas of diminished vitality can be found in the "diagnosis" of neurasthenia, a disease popularized by George M. Beard and others during the last decades of the 1800s.

Neurasthenia, generally viewed as the late-nineteenth-century counterpart of hypochondriasis,[102] created a diagnostic entity from such varied symptoms as "sick headache," noises in the ear, atonic voice, deficient mental control, bad dreams, insomnia, nervous dyspepsia, vague pains, flying neuralgia, and hopelessness.[103] At the same time it reinforced in the minds of many the protean nature of nervous complaints. The suggested pathology was an "impoverishment of a nervous force," and the varied treatment regimens inevitably included tonics. In his manual of domestic medicine (*Our Home Physician*, 1875) Beard noted a recent revolution toward tonics: "In our method of treatment a great revolution has been wrought than in the types of disease. Instead of bleeding and calomel, tartar emetic and low diet, we now give tonics and stimulants—iron and quinine, strychnine and arsenic, cod-liver oil and whiskey, air and sunlight, passive movements, general electrization, abundance of sleep, and a large and palatable variety of nourishing food."[104] By the end of the century a vast choice of tonics existed, variously classified as gastric, blood, and general tonics, all strengthening "the tone of the body generally, or part of it."[105]

Other approaches to treating nervous disorders discussed in the nineteenth-century medical literature, especially home medicine books, included the use of blood purifiers: "There are occasions . . . when the right thing to do would be to take immediate steps to use a blood purifier," remarked one almanac author.[106]

Mr. Bass's recommendations for "nerves" reflect many of the approaches just noted: constitutional treatment (using tonics and blood purifiers), specific remedies such as nervines, and exercise and "getting away from it all." His blood purifiers have been discussed earlier; his tonics and specific nerve medicines are considered here.

Above almost all else Bass places considerable value on tonics, and he has a number of general "all-purpose" bitter ones. His description of them underscores his mechanical approach to physiological processes: "Tonics are good for kidney and liver, and they help digest your food by furnishing something that takes the place of bile in your gall bladder. Digestion needs a bitter substance, so much of that bitter bile has to get into the stomach for the food to digest. The bitter medicine cleans off the liver like the septic tank and helps the bile. That's why bitter medicine does us so much good. Tonics also make a good, red, healthy bloodstream. They make you feel good."

The bitter plants (often called "bitters," as were the alcoholic preparations once commonly made from them), such as yellowroot, dandelion, gentian, and goldenseal, generally have been regarded as tonics. They are commonly taken as teas but, as with other herbs, Bass prefers the "team" approach of a compounded remedy. Since around 1980 he has been making and selling BH Tonic. The formula varies at times, but generally comprises the following items: two ounces of angelico, or boarhog root ("good tonic for run-down people"); two ounces of boneset (used as mild laxative); two ounces of wild cherry bark ("God did not make anything better"); and two ounces of yellow-root ("a tonic; if I just had to have one herb I would have yellowroot"). These are combined and boiled in a gallon of water for one hour. Then one tablespoon of cayenne pepper is added ("that's what people like, cayenne pepper. It's a stimulant, and a whole lot quicker than whiskey"). Occasionally two ounces of ginseng and dandelion are added. The recommended dose is one tablespoon three times a day.

The local popularity of the tonic, particularly among blacks, is considerable, partly because of its reputation as an aphrodisiac. ("Word about it has spread quickly," and "women buys it too.") Bass believes the BH Tonic improves "all-round tone." He has never recommended an aphrodisiac as such, but recognizes that, apart from boarhog root, other tonics such as bloodroot and ginseng are often purchased from him specifically "to help nature."

Not all "tonics" employed by Bass are bitter. Many are better known as blood purifiers (like sassafras and sarsaparilla) or liver medicines (like mayapple), which he thinks improve the function of the liver and bile, and hence of the body as a whole.

Others, like the angelico in the BH Tonic, can be placed in the once-popular group of "aromatic stimulants." These included a large number of volatile oils such as anise and dill from the family Umbelliferae (Apiaceae) or peppermint and pennyroyal of the Labiatae (Lamiaceae) family. It is of interest that Bass is unaware of the concept of a stimulant action for many plants; he views many essential-oil-bearing plants as generally having a sedative action.

Apart from general tonics, Bass recommends specific "nerve tonics." His main ones are maypop, skullcap, peach leaves, bay, and black cohosh. He suggests that a mixture is best; for instance, catnip "mixed with maypop, sage, or peppermint, skullcap, and peach tree leaves creates one of the finest nerve tonics you can use."[107] Bass recognizes that not all nerve tonics have the same action; some, like maypop and peach leaves, are sedatives, while others, like sage, are stimulants.

Vinegar ("poor man's smelling salts") is also a stimulant for faintness, especially among those feeling generally miserable. In practice, however, Bass often does not make a clear distinction between sedatives and stimulants, for he holds the concept that everything that adjusts the carburetor will restore balance. Medicines like catnip, sage, and peppermint are of special interest because the sedative action is, he says, mediated through the stomach, a notion which is apparently a legacy from the early decades of the nineteenth century, when the stomach was thought to play a key role in producing certain nervous disorders.

Nerve medicines provide a good illustration of the nineteenth-century demise of many botanicals within regular medicine under the growing impact of chemical remedies. As far back as 1879, Austin Flint's standard medical textbook stated in a section on neurasthenia: "The preparations of phosphorus are perhaps useful in promoting the nutritive processes, which are recuperative. The hypophosphate of lime, and the phosphide of zinc are eligible preparations." [108]

Flint also might have mentioned that chloral hydrate, paraldehyde, and bromides were widely used for many nervous conditions. Later, in the early years of the twentieth century, barbiturates were added to the growing chemical armamentarium for nervous disorders. They remained the most conspicuous type of hypnotic and sedative medicines until recent decades.

Recent publicity given to Valium and tranquilizers in general reinforces the awareness of Mr. Bass and others of chemical drugs and side effects. He has stressed a number of times that the old-time medicines, those once prescribed by doctors and sold over the counter and still recommended by him, are mild and safe. He stresses, too, that he gives nothing like morphine, a reflection not only of his general fear of dangerous medicines, but also his dislike as a child of the popular opium preparation paregoric.

Assessments of the effectiveness of the remedies for nervous disorders are especially difficult because of the broad spectrum of symptoms that have been labeled "nervous." The diagnosis of a "run-down condition," for instance, is vague, and almost certainly factors other than medicines (for instance, merely talking to Mr. Bass) are behind the apparent improvements in many a patient's condition. Further, it seems clear that outdated theoretical considerations have been a major factor encouraging the use of some remedies. That fetid medicines are good for the nerves is one example, although evidence exists that some do have sedative actions.

Tonics, too, are problematical. Although "bitters" have been used widely—a number of laboratory studies in the early decades of this century suggested that they improve the appetite and perhaps increase gastric secretion—the relevance of tonics to "nerves" may be merely an improved sense of well-being. On the other hand, the concept of tonics has undergone some revival recently with the view that certain plant constituents acting as adaptogens (e.g., in ginseng) can help the body withstand stress. A tendency also exists to argue that taking tonics over a long period of time may even reduce plasma cholesterol and hence prolong life.[109]

The topic of aphrodisiacs is of special interest because of the many substances with that reputation that are totally devoid of pharmacological action. "No pharmacotherapy is known that has been experimentally substantiated. The therapeutic results in controlled studies were no better than placebos," is one recent comment. Even hormonal preparations generally are of doubtful value. No grounds exist for thinking that the local popularity of boarhog root and bloodroot has any physiological basis, but local testimony is noteworthy. Scientists at least recognize the powerful allies of suggestion and cultural factors.[110]

Issues of suggestion and culture are central to the widespread interest that has arisen recently over the relationship between folk healing and psychiatry. It has generally been argued that treatment of a wide spectrum of mental ailments is aided by folk practices that are set in culturally accepted belief systems. This is an acceptable interpretation for Mr. Bass's success with a few of his visitors, but certainly not all.

The Liver; Biliousness

Requests for advice about liver ailments have gradually declined in numbers during the past twenty years or so, but, like many of his visitors, Bass still believes the liver plays a crucial role in general health. This is because he and his generation grew up believing that an upset, "sluggish," or "torpid" liver was the root cause of many ailments. Not only does he remember countless patent medicines sold specifically for the liver (e.g., Simmons's Liver Medicine and Carter's Little Liver Pills), but he also recollects that old-time doctors often prescribed medicines for torpid livers as late as the 1950s.

The liver has long been of central consideration in general health; it was particularly prominent in nineteenth-century medical thinking as part of the new clinicopathological approach to diagnosis, which correlated signs and symptoms of an illness with specific organ pathology. While this led to the attribution of more specific diseases to the liver than before, the long-standing notion that the liver affected, in a nonspecific way, the general constitution through a "deranged or torpid state" (or "burning sensation") apparently became more conspicuous; indeed it was sometimes described as lithemia.[111] In some respects nineteenth-century views echo those of physician John Symcotts, expressed in a letter written to a patient in 1633: "The crick of your neck, the pain of your toe, the swelling of your knees and the trembling of your joints which you call the palsy are all from one and the same cause—[a sharp humour of choler from your liver]."[112]

Over the years, treatment for many liver problems commonly included ensuring an adequate flow of bile. As James Johnson wrote in 1818: "I have already demonstrated that in ninety-nine cases out of one hundred [of diseased liver] there is a deficiency or irregularity, together with a vitiation of the biliary secretion."[113] Calomel, a mercury compound, was one of the most popular of many treatments recommended for this during the first half of the nineteenth century, and it is still known to Bass. Botanical alternatives included many bitters, such as gentian, cascarilla, calumba, and dandelion.[114]

In Bass's younger days, self-diagnosis of liver ailments often rested on biliousness or on such symptoms as general malaise and vomit containing yellow bile. Biliousness is a loose collection of symptoms still recognized by Bass, but sufficient for a "diagnosis" is a sickly feeling and a headache or, more characteristically, a weak and dizzy feeling. The latter is sometimes described as a nonspecific ethnomedical ailment, but Bass believes that in "nine cases out of ten" it indicates the liver, and more specifically "blocked bile." Although biliousness was described by one physician in 1920 as a "cherished dogma of medicine no longer popular," it continued to be a common layman's diagnosis until the 1950s. In fact, some physicians were still prescribing calomel for the liver as late as the 1950s.[115]

One other symptom of "liver problems" Bass remembers, though he has not heard anyone mention it for a long time, is a bitter taste in the mouth, especially in the mornings. A bitter taste signaled the liver, in contrast to, say, a sweet or sour taste, which was indicative of gastric upsets. If diagnosis by taste is generally forgotten nowadays within Western medicine, it is still part of Chinese practice.[116]

Mr. Bass's approach to treatment is to stress the need to keep bile flowing. ("You have to open up the liver, just like a gas line.") Apart from bitter medicines (e.g., ratsvein and knotweed) he is always ready to recommend the laxative mayapple, though he rarely supplies it because he feels it is too strong. His confidence in mayapple for liver trouble rests not only on past regular medical advice, but also on domestic practice reflected in recorded folk beliefs.[117]

Bass's liver medicines are perhaps better described as bile medicines insofar as he does not really conceive of most of them acting on the liver as a whole. He has not acquired any firm appreciation of specific liver diseases, except cirrhosis—a term he associates (like many medical writers in the past) with such symptoms as jaundice, pain at the site of the liver (assumed to be linked to its hardness), and almost any illness associated with alcoholism. General liver remedies are considered to ease such symptoms. Few are considered to possess any specificity, and Bass suggests only two: wild cherry bark he has "known all his life," and red oak bark. The latter acquired some local popularity during 1985, but the various testimonials apparently do not rest on a pathological diagnosis of the disease, and no scientific evidence suggests that the two remedies have any relevant pharmacological effects.

Bass's faith in the value of certain herbal remedies for general diseases of the liver has been reinforced by reports he has heard (via popular articles) that silimarin (a mixture of compounds) isolated from the seeds of the milk thistle, *Silybum marianum* (L.) Gaertn., is a useful antagonist to general liver toxicants such as carbon tetrachloride. This is one of a growing number of plants attracting interest for antihepatotoxic effects, at least in laboratory studies. Whether the constituents can account for its reputation for treating jaundice is undetermined.[118]

Bass occasionally has recommended a general remedy for presumed liver ailments that is not administered internally but in the form of a poultice over the area of the liver. Seemingly this is a legacy of a notion of a "chill on the liver," a popular lay idea when Tommie Bass was growing up, which was considered the cause of a wide range of symptoms best characterized as a general feeling of unwellness.

A conspicuous feature of Bass's views on liver medicines is that he believes they are also valuable for the kidneys. An association between the liver and kidneys is well established in Bass's mind in an intriguing way. Medicines, he says, that act on the liver help clean the blood by sieving bile from it. In consequence, the kidneys' role of cleaning the blood is made easier.

Kidney and Bladder Disorders

In turn, Bass considers that innumerable kidney medicines (most of which are considered diuretics) help the liver. Bass and his visitors identify kidney problems on the basis of various symptoms, some accepted by physicians as well. These include "burning urine," blood in the urine, and loin or, more especially, lower back pain. A very subjective notion—too much or too little urine—is also widely held; this, which can be described as an ethnomedical concept, is part of the long-standing view that almost all urinary problems are linked with the kidneys. In a similar way, bed-wetting by children is readily seen as requiring a kidney medicine. Self-diagnosis of a kidney ailment is especially commonplace; few of Bass's visitors trouble a doctor unless a persistent pain or burning sensation is present.

Mr. Bass's preferred treatment for all "kidney" problems is corn silk. If unavailable, his order of preference of substitutes is goosegrass, witchgrass, and smartweed (any of the varieties). He adds: "Mullein is good too. Mix it with yellowdock and it will work on the bladder." If peach leaves are added, he says, the medicine is improved. ("We always use them with kidney medicines. It helps to calm you down.") It is noteworthy that peach leaves were specifically recommended in the nineteenth century for bleeding from the bladder, for which Bass's preference is red oak ooze.[119]

A specific problem brought to Bass is difficulty with the prostate, recognized by a slow rate of urination. "I guess it's the number one trouble," says Mr. Bass. "Many don't realize how serious it is until the doctor gets hold of them and wants to ream it out." Apart from use of "kidney" medicines, Bass says, the main thing for treatment is an astringent tea made from redroot, hyssop, wild alumroot, or bloodroot. "We don't claim it will cure, but it is worth trying before an operation."

Bass's kidney remedies also are currently employed by many herbalists. These remedies—along with the once-popular colchicum, broom, juniper, turpentine, and copaiba—were used by regular physicians until eclipsed in the early years of this century by new diuretics and chemical antiseptics.[120] In turn, the latter—and some surviving botanicals—were pushed aside by antibiotics. Assessing the effectiveness of herbal remedies is not easy because none have been subjected to modern clinical trials; they were merely left behind by new, "stronger" medicines. Making informed judgments from the historical record is difficult because of uncertainties of diagnosis and usage, including for menstrual problems and syphilis. Concerning the latter, many diuretics were said to be antisyphilitics, and, conversely, remedies for syphilis (including blood purifiers like sarsaparilla) were often assumed to be diuretic, at least in part.[121]

Despite uncertainties over the value of many diuretics, their constituents—for example, xanthine alkaloids, caffeine, and theobromine—clearly explain their diuretic effect; as perhaps do the irritating properties of turpentine and the volatile oil of juniper. In some cases (e.g., digitalis) the diuretic action is really a cardioactive property, whereby excess fluid (edema) is eliminated as the result of improved action of the heart rather than the kidney.

For some herbs the reputation as a "kidney" medicine may be due more to anti-infective than diuretic action. Apart from antibiotic effects, anti-infective action can arise from such diverse properties as changing the pH of the urine to affecting bacterial adherence to mucosal surfaces. The effects of, say, redroot or saw palmetto on "prostate" problems may be associated with counteracting infections that contribute to difficulties in urination rather than due to a reduction in the size of an enlarged prostate gland.

Some herbal "diuretics" of doubtful efficacy—unknown to Bass—may have acquired their reputations as a result of being given in a large volume of liquid in the form of a tea. Alternatively, some reputations may have emerged, at least in part, based on the theory that "hot" medicines had a general deobstruent action, including on the kidneys.[122]

Eyes and Ears

Traditional treatments for eye ailments are generally less called for today than in the past. In fact, during recent years Mr. Bass has rarely been called upon for eye problems ("although many people wear glasses they do not often see me about eyes"). In part this reflects comparatively recent changes. "Red" eyes are now treated with anti-histamines and vasoconstrictors obtainable from the drugstore and antibiotics prescribed by the doctor. Nevertheless, Bass's help is still occasionally requested and, although he hardly makes distinctions between deteriorating vision, "red eye" and eye infections, and "tired eyes," his suggestions again reflect nineteenth-century regular and domestic medical practices.

In the past an extraordinarily wide range of treatments have been applied to sore eyes and eyelids (in 1922 seventy plant remedies were reported to be still in use in Belgium).[123] Bass has many suggestions for poultices—said to be good for styes—but recommends only a mucilaginous preparation of sassafras pith or, more commonly, eyewashes (once generally known as collyria). Washes containing mineral substances (e.g., lead, alum, and boric acid) were probably the most widely used treatments in the nineteenth century, and Bass usually recommends boracic acid solution when asked for advice over the telephone.[124] If it is not available to the caller, he might suggest a little olive oil in water.

Occasionally Bass recommends a wash made from botanicals, some fairly well known in the past: "When eyes burn and smart, take a handful of peach leaves and boil them in water. That's the way old Doc Nelson recommended. He made the stuff by the gallon." Alternatives to peach that have been popular in the past include eyebright (for which Bass collects substitutes; see "Eyebright", volume 2), china-berry, redroot, goldenseal, and yellowroot. The prescription is: "a handful of herb in a gallon of water, just boiled, and the eyes bathed two or three times a day." Sometimes a little boracic acid might be added. When asked about tired eyes—an idea not new to the twentieth century, but one popularized in recent decades—he suggests eyebright because it is mild.

Past rationales behind the use of such eyewashes are rarely discussed in detail in the medical literature, nor is it always clear whether a plant is more effective as the expressed juice given as

drops or as a wash.[125] In the framework of Galenic medicine, while
"hot" or "cold" medicines were employed according to the ailment,
it appears that some of the most popular eye medicines—whether described as hot or cold—were mildly astringent, demulcent, or bitter.
Suggestions have been made recently that some of these materials
have antibacterial properties, but the clinical relevance is generally
unclear.[126]

Bass is asked about ear problems, generally earache, much more
frequently than he is about eyes. Giving advice over the telephone
to a distraught mother about a child's earache has been a notable
service to his community. Until well into the nineteenth century a
twofold approach existed to treating many major and minor ear problems: constitutional and local. The constitutional frequently included
dealing with inflammation—real or merely suspected on theoretical
grounds—often by bloodletting. The use of cathartics was also commonplace, sometimes rationalized on the grounds that the stomach is
the center of "sympathy" for the whole body.[127] Bass still appreciates
the constitutional approach when he says a tonic should be given to
anyone with persistent earache.

Local application has always been by drops or irrigation by syringe.
Countless substances have been recommended for earache. By the
1830s, however, many, such as cajeput oil, camphor, opium, onion
juice, oil of clove, tincture of castor, and eau de cologne, were being
criticized as too irritant. Bass recognizes that only "safe" substances
can be put in the ear and recommends sunflower oil in which the
seeds from peach pits have been warmed, onion juice, garlic juice,
or prickly ash bark warmed in any oil as treatments for earache and
deafness. He has received countless favorable testimonials for such
treatments. A 1983 letter reads: "Tommie, Uncle John said tell you
that earache drops you sent him done a good job on his ear. For two
years he was deaf in his left ear. After using the drops for two weeks
he can now hold his hand over his good ear and hear out of his once
bad ear." (The loosening and removal of wax was almost certainly the
reason for the improvement.)

If drops of medicated oil are unsuccessful, Mr. Bass says that applying heat (e.g., a cloth wrung out with hot water) is helpful. Certainly
this is a long-established method, as is the application of a boiled
onion to the outside of the ear, a method known to but not recom-

mended by him.[128] Another old-time remedy remembered by many people involves taking a bess bug (a beetle also known as a "pinchin" or "bessie bug"), breaking off the head, and allowing a drop of blood to fall into the painful ear. If Bass is doubtful about its efficacy, others, he says, still believe in it.[129]

Female Complaints

Relatively few requests for help with "female complaints" reach Bass directly from the sufferer. More often the husband asks for help. The expression "female complaints" is employed, nowadays somewhat euphemistically, for a range of gynecological disorders, but mostly menstrual irregularities, menopausal discomfort (especially hot flashes), and vaginal discharges. Occasionally the expression also covers unwanted pregnancies.

Special medicines "for females" received increasing publicity in the eighteenth century with the marketing of such proprietary medicines as Hooper's Female Pills. Knowledge of their constituents is scanty, but many probably included "antihysterick ingredients," reflecting a long-standing belief that female problems embraced a nervous component; by the nineteenth century, however, Hooper's pills contained basically iron and purgatives.[130]

Behind the vigorous nineteenth-century marketing of female medicines were countless discussions in all types of medical literature on female complaints. The biological nature and social role of women and the attitudes of physicians to women were debated with intensity, sometimes amid such glib generalizations as "the Almighty, in creating the female sex, has taken the uterus and built up a woman around it."[131] Despite emotive views and a sense that female problems were too frequently diagnosed, the incidence of gynecological ailments—real or imagined—was high, and the vagaries of reproductive organs were considered to be the root cause of many problems. Mr. Bass still believes this.

One legacy of the past found in Bass's practice is knowledge of a wide range of female remedies recorded in the regular and Eclectic botanical medical literature of the nineteenth century and in the promotion of patent medicines. Many remedies possess marked astringent action—ostensibly intended to control secretions—and others have reputed sedative or uterine actions.[132] This is a reminder that nineteenth-century female therapy was more than the widely recorded bleeding, use of cautery, and other vigorous methods; it also included a wide range of botanicals.[133] Bass's favorites are bethroot, squawvine, Solomon's seal, black and blue cohoshes, pennyroyal, mistletoe, and any "kidney medicine such as smartweed."

He stresses that the first three have the "authority" of Indian usage. Squawvine, he says, is a general tonic not specific for menstrual problems or hot flashes, though useful for them. "It is good, too, for the nerves; it can be taken regularly though not two months before term." Bethroot (birthroot) "acts a little different" to squawvine and is more for "monthlies" and perhaps as an aid to speed labor. Mr. Bass has not used Solomon's seal in any medicine, but has often recommended that it be tried "because of its Indian reputation."

Bass believes that black cohosh, while not closely associated with Indians, has a long history as a "woman's medicine." Although he has known about red maple as a tonic for a long time, he only recently has heard testimonials that it relieves hot flashes.

Pennyroyal is not usually described as a "female medicine" as such, but it is widely regarded as an abortifacient and emmenagogue (to encourage menstruation). Bass has never recommended it (except to be put in a dog's bed to ward off fleas) because he is fearful of misuse, that is, producing abortion. Another reputed abortifacient known to but not recommended by him is mistletoe. Again, he feels it is too toxic for general use, and also "people shouldn't know about it." The only time he has employed it was as a heart medicine for two elderly neighbors.

Bass's knowledge of "female remedies" is only a small part of a vast number of plants recorded in the past as emmenagogues and abortifacients (most served both purposes). Knowledge of these extends back to classical times and is conspicuous in sixteenth-century herbals;[134] many were reported in Christopher Sauer's eighteenth-century American "herbal." Out of 266 plants considered by Sauer, 97 had reputed emmenagogue properties. Sauer's caution about the dangers of certain plants—which included rue, parsley, savin, mugwort, pennyroyal, and tansy—suggests considerable experience in their use. On the other hand, the past reputation of many emmenagogues and abortifacients is not consistent and has been increasingly questioned since the nineteenth century. In 1848 C. D. Meigs's influential *Females and Their Diseases* stated flatly that emmenagogues will not cure amenorrhoea. His therapeutic approach was more constitutional in nature, paying attention to food, exercise, and other regimens ("perhaps you would prefer to call a foot-bath, or a suffumigation by the name emmenagogue"), or treating illnesses assumed to be the underlying cause.[135]

Because the reputations of many emmenagogues have been linked to notions of hot and dry and associated deobstruent action (the latter often called stimulant action in the eighteenth century), suspicion must exist that in many cases an emmenagogue's reputation rested on theoretical rather than empirical grounds, and perhaps also on analogies with plants that produced positive effects. Apparently there is a physiological basis for at least some plants acting as abortifacients. Substances that have "irritating" actions on the uterus or actions influencing contractions of the uterus (the latter sometimes called ecbolics) are reported for many plants. However, a generally toxic action on the mother and fetus is generally considered to account for abortions with tansy, rue, apiol (from parsley), and savin.[136] Bass has little recollection of abortifacients administered vaginally, except for the use of plantain root.[137]

Innumerable physiological explanations for the general action of "female medicines" on various menstrual irregularities, premenstrual tension, and so on have been put forward and discarded; nowadays it is felt that diuresis and actions on prostaglandins may be at play in some instances.[138] Evidence of specific actions (direct or oxytocic) on the uterus that are clinically significant (e.g., ergot) is meager. In part information is limited because interest in botanicals for females declined among physicians following the disillusionment with existing therapy during the second half of the nineteenth century. This was linked with the rising popularity of chemical remedies and, later, the introduction of sex hormones during the 1930s and 1940s.[139]

Bass tends to view "female medicines" as "regulators" that restore balance rather than have a specific pharmacological action in, for instance, excessive menstrual bleeding or amenorrhea. Restoring balance can, he thinks, also relieve painful menstruation (dysmenorrhea). He has no specific recommendations for this, but considers that a nerve medicine (e.g., skullcap) should be taken with the female medicine.

In contrast to the lack of specificity for most medicines, Mr. Bass recognizes that such astringent medicines as bethroot, witch hazel, and raspberry have been regarded as valuable in controlling excessive menstrual flow, uterine pains, and vaginal discharges. These are recorded for both internal and external administration. When asked, Bass says that white oak tea would be an effective vaginal douche, but he has never recommended it.

Bass has acquired relatively little information on herbs for expectant mothers and for managing labor or postpartum recovery. He has, however, helped to make popular a tea made from peach leaves to treat morning sickness. He says this is better than peppermint or wild yam because it has sedative properties. He is also ready with suggestions for postpartum recovery, which include "getting the womb back in place." He knows about raspberry, long recorded for this purpose, but tends to recommend the readily available squawvine, black-haw, or white plantain.

He is familiar, too, with the problem of insufficient milk in a nursing mother. Until the 1950s Bass was asked about this problem fairly often, or was requested to supply a plant already known to the visitor. Plants with a reputation for increasing milk flow (called galactogogues) known to him include fennel, dill, devil's shoestring, chickweed, and slippery elm. While no published record has been found on chickweed and slippery elm, his suggestions mirror the diversity of the many items recorded in the past.

By around 1900, within regular medical practice, galactogogues were generally viewed as useless; nevertheless, the reputations of many, especially fennel, persisted within the popular tradition. Recent scientific studies have provided clinical evidence that some do work; suggested biochemical explanations have been put forward to account for the action of, for example, anise and fennel,[140] but the commonest explanation suggests that some galactogogues flavor the milk, which in turn encourages suckling.[141]

Diabetes and Blood Pressure

Diabetes and high blood pressure, more than many other ailments, raise questions about the safety of herbal remedies used for serious problems needing long-term, careful monitoring.

A striking feature of Mr. Bass's practice is a group of about twenty visitors with diabetes, all with adult-onset (type II) disease. Diabetes, which had a big impact on the public mind after the introduction of lifesaving insulin in 1921, provides an interesting illustration of trends in herbal medicine. Bass says that he never heard about diabetes when growing up. "About 1925 the diabetes got around and people started talking about it, you know. People told me about all sorts of herbs to try, and I guess new ones. Anything good for the blood could be tried for sugar. Queen-of-the-meadow was highly recommended for it." Nowadays, his favorite diabetes remedy—based on many testimonials from visitors over the years—is huckleberry (see "Bilberry", volume 2), which he first heard about "sometime in the 1940s." Nonetheless, he commonly uses Queen Anne's lace because it is readily available. Some visitors prefer other medicines "for sugar," including yellowroot, which is not recommended by Mr. Bass for that purpose.

"Sugar and high blood run together," according to Bass. Even so, as discussed earlier, Mr. Bass understands the terms high blood and sugar to mean high blood pressure and diabetes, respectively, rather than concepts of thickening, thinning, or sweetening described in other studies on popular medical beliefs.[142] On the other hand, he seems to cover these notions in recommending a blood purifier for both complaints. For high blood pressure he has long used the well-known purifiers sassafras and sarsaparilla. Boneset, too, is acceptable. In recent years he has employed huckleberry (though he views this as more effective for sugar). Mr. Bass considers also that "improving" the blood can help and sometimes recommends yellow dock, which he believes contains iron.

In line with much of his thinking, he says a compounded preparation is preferable. Of a number of recipes, the following is typical.

For a gallon of tea:

one teacup redroot (for sugar)
one teacup wild cherry bark (tonic and sedative)
one teacup sassafras (blood purifier)
one-half ounce yellowroot or one-half of goldenseal (as tonic and for sugar)
two teacups huckleberry leaves (for sugar)

Boil for twenty minutes and strain. One teacupful to be taken three times a day. Once made, the medicine should be refrigerated.

In recent years Bass has tended to add a sedative to treatments for high blood pressure (e.g., skullcap or passionflower), in line with what he has heard about stress bringing on high blood pressure.

A new twist to the sugar–high blood story has emerged recently in the considerable number of Bass's visitors who complain of hypoglycemia. Most do not have a diagnosis from a physician, many of whom see hypoglycemia as a controversial diagnosis and do not accept it. Various reasons have been put forward for the widespread belief in the disease, which is diagnosed from a range of symptoms of which tiredness, weakness, and dizziness are prominent.[143] However, it seems that a major factor behind the relative popularity of hypoglycemia among Bass's visitors is that "low blood" has been translated (one might say modernized) into hypoglycemia. Some support for this comes from Bass's suggested treatment, which is characteristic of that used for low blood (a thinning of blood) in the past, namely, the use of tonics and building up the blood with iron and meat.

While many plants have been reported to lower blood-sugar levels, and some have been demonstrated to be active hypoglycemic agents,[144] few, if any, have a long, well-established reputation. In the nineteenth century and earlier, vegetable substances in general were recommended for diabetes, either as a dietary vegetable regimen or in the form of large volumes of diet drinks; if hypoglycemic agents were present, their particular value was not appreciated. Such "specifics" recommended before 1900 as gall and opium have no known physiological action on blood-sugar levels,[145] and neither do astringent medicines such as alumroot, at least not on the basis of their tannin content.[146] It seems that this reputation rested partly on the concept of blood purification.

Since many alleged hypoglycemic agents are also regarded as diuretics (e.g., wild carrot, dandelion, and pipsissewa, all well known to Bass) the significance of the concept of like curing like should be considered. On the other hand, some plants with demonstrable hypogylcemic activity (e.g., blueberry) may well have a long history of use in domestic medicine. That the inconsistent reputations of many diabetes remedies rest on differences in preparation is possible but only subject to speculation at present.

Remedies reputed to treat high blood pressure present as many difficulties as diabetes remedies in terms of determining whether the historical record offers evidence of effectiveness. We suggest that many have acquired a "carry-over" reputation from their use as blood purifiers. However, modern studies have shown that a number of plants have hypotensive action (e.g., see "Veratrum", volume 2). Some herbalists correlate this with their reputations as blood purifiers, but there is no reason at present to think that such an association is anything but coincidence.[147]

Obesity

Many of Mr. Bass's diabetic visitors have concerns over weight problems. For this his treatment has become well known in his area. A local fashion has been created, reflected not only in countless visitors but also scores of letters, such as the following:

> I read about your hebal medicans in the Anniston Star, and decided to write you. I'm interested in one in particular, "the chicweed." What does it look like? Dose it grow this far South? I would try it since nothing else helps me. I'm over-weight to the point my blood pressure is uncontrolable. Diets and pills dont help. Do you have any on hand, if so, would you send me some. I will be happy to pay you. Also would like information on how to identify the chickweed. I'm 100 lbs. over-weight if that will help you to determine how much I need to reach my goal of 150 lbs. I will not hold you reponsible if it does not work. I'm very serious about it. Also would like a jar of your salve. You can call me collect any evening after 6 p.m. if you need to talk about this.

Bass's primary reducing remedies are Queen Anne's lace, goosegrass, and chickweed. Local testimony on their effectiveness is considerable. Queen Anne's lace and goosegrass have a well-documented diuretic action which accounts, at least in part, for their reputation. In this, Bass is following a practice of using diuretics—often producing an initial weight loss—not uncommonly employed by physicians until recently and still found in many weight-loss programs.[148]

Medicines for the Heart and Circulation

Mr. Bass is very cautious about heart treatments. When a visitor arrives with a "heart diagnosis" from a doctor, he prefers not to intervene, except to suggest that a blood purifier can always be helpful; he associates heart attacks, at least in part, with thick blood. Thick blood also is considered the cause of many circulatory problems like cold feet, and he follows common herbal practice in giving hot or cordial medicines to stimulate the circulation. His favorite is cayenne pepper, but he remarks: "Sedatives like sage tea can be helpful. Old-timers said stimulants and tonics like cayenne pepper or ginger tea are good. Wild cherry or any blood purifiers would help by purifying and thinning the blood. That will help the heart. Other things like chickweed cleanses and thins the blood by getting the fatty substance out of it." On the other hand, if he is asked about a racing heart or palpitations in a female, he suggests that it might be part of "female trouble." This is one reason why he suggests black cohosh, though also he believes this plant acts specifically on the heart. Other "specific" medicines are "hawthorn, but now garlic is becoming famous." He also knows about the direct "strengthening" action of such plants as digitalis and lily of the valley, but he says these are too strong for a herbalist to use.

Mr. Bass thus steers away from such cardioactive plants as digitalis, although he will use hawthorn. Current scientific knowledge of most other herbs with reputations for improving the heart—which illustrate the pervasiveness of notions of blood purification and stimulation of the circulation—offers no chemical or pharmacological justification for their widespread use.

Gastrointestinal Ailments

Despite the commonplace nature of many gastrointestinal ailments, Bass is not asked about them as much as might be expected. This appears to be due to dependence on over-the-counter medicines, particularly, he says, since the 1960s. Nevertheless, a host of queries come his way, including some for which no over-the-counter medicine is generally available. An example of this is a coated tongue in the morning, for which he might recommend alumroot.

Constipation and diarrhea. Of all the gastrointestinal problems that plague mankind, constipation has probably occasioned the most frustration and worry. A wide array of laxatives and the more powerful cathartics have been used through the years. It is an area of treatment beset with fashions and fads—such as enthusiasm for "cleaning" the bowels—which have waxed and waned through the years. Some of the best-known botanicals are laxatives: aloes, buckthorn, cascara, castor oil, colocynth, jalap, manna, podophyllum, psyllium, rhubarb, and senna; although many others have been used. In 1856 Appalachian root and herb dealer C. J. Cowle wrote to well-known patent medicine manufacturer A. J. Ayer: "You make a cathartic pill—we want to supply the material for them or at least a part of it—we can supply mandrake [podophyllum], bindweed, Euphorbia species, pokeroot, butternut and some others."[149]

During the early years of this century, when Mr. Bass was first learning about herbs, considerable attention was paid to cleansing the system because of fear of "focal infections" in the gut producing general illness, and there was much talk about lazy colons. He certainly has sharp recollections about laxatives:

> Back in the old days, we were on the farm, the menfolk worked in the fields and they could take a laxative at any time. It was the same for women and children who worked around the barn and could go anywhere. In that time, the toilet paper was corn cobs. There was generally a pile of cobs in the barn. Generally speaking, the laxative was taken at night. Nowadays, living under the conditions we do, it's not easy to take laxatives, for when nature is ready to do things, there is no opportunity. The warning that we needed a laxative was when you stood up and felt dizzy, or if one was sick in the stomach. Now the doctor, the way he told was the color of the tongue. If the tongue was yellow, he said you had a torpid liver and you needed a laxative. If the tongue was white you might need a mild laxative. The old favorites in the home were things like Vega-Cal, Black Draught, Hitchcock's powders, Simmons's Liver Powder, calomel, Epsom salts, castor oil.[150]

Like many people, Bass thinks that "regular" bowels are important and suggests that doctors do not emphasize regularity enough. Yet because of this and the widespread use of over-the-counter laxatives, it is perhaps surprising that laxatives do not loom large in Bass's present practice; in fact, he does not push them and tends to recommend only "mild" senna tablets or prune juice, reflecting a view that too many laxatives can cause constipation.[151]

If necessary to suit a visitor's preference or whim, Bass sometimes provides such other plants as boneset, box, calamus, cascara, hyssop, butternut, and walnut. Of these, only box, cascara, hyssop, butternut, and walnut are well established. Mr. Bass says they all act as mild laxatives in small doses and as strong purgatives in large doses, whereas mayapple, black Indian hemp, Culver's root, goldenseal, and Virginia snakeroot are purgative in small doses, and some plants like psyllium are comparatively gentle in all doses.[152]

The story of laxatives has many noteworthy general features. Although many Appalachian informants say they do not use laxatives because they eat a lot of locally grown apples, many of Bass's visitors have developed the habit of adding bran to food. This follows recent publicity about high-fiber diets, which affect, among a number of other gut functions, the consistency and bulk of feces. When Bass started to recommend bran, whole-wheat bread, and so on around 1985, he felt he was helping people avoid too many laxatives. On the other hand, much recent herbal literature has encouraged the belief that laxatives should be taken regularly to remove toxins from the body; the long-standing notion of the importance of inner cleanliness has come full circle.

Bass is asked more often about diarrhea than constipation. "Lots of people," he says, "have chronic diarrhea." He recommends any astringent tea but especially blackberry, since it is easy to get, or the roots of any other edible berry, for example, raspberry and huckleberry. In addition, he might recommend redroot, wild alum, persimmon, or white oak. Interestingly, he remembers that old-timers sometimes recommended an overdose of laxatives for diarrhea on the basis of cleaning out the system. For "flux" (rampant diarrhea) he remembers his mother giving him tablespoonfuls of castor oil mixed with five to ten drops of turpentine.

Indigestion and stomach upsets. "The first thing I would recommend for indigestion in the summertime is peppermint tea," says Mr. Bass. "One could also use teas of spearmint, anise, heal-all, horsemint, ginger, or catnip." He adds that they act on gas, too. This long list of aromatic indigestion remedies reflects the widespread nature of the problem and the ongoing discussion on causes and treatments. In the nineteenth century "dyspepsia" was considered the root of various chronic medical problems, and numerous factors—from hot bread to nervous energy—were blamed.

Many medical books—for physicians or laypeople—include remedies analogous to Bass's, and rarely is a clear distinction made between "indigestion" and, in the context of swallowed air, "gas." American authors Capron and Slack (1848) indicated the value of paregoric for "wind," but added "whenever there is fermentation in the stomach and bowels, it will be proper to make use of warming and soothing teas and essences, such as pennyroyal, peppermint, tansy, spearmint, hop, poppy, red pepper, and ginger." [153] Carminatives were felt to help with fermentative actions, while antispasmodics, which reduced the mobility of the stomach, were indicated for "wind" or air, but in clinical practice the distinction was rarely maintained. [154]

Bass has an array of comments about nonaromatic remedies for stomach ailments. His suggestion that sourwood is good for acid stomach is an example of treating like with like (acid with acid). He views wild cherry bark as a general sedative, and apple bark has acquired a reputation apparently unrelated to any sensory property or active constituent. But perhaps his most popular remedies are bitters. These, he says—acting as tonics—can be especially helpful for long-standing problems. His favorite suggestion is yellowroot (particularly if an ulcer might be present), but he also recommends dandelion or yellow dock as "not too harsh." If a harsher remedy is wanted (when milder plants fail), goldenseal is used. [155] Mr. Bass believes that some of the value of the bitters lies in improving the constitution in a general way.

Hiccoughs. Bass occasionally receives a telephone call about protracted hiccoughs. Over the years his standard recommendation has been two tablespoons of apple vinegar and a little lemon juice in a glass of water. More recently he has heard that swallowing pineapple juice is helpful. This was "confirmed" by testimonials from three visitors who said it "worked within a few minutes."

Bass recognizes that hiccoughs are often difficult to stop and that "hundreds of remedies exist." Almost anything has been administered internally, he says. "Water is perhaps the best known, sometimes taken in seven or nine swallows."[156] If one does not work, he suggests "just try something else." When medicines fail he might mention applying pressure to various parts of the body, such as behind the ears, or shaking the arms, methods once popular in his region.[157]

Sick Children

This account of human ailments closes with notes on some children's problems. While Bass has received fewer and fewer requests during the last twenty years or so—parents are using medical practitioners more regularly for pediatric complaints—he still receives many telephone calls from worried mothers, who commonly compare his ideas ("they're similar to grandmother's") with those of the pediatrician or family practitioner.

Colic (or wind) and teething prompt the most calls, and Bass has many suggestions to offer. These only partly reflect medicine of the recent past, because during much of the nineteenth century many regular practitioners and laypeople relied more on opium medicines and calomel, although preparations of magnesia and chalk were also common. Of the many well-known plant remedies, which include asafetida, anise, dill, onion, and Sampson snakeroot, Bass says that far and away the most effective is catnip. "It not only relieves wind," but also possesses mild sedative properties. Indeed, catnip was at one time a veritable panacea, including, says Mr. Bass, for teething.

Until the early decades of this century, teething was considered a potentially serious time in a child's life, and Mr. Bass has heard of countless remedies. These include many "superstitious remedies," especially such easy-to-use ones as hanging a rabbit's foot around the neck, a much less expensive version of the elaborate coral and silver amulets common until well into the second half of the nineteenth century.[158] Catnip is Mr. Bass's prime recommendation, but he says that mothers generally do not give enough and hence "try everything else."

Hives is another fairly common ailment for which advice is requested. Mr. Bass and numerous visitors understand this to mean not the regular medical diagnosis of urticaria or nettle rash (whitish, pink, or red elevations attended by itching, stinging, or burning), but instead a feverish "breaking out inside the mouth, and sometimes all over." Catnip is again the favorite remedy, though peppermint or spearmint tea are also used. Other alternatives Bass recommends are tag-alder, cotton seed, elderberry, mistletoe, and onion.

Some confusion exists between hives and thrush (or thrash), a breaking out in the mouth. Thrush, however, is considered more akin to a sore mouth, and in line with this Bass recommends yellowroot or goldenseal. Although very bitter for children, "they are better than many new remedies." If a child refuses to take them, astringent remedies like alder, red oak, and persimmon can be tried.

For most feverish conditions—including such common children's ailments as measles, mumps, and chicken pox—teas such as catnip are given to "bring out" the rash or a "breakout." Blood purifiers like sassafras and tonics are often given at the same time. Very occasionally Bass is asked about fits in children, either epileptic or those associated with high fever. Recommendations are the same whatever the cause: "skullcap, peach tree leaf, or passionflower (best combined together: one part skullcap, two parts peach, and two parts passionflower), or anything that's good for the nerves."

Bass has heard of using "cooling herbs" (though he does not use the term) such as chicory, sorrel, and purslane for treating high temperatures. These plants were often recommended well into the nineteenth century. Mr. Bass had no early experience of anyone using them and has not tried them. However, he recommends lemon drink, another cooling remedy of the past.

About "twelve times a year," Bass is asked about croup. "An old croup remedy," he says, "is boneset, but most old-timers would give about two or three drops of turpentine on sugar; some would use kerosene instead, since it was handier. But croup is pretty hard to treat and I recommend the doctor."

Bass is also very cautious about whooping cough: "I wouldn't want to recommend anything. People should have shots. It's a hard thing to deal with. It used to run its course you know. I have recommended a cough medicine of heartleaf (wild ginger we call it) and make a syrup out of the leaves. But I have not been asked about it recently."

A problem Bass is still regularly asked about is bed-wetting in older children (enuresis). "The quickest thing I'd recommend is corn silk, but if I didn't have that, teas of watermelon seed, pumpkin seed, St. John's-wort, mullein, yellow dock, would be good. All astringent teas would be good." The employment of diuretics (e.g., watermelon seed, St.-John's-wort) for enuresis is well established in folk literature and they were mentioned often in the regular medical literature in the past. In fact, the history of the treatment of enuresis is littered with discarded suggestions for medical treatment. Many of these, however, were pushed aside in this century through the belief that psychological approaches were more efficacious, though even these have often been of limited value. For Bass, the use of diuretics for bed-wetting is rationalized on the basis that the action on the kidneys helps to restore balance or normal function.

Requests for help with the last condition mentioned here, worms, are rare nowadays compared with the years prior to the 1950s. Nevertheless, past treatments are far from forgotten in the region, testimony to the onetime high incidence of the problem. When diminutive Mr. Bass reminds older visitors that he is a "wormy fellow," an immediate association with childhood worms generally is made.

Innumerable remedies have been suggested in the past, and many are known to Bass. These include some, like Epsom salts, which appear to possess only purgative properties. Up to the 1940s children less than ten years old in the Mackey-Leesburg area were generally given a routine worm medicine in the spring. Jerusalem oak was probably the favorite, though he says pinkroot was probably better. Others, less frequently used, were black walnut bark, chinaberry (for pinworms), male fern (for tapeworms), and pumpkin seeds. Mr. Bass has plenty of other suggestions, as noted in the monographs in volume 2. The particular regimens mentioned (e.g., dosage and whether a purgative is also given are worthy of note) for variable practices can certainly account for variable reputations.

Despite the decline in the number of requests for help with all children's complaints during recent years, Mr. Bass still provides a service in this area. His answers—even if not acted on—always elicit interest, not the least because they reflect versatility, economy, and (generally) safety. Of course, there is no sense that they do more than ease symptoms (except in the case of worms), but neither is there evidence that his role occasions delay in obtaining regular medical advice.

Animals

No consideration of Bass's practice would be complete without some comment on veterinary medicine, another of his many services to visitors. His knowledge of animals, tame and wild, is extensive through years of farming, trapping, and backwoodsmanship. He loves to talk about "looking after the stock" when he was a child. He learned a considerable amount about treating animals with herbs: crossvine when they were "run-down," along with the roasted bark of poplar roots and ratsvein. White ash bark was used for "the kidney and to give them [mules and horses] appetite." The employment of horse liniment was commonplace—Dr. Lee Geer's liniment, the National Remedy liniment, and lots of homemade liniments. That some of this experience was soon translated into human medicine illustrates his confidence that men can learn about medical plants by watching which plants animals eat for specific ailments.

Nowadays Bass is rarely asked about treating livestock, but, as part of the neoherbal movement, questions about domestic animals are on the increase.[159] The four problems most commonly asked about are mange, fleas, worms, and distemper. For mange, perhaps now declining in the area, he has fervent belief in a formula once published in the local *Coosa River News*. It is a greasy ointment containing sulfur, pine tar, carbolic acid (phenol), and lard. Mr. Bass advises "don't rub it in, just gently diffuse the hair. Wash hands to avoid blisters. One application is usually sufficient." The same ointment will "get rid of fleas, but all you generally need is pennyroyal."

"Pennyroyal is really easy to grow and everyone who has dogs and cats should have some. Fleas, mosquitoes, and things just can't stand it. Make a tea out of it and use a spray—it'll run them off. Sassafras tea is an alternative, not so effective, but it is a wonderful wash for animal hair." Mayapple is used occasionally: "Just boil the roots and make a strong tea and it will cure the mange, too."

Of many plants recommended for worms, Bass's favorite is black walnut: "A friend of mine, her dog was wormy. It was up in years and almost had the brain staggers. And she took to giving him black walnut and he's out running rabbits." Jerusalem oak and wormwood are alternatives. Mr. Bass recommends that they be made into a bread.

Distemper is one problem that causes concern, and Bass generally recommends a visit to a veterinarian. However, since "distemper is like a cold," he suggests that catnip for cats and boneset for dogs is helpful.

Chinese medicine is like mine.

In the Mackey-Leesburg community and the surrounding area, Mr. Bass has given ease for over forty years. He has listened to and advised the ailing in body and spirit and treated myriad minor and some serious ailments during five decades of social and medical change. His life is viewed by many visitors as one of few constant features in the area.

We have considered how Bass acquired his herbal knowledge against a background of minor complaints and self-treatment that continue to provide him with much specific information, confidence in the use of herbs, and mutual understanding with visitors. We have shown that many of his concepts can be seen as a continuum of the regular and domestic medicine of the past, though not without changes. Some concepts and practices are readily traced to early colonial times and before; others are more recent, and some originated in the twentieth century. We have emphasized, too, that Bass's practice also is shaped by his personable character and extensive general knowledge of plants, which attract visitors with diverse attitudes, interests, and ailments. This review and summary of the diverse features of Mr. Bass's practice prompt consideration of some general issues about traditional medicine, including research strategies.

BELIEF AND DOUBT IN THE EFFICACY OF HERBS

We have implied that much of Bass's success in giving ease cannot be explained by current knowledge of the pharmacological actions of most herbs. Yet among many reasons for visits to Bass—from economic considerations to fear of side effects of regular medicines—there is a fervent belief in the value of herbs. Additional comments on this are appropriate in the context of worldwide usage.

Throughout the Appalachians confidence in herbs remains widespread, especially among those sixty-five and older. "People in the mountains still use a lot of herbs," one elderly citizen recorded in 1986. "Back when I was growing up we lived twenty miles from the nearest doctor. You had to depend on survival and learn a lot about herbs." However, while many people in this age group in the Appalachians occasionally employ herbs, most use relatively few, perhaps only yellowroot, sassafras, catnip, and poke.[1] This is due more to changing life-styles than a lack of faith. Many continue to try herbs now being sold as health foods. On the other hand, less faith in herbs (often none) is found among the generations born in the Appalachians during the 1930s and 1940s, especially those who left their rural homes for industrial jobs. In contrast, many people born in the 1950s and 1960s have become enthusiastic participants in the neoherbal medicine movement. Certainly, with the growth of this movement, current Appalachian interest in herbs can be called a living force.[2]

Herbal knowledge among older Appalachian people was acquired from the popular tradition, with its strong input from professional medicine, experience in use, and testimonials. The latter, when delivered by friends and relatives, have been particularly important, especially if reinforced by the belief that God placed medicinal plants on Earth for all ailments. People who do not invoke religious explanations for the effectiveness of herbs frequently talk about natural herbs helping the healing power of nature. Some, too, tend to believe in the effectiveness of herbs alone for treating minor ailments and the necessity of the combined powers of God and herbs for more serious complaints.

Another factor promoting confidence in herbal remedies, conspicuous among those who buy items from health food stores, is the magical aura of "exotic" or overseas plants such as gotu kola. Indeed, the worldwide use of herbal medicines is comforting knowledge for many, including Mr. Bass. Few people in the area have detailed knowledge about traditional medicine overseas, but the small amount of information reported in popular magazines and newspapers is strong reinforcement.

While extranatural influences (including witchcraft and black voodoo as practiced in the United States) are commonly viewed with disbelief in modern Appalachia, concepts such as the balance between
hot and cold—a legacy of humoral pathology—infiltrate Bass's practice. Close questioning has revealed that some visitors are vaguely
acquainted with it, perhaps because it can be readily assimilated into
existing popular ideas of feeling hot and cold. (By this we refer to
physical perceptions, not metaphorical or theoretical notions.) Certainly belief in the therapeutic value of applying hot or cold has a
long history in Western medicine and today is used to rationalize the
commonplace practice of reducing temperatures, say, with aspirin,
and efforts to prevent cold and damp air from reaching the body.[3]
More significant concepts in supporting or reinforcing belief in herbs
embrace ideas (noted also in Bass's practice) such as blood poisons
or "the blocking of body tubes."

Clearly, a spectrum of general factors exists for sustained popular
interest in herbs, especially those long discarded from regular medicine. In addition, specific factors—ranging from promotion by botanic
practitioners to new theories and chemical evidence that bolster a
dwindling reputation—can be relevant to particular plants.

Modern scientists' attitudes toward herbs are diverse but, on the
whole, skeptical. Reasons range from the unacceptability of testimonial evidence supporting the efficacy of an herb—on the basis that
evidence from a single or a few cases is often misleading, especially
as the experience of the observer is usually unclear and cannot be
quantified—to the opinion that even if physiological effects exist,
incompatibilities all too often occur in compounded herbal preparations.[4]

On the other hand, there are those who consider that clues arising
from years of testimony are often dismissed too readily. This view
is frequently bolstered, somewhat superficially, by reference to the
continuing wide usage of such remedies as digitalis (for certain heart
ailments) and such plants introduced relatively recently as rauwolfia
for hypertension and *Catharanthus roseus* (Madagascar periwinkle)
for certain leukemias. Reference is often made, too, to a report that
25 percent of all prescriptions dispensed from community pharmacies in the United States between 1965 and 1980 contained active
principles extracted from plants.[5]

On the whole, the lack of enthusiasm among most scientists for studying plant remedies and their constituents arises mostly from disappointment over the relatively few new drugs found after years of intensive research. Few clinically useful active principles more effective than drugs already in use have been discovered, while new understanding of existing practices (e.g., the antibiotic action of chewsticks, due, in some cases, to tannins coagulating bacterial protoplasm) offers little of value to modern Western medicine.[6]

Another reason for doubts about herbs is that many studies claiming efficacy on the basis of chemical constituents have been overoptimistic, or, at least, the precise relevance to clinical practice has not been demonstrated. Numerous scientists argue that the only acceptable evidence is from double-blind clinical trials—an essential component in the modern scientific testing of medicines that has rarely been undertaken on herbs.

Proponents of herbal medicine—or at least those sympathetic to it—respond in various ways. Most accept that recognized scientific methods have to be followed. In fact, aspiration to scientific respectability is a conspicuous response to much criticism of alternative medicine, and more and more studies on alternative medicine employ "standard" scientific methodology and try to distinguish and investigate the specific contributions of innumerable variables affecting the healing process.

In contrast, many who promote the value of herbal medicine argue that herbs must be evaluated in the context of the "field," the total range of conditions under which they are collected, prescribed (as extracts and often in the form of compounded preparations), and used (sometimes for long periods of time). In addition to the argument that field conditions have to be considered all together, many (including some of Mr. Bass's visitors) argue that the use of animals for testing herbs is inappropriate; in other words, they question at least some standard scientific methods. In fact, the questioning of scientific methods takes many directions; perhaps the most constructive is to appreciate the value of standard scientific approaches but also to recognize the limitations.[7]

However desirable field studies rather than standard approaches may be, the former rarely are undertaken because of the difficulty in replicating the many variables (for instance, employing a tea made from a fresh plant) as well as the attendant experimental cost. Evaluating herbs will continue to depend heavily on the presumed action of isolated constituents and on pharmacological tests—which may miss activity because of inappropriate laboratory conditions—supplemented by clinical observations and data from the historical record.

In this context major limitations must constantly be borne in mind. There is, for instance, insufficient knowledge of constituents, and assessing relief of symptoms—a role for many herbs—has a large subjective component, as in sore throats, clearing the throat and respiratory passages, indigestion, stimulating the appetite, bringing down mild fever, soothing aching muscles, diarrhea, bladder infections, and skin complaints. There also is the influence of theoretical considerations. These may apply more to uses that failed to become mainstream by not surviving the test of experience. Many instances of this are associated with the concepts of hot and dry qualities, though such concepts did frequently rationalize well-established pharmacological actions.

OTHER FACTORS AFFECTING TREATMENT

Although new chemical and physiological knowledge may ultimately justify the reputations of more and more medicinal plants, present information suggests this is unlikely in many cases, thus underscoring the question of whether factors other than the plants themselves account for the reputation of a particular plant.

While we have said much on the role of theory, in summarizing this and other points raised in earlier chapters (such as the common understanding between Mr. Bass and many visitors), we must also consider what is called the placebo action. Many see this as critical to understanding traditional practice, although others consider it unhelpful because it is an imprecise, nonscientific concept used to explain imprecise data. Nevertheless, the phenomenon is well established and far-reaching, and it cannot be ignored.[8]

While the various descriptions and definitions of placebo action reveal numerous differences of opinion about its scope, all views identify a specific response (apparent cure or improvement in symptoms) linked to suggestibility and inexplicable in terms of known physiological or pharmacological actions of the medicine or other treatment.

Interest in placebo action has mushroomed and sharpened in recent years, largely through the development of sophisticated clinical trials and broadening investigations into the behavioral and social factors at play in treatment.[9]

Placebo action is widespread in all manner of therapy, not only with drugs but also with surgical and nursing procedures.[10] Even drugs with specific actions (e.g., digitalis, on the heart) have been shown to produce placebo effects additional to the known pharmacological response. The variable incidence of placebo responses—frequently considered to be around 30 to 50 percent of cases—can reach up to 100 percent in different populations, diseases, and treatment conditions.[11] The complexity of the phenomenon is compounded by some patients, known as negative reactors, who develop an unanticipated worsening of their medical problems when given a placebo (then known as a nocebo).

It has long been argued that a complex matrix of factors accounts for positive placebo responses. In trying to isolate and understand the variables, most studies consider factors within five broad areas, though, as listed here, they should be viewed as interwoven rather than discrete entities:

1. the patient's personality, existing medical and drug history, expectations, and attitudes
2. the physician's personality, attitudes, and expectations
3. the treatment setting and the form and manner in which the medicine is administered, and whether the patient perceives any effect, even if not the desired one
4. the milieu of home, work, and social setting [12]
5. specific metabolic effects attributed to certain "placebo" actions [13]

Much has been written on the psychological characteristics of people most likely to show positive placebo responses. They have been described as immature, eccentric, inadequately controlled, dependent on outside stimuli, and anxious, as well as elderly, uneducated, and of a generally nonintellectual outlook. Yet the conclusions from many studies are contradictory, suggesting that individuals do not respond consistently to placebos; certainly consistency is apparently absent for sex, intelligence, socioeconomic level, race, or personality type. On the other hand, such attendant circumstances as anxiety, desire for drug treatment, and trust in a physician do predispose individuals toward a positive response.[14]

Results of studies on a physician's or therapist's role in encouraging placebo responses also are confusing. However, there is consensus that the practitioner's faith, belief, enthusiasm, conviction, commitment, optimism, interest, expectations, skepticism, and pessimism about treatment can be significant factors.[15] It also is important for a practitioner to mobilize a patient's hope and optimism, which is another way of saying that good physician-patient relationships are important.[16]

We cannot detail here the other innumerable factors considered to shape placebo action, but summarize that placebo responses are complex and inconsistent, even amid the relatively standard conditions under which powerful drugs are employed within regular medicine.[17] Almost all investigations of the placebo response have been undertaken within the framework of regular medicine, but many investigators believe that placebo reactions are more numerous with modern over-the-counter medicines. The history of medicine is commonly and glibly seen the same way, supported by the view that cultural factors (e.g., healing ceremonies) encourage a positive therapeutic milieu.[18]

Part of the difficulty in assessing placebo response—distinguishing it from reproducible physiological effects—is that there is no generally accepted theory, and hence no understanding, of placebo action. Many theories are little more than descriptions that offer few suggestions about underlying mechanisms.[19] We believe that a basic consideration for any explanation of placebo action must take into account the distinction between disease and illness commonly made by anthropologists and sociologists. It has been said that a key axiom in medical anthropology is the dichotomy between these two aspects of sickness.[20] *Disease* is defined as a measurable physiological and psychological disorder, while the term *illness* refers to how people respond psychosocially to diseases.[21] Illness, then, is the sum of responses to disease resulting from individual attitudes shaped by cultural factors and social circumstances. The success of much traditional practice, it is argued, is because its practitioners are able to relieve the illness by paying special attention to psychosocial factors through an appreciation of personal worries and concerns and the social and cultural parameters of a community. This is supported by the view that traditional practitioners treat primarily three types of disorders whose severity is difficult to evaluate: (1) acute self-limiting (naturally remitting) diseases; (2) non–life-threatening, chronic diseases; and (3) secondary somatic manifestations of minor psychological disorders and interpersonal problems. Specific treatment of disease pathology often plays a small role in the overall treatment of these disorders.[22]

If social and cultural factors affect primarily patients' responses to a disease, the relief of, say, anxiety through reassurance can nevertheless directly affect the disease pathology, or at least symptoms, and thus contribute to an observed placebo action. It is well known, for example, that attitudes inculcated by a patient's culture can have dramatic influences on responses to pain.[23]

As one looks at Bass's practice again, the distinction between disease and illness—an abstract one—is clearly not appreciated by visitors. Unquestionably, without detailed, long-term studies on the visitors, the illness component of a medical problem is difficult to assess, as is its form and how large a role it plays; some observations nevertheless suggest that it is a significant factor in his practice.

Bass holds the view that "50 percent of visitors are not really sick." This does not mean that aches and pains are absent, but indicates his belief that some exaggerate the severity of their disorders—something, he says, which is much more noticeable in recent years. While this may reflect declining stoicism—a cultural facet of illness—many of Mr. Bass's visitors clearly want something to be done at once. Such urgency, combined with the fact that Bass is easier to see than a doctor, accounts for numerous visitors "dropping in" as neighbors do. A visit to Bass also allows concerns and fears to be expressed without dependence on a physician or involvement with the often fearful institutional aspects of medicine.

The urgency sometimes suggests a worry that a serious ailment exists behind the symptoms, worry often expressed behind such comments as "I don't feel too good, I don't feel too bad," especially when visitors also admit that their doctor "cannot find a cause." Worry or stress may produce or accentuate a symptom, something that Bass has discerned more and more over the years. Whether this reflects a trend to "medicalize" many aspects of life in recent years or is the biological manifestation of stress (or a combination of both) is open to discussion. The extent and impact of stress are always difficult to assess. While little evidence of stress was discerned in our structured talks with Bass's visitors, stress constantly occurs in all walks of life in the forms of marital problems, bereavement, and so on. Responses to stress have been discussed widely in recent years and some of its medical manifestations, such as peptic ulcer, hypertension, and some heart problems, are well known. Although it is perhaps too easy to attribute a wide range of sequels to it (forgetting that responses to stress are variable depending on the psychological characteristics of the individual, the physical environment, social support, and cultural background), and although stress is not conspicuous in Bass's practice, he may play a larger role than we ascertained in helping to ease worries and anxieties. It has been shown that family and other social supports can relieve stress, which, on the other hand, may be worsened if a person is out of step with cultural norms. Mr. Bass's role is analogous to that found among good neighbors, close friends, and those with special training in providing a sensitive ear, sympathy, and support, such as pastors and counselors.[24]

It must be said that the concept of placebo can be invoked too readily as a reason or excuse to dismiss apparent cures, because a tendency exists to view placebo action as "unscientific." Possible measurable physiological responses—like body defense mechanisms—are often not looked for, and identifiable, if subtle, cultural effects may not be considered.[25] For instance, the question arises in Bass's practice whether the reputation of boarhog root, with its background aura of superstition, should be considered in the same way as wild cherry bark. The latter, backed by a long pedigree of medical testimony, has long been known for its active principle, hydrocyanic acid, though this cannot account for much of its reputation. Criticisms of the term "placebo" generally embrace the view that the term creates too narrow a focus in explaining therapeutic action.

Yet however we interpret aspects of the healing process that cannot be explained by known physiological actions of drugs, several characteristics of Bass's practice match those recorded elsewhere as encouraging placebo responses. Obviously not all the factors listed below, summarizing many points made in the previous chapters, are relevant to each visitor and visit. The particular attitudes at play in each case depend on visitors' attitudes, beliefs, anxieties, ailments, and frustrations, and on the herbs used. The list does not indicate order of importance, merely the many components in the matrix of social and cultural forces, often reinforcing each other, that can impinge on a visitor's mind. Similarities exist with circumstances listed for traditional practices in other countries.[26] Those who consider the authority of a practitioner as the major force in a placebo response can interpret a number of features to support that opinion.

1. The shack, porch, or yard serves as a place for friendly, informal meetings where no restriction is placed on time. Visitors can "drop in" to get Bass's opinion, which may be the second or third opinion they have obtained on a particular medical problem. Additionally, visits are memorable because of the atmosphere of the place, with its many shacks and the large amount of junk inside them and in the yard. Often friends or relatives arrive with the visitor, and if more people arrive they may join the group. Talk about health and community problems is certainly welcomed by many people. Furthermore, visitors sometimes leave with vegetables from the garden, adding to the feeling about Bass's caring disposition. While he does not consciously set out to relieve the psychosocial aspects of an illness, this can occur.
2. Bass is sometimes viewed as a healer in the context of his charisma and a visitor's religious and other experiences.
3. Other factors that help foster good relations range from a shared appreciation of folk beliefs to nonthreatening visits; something helped by the fact that no time is needed for making a diagnosis— for many people one of the most frightening aspects of a visit to a doctor.
4. Bass's reputation as an authority on herbs is soon apparent in a conversation with him. Furthermore, news of successful results circulates among friends and relatives. Close kinships among many people help spread the news, just as the kinships provide support in illness and during personal problems. Meshing with local success stories is a long tradition of herbal medicine. Many visitors, even those who know little about herbs, appreciate that grandmother probably used them, hence they must be effective and safe.
5. The first herbal medicine is frequently given away on a "free trial" basis, which impresses and encourages many visitors. Prices there-

after are inexpensive, an important consideration for many visitors.

6. Beyond the free sample there is often a "satisfaction-or-money-back guarantee," even for commercially prepared items. At the same time, expectations of the efficacy of herbs are not as strong as with antibiotics or prescribed medicines. Disappointments over failures are consequently readily accepted, which is significant since discrepancies between expectations and outcomes can have a major role in health care and a sense of well-being.[27]

7. Visitors are sometimes advised to collect their own plants, or at least to make their own teas, and thus become involved in their own therapy.

8. Belief in the effectiveness of many medicines is often linked with their marked sensory characteristics (e.g., bitterness or astringency) or pharmacological activity (e.g., laxative action) and physiological effects. This makes them "active," rather than "passive" (or inert) placebos. Additionally, some theories of disease and drug action (e.g., notions of blood purification and mechanical views of the body) have not only contributed to the persistence of belief in herbal medicine as it has become more and more a fringe activity during this century, but also continue to lend support for the use of many herbs.

Apart from physiological theories of disease and drug action, it is often said that the symbolic aspects of drugs contribute consciously and unconsciously to their popularity. Some anthropologists see the role of symbolism as an essential component of healing.[28] Certainly many facets of Bass's practice can be interpreted as having symbolic meaning; indeed, some people may see him as the most powerful symbol, one of rugged individualism reminiscent of the "good old days" of the pioneers. In addition, many visitors see the herbs as good and wholesome, a view encouraged in recent years by the promotion of herbs as health foods and the Protestant ethos so prominent in the region. A few herbs, like St.-John's-wort, still have strong biblical associations, while others such as squawvine have a well-known Indian pedigree. It is not clear how much of this (and other) symbolism is significant; our discussions with visitors suggest clearly that when symbolism is at play, it is a factor which varies according to the eye of the beholder.

The cultural factors considered to contribute to a placebo action raise the question of whether Bass's remedies—at least some of them —might have been more effective in the past when attitudes were often very different. Nineteenth-century patients, for instance, had— in a personal and cultural sense—different illnesses than nowadays; for instance, they saw today's treatable infectious diseases as almost invariably fatal and considered hospitals places where people went to die. In such contexts placebo responses to blood purifiers or internal antiseptics could well have been greater then than today. Evidence exists that the power of imagination in therapy has long been appreciated and at times exploited.[29] All this may have contributed to a reputation that is no longer justified. Theories of placebo action, especially if they recognize conditioned responses, justify the view that the strength of placebo action varies according to circumstances.

The thrust of these comments, and the study as a whole, is a reminder that treatment, including what is called the therapeutic relationship between patient and practitioner, is multifaceted and complex. Mr. Bass's practice—its setting and the herbs, be they physiologically active or not—illustrates this well as it serves a variety of visitors and their attitudes, beliefs, and changing needs.

Indeed, this is the cardinal feature of the practice, and its strength.

SOME ISSUES AND DIRECTIONS

The account of Bass's practice raises issues relevant to the employment of herbs and health matters in general throughout the United States and in other industrialized and nonindustrialized countries. The openness of his medical care and its multifaceted nature serve as a reminder that traditional medicine prompts an array of current opinions, some firmly based on data and others based more on subjective grounds. Since some of the opinions and attitudes can affect health care services in various ways, we raise a number of issues for discussion.

Persistent Beliefs

Throughout our account we have been concerned with the persistence of knowledge about plants, as well as of certain beliefs and ideas concerning disease and treatment which still affect medicine in many ways.

The persistence and disappearance of beliefs have attracted a great deal of attention from students of folk life and anthropology. While it is easy to say that beliefs continue from one generation to the next through the oral tradition, many argue that the beliefs must be reinforced in each generation; otherwise they fade. Some see this reinforcement as coming from the social functions of folk beliefs, which range from helping to establish social conventions to creating channels of communication. For folk medicine, however, professional medicine also has served an important role in sustaining domestic or folk practices. Even today the pervasive influence of the authority of professional medicine can be seen among those who practice herbal medicine in the Appalachians. Many, like Bass, place their greatest faith in the plants they call "official medicines"; namely, those which have been or remain items of wholesale commerce and hence are used or believed to be used by regular doctors. Bass places less interest in what he calls—almost in a pejorative sense—"folk medicines." Often such medicines are associated with past uses by blacks and "poor white sharecroppers." One example is broom-sage, which was widely employed in the South until the 1930s. Yet even this plant, perhaps never mentioned in the regular medical literature, is part of the "herbal family" of grasses, all known for kidney actions.

We have made clear that there is validity to the distinction between ethnomedical and biomedical concepts of disease, and that there is a tendency to "modernize" ethnomedical ideas, to make them more scientific and hence more socially acceptable. This, too, encourages the persistence of long-standing ideas, albeit often with some modifications or new nuances. In the account on snakeroots (volume 2) it is noted that persistent faith (even today roots are carried for first aid) is sustained through continued belief in "toxins" and the need for blood purifiers, even though widespread doubts about the effectiveness of snakeroots already existed by the eighteenth century.

Any consideration of the persistence and variability of beliefs needs to look at the extent to which magical associations are at play. While it is difficult to be precise, various instances (e.g., black snakeroot and Solomon's seal) have been noted. More problematic is the role of symbolism and such beliefs as "being in accord with nature." Space does not allow consideration of these factors, but it is important to appreciate how difficult it is to assess the extent of their influence. This is partly because their role is generally interwoven with theoretical and other support for the use of a plant.

It is noteworthy too that long-standing beliefs about the body and disease are probably more pervasive today than is generally imagined, and they contribute much to shaping attitudes toward and confusion about regular medicine. They can have direct effects on physician-patient relationships and present many difficulties in health education. A number of studies, for instance, have shown how beliefs about menstruation affect attitudes toward birth control methods, just as concerns about side effects of drugs affect compliance with physicians' prescriptions in a negative way. This study is another voice arguing for the inclusion of medical anthropology in curricula for health care workers to make them better aware of cultural factors that shape medical care.

Wholistic Care and Other Issues in America

Disagreement and debate have recently raged, particularly in America, over wholistic (or holistic) approaches to medical care. Such approaches focus as much on maintaining health as on treating disease, and argue that the cultural and social factors we have mentioned, plus various environmental factors, are central to medical care. Interestingly, the concept of wholism has been applied beyond specific health matters to the analysis of social and cultural phenomena.[30] We have no intention of discussing this, though our account of the many factors that shape Mr. Bass's practice supports the view that social boundaries are rarely precise, and that it is necessary to study functional relationships between social groups (a wholistic approach) to understand continuity and change, especially as it relates to health care.

Visitors who say that Bass practices wholistic medicine generally echo the assumption that all alternative systems of medicine (for instance, homeopathy, chiropractic, and acupuncture) are wholistic compared with modern regular medicine. Critics of regular medicine often see it as nonwholistic in both a broad cultural sense (that is, its technology has isolated it from other social systems) and a personal sense (it ignores, for instance, the constitutional effects of disease,

religious and other beliefs, and dietary habits).[31] Wholistic medicine
and debates over medical technology have been called a modern dialectic. The medical profession has been chastised for impersonal care,
often for violating the concept of patient as individual, a sentiment
mentioned by Bass's visitors ("you feel like a black box").[32]

Rejoinders to such criticism, usually from the medical profession,
express disquiet with alternative medical practices, especially by emphasizing the vagueness of many "wholistic" practices and a lack of
critical (usually meant as scientific) reasoning.[33] A good deal of this
is just; it certainly is wrong to assume that Bass's practice and others
like it provide wholistic care all the time. While cultural factors bring
visitors and establish lines of communication, much of his practice
is by mail and telephone, often with people he does not know. Nor
does Mr. Bass have a consciously wholistic approach. He does not
ask questions about, for instance, beliefs and personal and family
problems, though sometimes he has insights into these.[34]

Another reason for caution in applying the label "wholistic" to
many alternative practices is that practitioners themselves sometimes
apply the concept only to the herbal remedies, not the practice. The
notion of wholeness is commonly linked to the belief that natural
things in themselves are good, part of a "divine plan."[35]

Our comments, too brief to convey the complexity of wholism,
nevertheless underscore that, while confusion exists over the concept, it can provide perspective on approaches within regular and
other medical practices. Unfortunately, despite a growing appreciation of wholistic attitudes among American physicians, nurses, and
other health professionals, sensitivity toward wholistic care and a
recognition of the public's demand for it is nowhere near the level
found in, say, West Germany, where alternative medical practices are
generally better accepted among health professionals.[36] If Mr. Bass's
practice is not as wholistic as is sometimes assumed, its very nature
at least offers what some commentators describe as a characteristic
of alternative medical practices—a ready setting for the expression
of personal existential feelings; this, for many people, is the essential
component of wholism.

Another issue concerning regular versus traditional care that merits
comment is raised by Bass's rural circumstances. It has been said that
practices like his will disappear as regular medical services improve

in rural areas, although in fact his has prospered. A major issue in America during recent years has been the shortage of medical facilities in rural areas and the quality of existing care, which is generally considered poorer than in urban situations. Specifically, the needs of Appalachia have occasioned much discussion on both achievements and failures.[37] Failures can be particularly instructive in highlighting cultural issues, as in the case of a clinic in the small Tennessee town of White Oaks. When the clinic was closed in 1976, after operating for five years, much bitterness among local inhabitants was aroused toward the Appalachian Regional Commission because local sensitivities had not been taken into account in developing the clinic in the first place. According to the local people, "Every day was a step toward the other people running the show." "As you got professional people, they started to talk to themselves, and not to the ordinary people. When the government stepped in they spoke to the professionals." "We'd rather close the door than be ruled by people who do not have compassion for the community."[38] It is not just the question of facilities but the attendant philosophy that is important. Such episodes not only taint physician-patient relationships, but they also propel lay interest in self-treatment and alternative medicine.

Because herbal medicine has such a following, much more attention should surely be given to the friction it can create between physicians and patients. Sometimes the friction is not obvious, as when patients avoid telling their physicians that they are taking herbs, often for fear of frank opposition and criticism. Such circumstances, obviously undermining good physician-patient communication, support arguments that physicians should possess greater understanding of— not necessarily agreement with—traditional practice.[39]

We recognize that the training of physicians and other health care professionals produces conceptual and professional difficulties in accepting traditional medicine and, through encouraging stereotype opinions, sees it as adversarial. This situation is recognized as an issue of worldwide importance. Much of the discussion on the problems of linking traditional practices with Western scientific medicine has focused on issues associated with the reductionist approach of scientific medicine, which is concerned with explaining metabolic processes, disease pathology, and drug action in terms of chemistry and physics. The unquestionable success of this approach in creating many of the medical advances in living memory is linked with choosing research projects with high potential for successful results ("the art of the soluble"). Such a framework, which allows little attention to medical sociology and medical anthropology, means that such notions as symbolism and patients' attitudes are often overlooked in present-day research in medical therapy; it hardly is conducive to wholistic thinking and a sensitivity toward the use of herbs.

Yet even given this conceptual framework, physicians need not view all herbal medicine as conflicting with or adversarial to regular practice. We have emphasized that Bass's activities often bear comparison with drugstore practices, at least when advice is readily available from the pharmacist. Most herbal medicines, like over-the-counter remedies, are aimed at providing relief, not cures. The monographs in volume 2 provide a great deal of data from which the reader may judge which plants can be used in this way and in what manner.

Of course, there are many who, even while accepting the non-confrontational nature of traditional herbal medicine and appreciating that the public will always look for cures, argue that herbal medicine's dangers (e.g., causing delays in visiting regular doctors) present problems that outweigh positive features. Many see the trend to protect the public, to control the ever-present threat from fraudulent and useless medicines, as a wise and necessary one. Notwithstanding this, comments such as "Traditional medicine in Appalachia is a Middle Ages survival . . . the ensemble of a practice and speculative medievalism beneath the changes of modern times" are always unhelpful.[40] Unsympathetic sentiments and frank opposition commonly arouse responses critical of the establishment and of the "arrogance of the elite."[41] Physicians and health care professionals have a responsibility to determine and understand patients' attitudes toward herbal remedies. Knowing whether a patient uses herbs can have many far-reaching consequences in disease management.

One consequence of understanding popular beliefs is the possibility of improving patient compliance. Discussions with countless users of herbal remedies suggest that if physicians knew more about herbal usage it might become clearer to them why there is such a distrust of chemical prescription medicines. Reasons for high levels of patients' noncompliance with physicians' recommendations are complex, and, despite many studies, no overriding association between psychological traits and noncompliance is generally accepted. Improvement in compliance, however, does occur when physicians show interest in the patients in such ways as by providing health education.[42]

In our comments we have referred to health care professionals as well as physicians; some passing comments are in order on two groups that can have a significant role in the interface between herbs and regular medicine: pharmacists and nurses.

One of the most paradoxical aspects of the present-day health care scene is that while some drugstores sell health food products similar to those available from other commercial outlets, only health food stores carry the herbs as roots, flowers, leaves, and so on, ready to be made into medicines. Community pharmacists in the United States regretfully have not taken greater professional interest in herbs or contributed to public education about their uses, unlike professionally minded pharmacists in many European countries.[43] Unfortunately, many factors, both economic and professional, have been behind the direction American pharmacy has taken, and they make it difficult to change. Pharmacy as a profession, like medicine, has been concerned primarily with medical science, and, by and large, current over-the-counter medicines are products acceptable to the medical profession. Pharmacy has not been as visionary as it might have been in looking for ways to exercise its professional expertise in self-care.

In contrast, one senses that the endeavors of the nursing profession during recent years, most conspicuously in America, have allowed many nurses to develop a catholic attitude to alternative treatments, usually in the context that a key role of nursing is providing a wholistic medical environment. Those who are concerned with directions in alternative health care will need to watch trends in nursing more closely than in other professional groups.

Our various comments about professional attitudes to herbs cannot be left without again mentioning the placebo effect. Many physicians and other health care professionals are distinctly uncomfortable with their lack of control over the placebo action. Some, too, raise an ethical issue of whether physicians should knowingly be involved in deception. Those who consider the deliberate employment of the placebo effect acceptable are often seen by others as taking a cavalier attitude to deception.[44] On the other hand, many physicians agree that the issue facing medicine "is not whether the physician should make

use of placebos, but how the omnipresent and sometimes powerful placebo effect can best be used."[45] Certainly physicians tend to
overlook the fact that they already prescribe considerable amounts of
placebo medication. As Helman says, "If six million gallons of cough
medicine are annually prescribed by doctors in the face of biomedical
doubt as to the pharmacological effectiveness, a case might be made
for the much wider use of harmless 'placebo' drugs—at least in those
conditions known to be trivial and self-limiting."[46]

One interesting approach has appeared in a discussion on medicines for minor respiratory disorders in an "official" British book on
medicines. The compilers state that although there is no scientific
basis for prescribing any of the preparations listed, it may be that
a harmless expectorant such as ammonium chloride mixture or a
demulcent such as simple linctus has a special placebo role. "Certainly this is preferable to the indiscriminate prescribing of antibiotics."[47]

So far we have discussed attitudes among health professionals. However, many see self-care as an issue for society as a whole to consider,
particularly the extent to which a variety of approaches to health care
are available for public choice. This subject looms large in the United
States as medical costs continue to rise and, of course, is also of special concern in developing countries where Western medicine exerts
a growing influence amid traditional practices. The question arises:
Does Mr. Bass's practice have any bearing on health care elsewhere?

At first sight, especially among those who consider that each traditional health system closely reflects the culture in which it is found,
Bass's practice may appear irrelevant to situations overseas, at least
in developing countries. Further, European herbal practices—and by
implication Anglo-Saxon practice in the United States—have been
described as "not really traditional" because they have been diluted
over the centuries by "official medicine."[48] Yet that view merely
underscores one characteristic feature of much herbal medicine or
self-treatment—its eclecticism and its roots in the popular tradition,
which, in the West, have continually been fed by regular medicine.
There is no doubt that at a descriptive, in effect empirical, level, Bass
shares many characteristics with traditional herbal medicine worldwide. These include a copious pharmacopoeia with widespread belief

in the efficacy of herbal remedies, much reliance on experience, regimens involving purification (including removal of blood impurities), obvious cultural and social factors at play behind the reputation of practitioners, and, often, criticism from regular medicine.[49]

It is especially interesting to compare Bass's practice with traditional Chinese medicine, and not only because of the increasingly widespread Western interest in Chinese medicine, at least in incorporating it into alternative medical practices. Also underscored is the hundreds of years of Chinese experience that "justify" the use of herbal remedies and natural living. Additionally, there is the well-known bicentric pattern of plant distribution of closely related species in eastern Asia and eastern North America.[50]

Bass's knowledge of herbs has a number of similarities to herbal knowledge described in the well-known *A Barefoot Doctor's Manual*.[51] Over five hundred plants are listed there, more than the number known to Bass, but, like his list, it contains a diverse range of medicinal plants. Some are used widely throughout China as much by the formally educated practitioners of Chinese medicine as by the barefoot doctors. Other plants have a modest or minimal reputation and, it has been suggested, are included more on theoretical grounds than on tried-and-tested experience.[52]

Common to both traditional Chinese medicine and Bass's practice is the heavy reliance on sensory characteristics, especially taste, to determine and explain medicinal properties. Bass's understanding of sensory properties is essentially the same as the Chinese reliance on tastes described as sour, bitter, sweet, pungent, salty, and insipid (the absence of taste).[53] In both traditonal Appalachian and Chinese practices a number of plants have reputations which appear to be best understood on the basis of sensory properties.[54]

Mr. Bass has no understanding of theoretical Chinese concepts such as yin and yang, the basic principles of the entire universe, or of hot and cold constitutions; however, the concepts fit readily into his notion that a main function for medicinal herbs is to restore balance, to regulate the system. In fact, the notion of balancing hot and cold is not new to Mr. Bass, for, as we noted, it was a basic plank of Western medicine until the seventeenth century and is still part of many herbal practices.

In the framework of balanced constitutions, a number of analogies can be seen between features of traditional Chinese medicine and Bass's practice. One is the employment of tonics to strengthen and improve the body. Another is the use of herbs to remove impurities (to eliminate "toxins"), although present Chinese practice tends to use diuretics as opposed to Bass's heavy reliance on blood purifiers and diaphoretics. The widespread emphasis on foods as medicine in Chinese practice is also reminiscent of Mr. Bass's knowledge, if not his everyday practice.

Yet, perhaps the most striking common feature between Mr. Bass's views and traditional Chinese medicine is the reliance on experience. Just as Bass says his practice rests on the years of testimony of visitors using his medicine, it is said that traditional Chinese medicine —at least the reputation of two or three hundred herbs—rests on experience "in the clinic." In a striking way this confidence in herbs is reflected in the nonwholistic approach of much traditional medicine, just as we have described nonwholistic features in Bass's practice. Many traditional Chinese practitioners spend no more than ten minutes with each patient. This is not to say that traditional Chinese practice is not wholistic in a physiological sense. A Chinese practitioner points out that in restoring balance (as in Bass's practice) he is treating the whole body, not merely the disease process.

Whither Traditional Medicine?

Similarities between Bass's practice and Chinese traditional medicine prompt questions about universal features of traditional care and whether in the foreseeable future health practices and the use of herbs in developing countries will follow the history of Western medicine; that is, a steady decline in usage, but with a variety of social and medical forces—stronger in some countries than others— sustaining the use of herbs amid a climate of opposition from scientific medicine. Facets of this can certainly be seen in China, although the recent emergence of a "new integrated medicine" providing institutional and theoretical—and hence "academically" acceptable— support for traditional practices is significant.[55] We are posing the question, asked many times: "Which way for traditional medicine?"[56] Our remarks offer comments on general trends and a brief epilogue on recent research trends.

Commonly, the question of direction in traditional medicine is framed in the context of the four principal motivations that lie behind the World Health Organization's concern with traditional medicine: (1) a belief that traditional medicine is compatible with the overall promotion of primary care; (2) a recognition that modern technology is not well suited to the needs of many poor communities; (3) an appreciation that traditional medicine is in tune with Third World nationalism; and (4) an awareness that traditional medicine is necessary if the WHO's ambitious goal of "health care for all by the year 2000" is to be achieved. It is hoped that, by encouraging the use of effective herbal remedies, the need for Western pharmaceuticals and the consequent high cost can be reduced.

Yet, even bearing these motives in mind, it has been said that "in one sense the [current] promotion of traditional medicine is an effort to redefine enough practitioners and therapies back into the realm of the officially acceptable in order to accomplish the task of providing health for all by 2000. Interest in traditional medicine is expressed primarily as a desire to achieve the integration of traditional and modern medicine into western-oriented public health programs."[57] Some would say this is a well-established strategy of orthodox medicine, that is, to incorporate and hence dilute some less extreme unorthodox positions while leaving others marginalized or on the fringe.

There can be no doubt that studies on the chemistry and pharmacology of constituents and occasional clinical investigations employing modern double-blind trials encourage the trend—consciously or unconsciously—to incorporate traditional practices within regular medicine. Further, a growing sensitivity within regular medicine to embrace wholistic approaches—associated with traditional practices —is not without significance alongside political and social factors in developing countries, which often favor scientific medicine over traditional practices. It has been said that interest in traditional medicine persists primarily because the supply of modern health care is inadequate, and that many "traditional" healers make extensive use of modern drugs.[58]

This is not the place to elaborate on the series of events that follow the planting of the ideals of Western scientific medicine in developing countries; some are beneficial while others are disruptive to social and family patterns. Anthropological studies have highlighted many local factors, but there is one general issue which merits comment here: the attitude toward quackery that is a conspicuous thread in the history of Western medicine.

The history of quackery is always a popular story, if only because it highlights people's foibles. Historians who write on quackery and try to understand its pervasive nature generally see it only in the context of greed and fraud perpetuated on the ignorant; namely, the common man or those who should know better, but whose critical ability is lost in the stress of illness.[59] Unfortunately, it generally is unclear in these writings whether the "quackery" under discussion is a straw man, or even whether there was a contemporary consensus that the practice was fraudulent. All somewhat unorthodox therapies tend to be classified as quackery, not necessarily on the basis of fraud but because they exploit fear and other factors that can be just as relevant in the context of regular therapy.

Historians must rely heavily on printed sources, which are frequently shaped by establishment views. The latter are always sharpened whenever the medical profession is worried about its social standing and authority with the public; questions then arise about whether certain attacks on quackery are primarily self-serving for the profession or are really necessary to protect the public. Writings on quackery are generally in line with a strictly modern-science approach to medicine. As this travels everywhere with Western scientific medicine, it has many ramifications. These include inhibiting discussion about any practice not seen to rest on the mantle of science (even those practices that rely heavily on nutrition and psychosomatic factors), especially when concepts are employed—such as herbs affecting vital forces—which are neither accepted by modern science nor amenable to study by its methods.

The conflicting social forces working either to establish more firmly the monolithic nature of modern medicine or to foster pluralistic medical services augur a long period of public disquiet, or at least confusion, over health care in all countries. Perhaps friction can be avoided in this context only if there is a general acceptance by the medical profession of a more pluralistic medical scene. While this raises well-known questions about individual freedom and the need to protect the public, it also must be considered that pluralistic approaches are seemingly a natural feature of most cultures and have emerged in response to diverse needs of individuals. Certainly the situation in countries such as West Germany deserves careful study, as does the common-law acceptance of alternative medical practices in Britain. We should question whether trends away from long-established pluralistic health care practices in many developing countries are appropriate.[60]

It often is said that even policies of corecognition are, in the long run, of little consequence, since alternative self-treatment medicines within the framework of scientific medicine will become more widely available in developing countries in the form of standardized, quality-controlled, Western-style medicines. This may be true, but many sequelae will follow (such as increased costs), even though some of the more expensive treatments may be no more effective for the type of self-care focused on in this volume.

Despite concerns about certain effects of Western medicine, it may be possible to harness Western elements to traditional practices and actually widen therapeutic effectiveness, both improving the safety of traditional practices and critically assessing trends toward greater commercialism. Perhaps, too, this may help to preserve various subtleties of traditional practices. Nowadays, most traditional practitioners in America and elsewhere are more than mere dispensers of medicine; they provide a nonthreatening, neighborhood service which straddles social and medical problems that affect various members of the community. Often the service, which blends inconspicuously into the multifaceted activities of a community and is recognized only when it is gone, underscores just how isolated modern medicine has become from community and social issues. One cannot help wondering how much the rapidly developing technology will continue to change it.

We believe that the history of health care, including the present-day scene of alternative practices, provides evidence of an enduring role in society and suggests a societal need for pluralistic health care. Concerns do exist over the quackery that arises readily in such situations, and few deny that the public needs protecting against overt fraud and dangerous practices, but societies have learned to deal with this in various ways.[61]

It is not easy to answer the question "whither traditional medicine?" But Mr. Bass's life and practice, by illustrating some of the fine texture of human nature and positive as well as negative features of one alternative medical practice, should raise many questions in the minds of those responsible for research into and organization of health care. We must search for the existence of diverse attitudes, and, if they exist, we must examine the reasons for them, the social functions of folk beliefs, the dynamic interface between regular and alternative practice, flexible patterns of health care and self-treatment, and how to maintain the delicate balance between the needs of society and those of the individual. "The lives of ordinary people have their own various ways of struggling for coherence, for a compelling faith, for social vision, for an ethical position, for a sense of historical perspective, for a meaning—a *raison d'être*."[62]

Notes

Introduction

1. It is appropriate to add that the present study is viewed as much as a contribution to community medicine as to self-care and traditional medicine. Patients' attitudes are central to many issues in community medicine, a discipline with complex roots in public health, hospital and health administration, and social medicine. Some frustration exists over the lack of conceptual unity in community medicine, but at least lay attitudes (spread through the community "grapevine") toward illness and self-treatment set a framework for much community practice.

2. This study is not specifically "about the Appalachians," though it contributes to Appalachian studies. Much debate and disagreement exist about how to view the people of Appalachia and about diverse interpretations by historians, sociologists, and others. For a useful summary, see R. M. Simon (1983–84). Studies which make clear that social conditions and forces conspicuous in Appalachia are not necessarily entirely unique to the region are in line with views in this account.

   Many topics mentioned by Bass have been noted in various publications on Appalachia; for instance, everything from apples to logging is recorded from the Rabun Gap area of Georgia, seventy-five miles distant from Bass, and published in the *Foxfire* series of books. Among much other relevant reading, T. Rosengarten's *All God's Dangers. The Life of Nate Shaw* (1974), an autobiography of a black tenant farmer from east-central Alabama, can be singled out. Nevertheless, Bass's recollections, with their colorful metaphors and considerable detail—always cardinal features of his conversation—add insight into diversity and change in the region.

3. See MacCormack (1982), quoting Fulder and Munro.

4. Atkinson (1978).

5. For example, World Health Organization Technical Report Series no. 622 (1978, p. 36). This significant publication provides a general survey and specifically con-

siders certain countries, e.g., Sri Lanka, Sudan, and Egypt; it is suggested that the WHO should cooperate with member states for the promotion and development of traditional medicine.

6. Of the many references to this theme, Foster (1978) provides a useful introduction.

7. Much debate exists over definitions of such terms as traditional medicine, folk medicine, primitive medicine, popular medicine, and ethnomedicine. These often are used interchangeably for practices that depend on plant remedies. We prefer the term herbal medicine for this study, both because it includes usage by regular practitioners and because it carries less pejorative or mystifying overtones than the other terms. Additional terms which produce a measure of confusion are Western medicine, regular medicine, and scientific medicine. Regular medicine is preferred here as implying medicine, whatever the quality, as practiced by licensed practitioners who have pursued a medical education within the framework of contemporary theory. For background discussions, see Press (1980), MacCormack (1982).

8. Talbot, "Folk Medicine and History" (1976, pp. 7–10), for example, takes some folklorists to task for paying insufficient attention to the long history of many plants and methods of collecting them.

9. Trying to understand everyday knowledge—how knowledge is constructed (the "sociology of knowledge")—has attracted increasing attention in recent years, stimulated partly by the perspectives of Berger and Luckmann (1966).

1. Medicinal Plants and Their Traditions

1. Moerman (1977, p. xi). A tendency exists in many studies of traditional medicine to accept statements about medical properties at face value as empirical statements, rather than to probe any "meanings" behind the statements. The historical record often suggests less empiricism than is assumed.

2. For some discussion on origins of the materia medica, see Ackerknecht (1973, p. 8). Erasmus (1961) stresses that people of both primitive cultures and developing countries are as capable of making frequency interpretations as are the educated elite of Western civilization. For pertinent discussion of the relationship between popular beliefs and the development of the life sciences, see G. E. R. Lloyd (1983).

3. Bass relates a story which reinforces in his mind the role of animals in identifying medicinal plants. It was told to him as if it happened locally, but as other versions are recorded, the possibility exists that it is a tall tale:

> It was up at the Lighthouse Restaurant in Cedar Bluff. I made a talk there and a man come around and said, "Tommie, I want to tell you something about the bugleweed you just showed us. I was down fishing on Terrapin Creek." He said he heard a noise out in the weeds. Well he looked out there, and I don't know whether he said it was a black snake, or some other kind of a nonpoisonous snake that was afighting this poisonous snake. Said it'd wrap itself round it, and in a little while this here poisonous thing would hit him

and that snake would run out there and eat something, and he'd come back
and fight him again; and he'd go back and do it again, and by jingos, finally
when it was all over this here nonpoisonous snake, he killed the poisonous
snake and just went crawling off down in the woods.

And the man said he went out there and by jingos that's what it was,
bugleweed. "I sure am glad you showed me that bugleweed," he said.

The Indians claimed bugleweed'd cure a snakebite. It would make you sick
and you'd vomit up the poison. Course the Indians had to do everything the
rough way.

The view that humans learned about medicinal plants from observing animals
is widespread; see S. Thompson (1955–58, 1:442). Siegel (1984) highlights "the
discovery of hallucinogens by observations on animals."

4. The above figures are from the following: classical materia medica: John Riddle
(personal communication); medieval manuscript herbals: Teigen (1980), Urdang
(1944, p. 36). For views, somewhat conflicting, on how representative were the
two editions of the London *Pharmacopoeia*, see Earles (1982). For American botanicals, see Rafinesque (1828–30, 1:ix). Although Cowen (1984) notes a basic
list of 550 American Indian plants and mentions Moerman's list of 1,288 species
(*American Medical Ethnobotany*, 1977), Moerman (1986) lists 2,147 species used
by American Indians. (The significance of many references to different species
within each genus needs study.) For U.S. pharmacopoeia botanicals, see Gathercoal and Youngken (1942); for British figures, see Phillipson (1981). For a list of
most popular remedies on the United States–Mexican border, see Trotter (1981).

5. One example is the activities of Stratford-on-Avon clergyman John Ward, who
practiced medicine and hunted for new remedies in the 1650s and 1660s. For a
review, see Frank (1974). Many examples of Ward's willy-nilly search appear in
the original diary. Other interesting examples can be found in the correspondence
of Sir Thomas Browne (1964, 4:85), and the celebrated seventeenth-century life
of Viscountess Conway (Nicholson, 1930).

6. The strength of the debates has waxed and waned since the issue was clearly
established in classical times. For introduction, via the attitudes of Galen, see
Temkin (1973, chap. 1). Countless examples of empiricism in therapy within the
framework of regular medicine can be given, but see J. T. Fisher (1811, pp. 3–7),
revealing a trial-and-error approach.

7. Instances include fostering beliefs recognized as superstitious, such as bad luck
arising from the failure to complete a job begun on Friday on that same day.

8. "Rampant" or "over-empiricism" is stressed by National Analysis, Inc. (1972) in
the context of current practices. The nature of the study was hardly designed to
determine cultural forces behind the apparent empiricism, but mentioned (pp.
60–62) are factors giving rise to "uncritical empiricism," e.g., unpredictability of
individual responses to medication and the influence of mind over body. These
factors were not identified in the setting of the present study. For discussion of
one example of the relations between theory and practice, see Warner (1980).

9. For some background discussions on reception of plants, see Risse (1984), who

highlights the importance of theoretical frameworks. For interesting comments that theory may have some effect on modern therapy, see Goodwin and Goodwin (1984), who argue an "efficacious treatment for a certain disease is ignored or rejected because it does not 'make sense' in the light of accepted theories of disease mechanism and drug action."

10. Shaping therapeutic practices has been illustrated best with bloodletting, which, for instance, changed from cautious to veritable heroic practices in the late 1700s and early 1800s. For background, highlighting such issues as the individualism of practitioners, see W. F. Bynum (1981), Risse (1985).

11. For example, Temkin (1973, pp. 111–14).

12. This is noted in chapter 7 in this volume. In the Anglo-Saxon tradition hot medicines are still used for colds but more often for "sluggish" conditions such as poor circulation.

13. For background to analogy in medicine and science, see L. S. King (1976), who argues that those who feel analogy was out of place are guilty of presentist interpretations; also, see Arber (1944, p. 223).

14. Compare with L. S. King (1966). The development of the doctrine of signatures in the sixteenth century is generally associated with Paracelsus (1493–1541) and Giovanni Porta (1535?–1615). The extent of earlier influence is not easy to assess, but for an example of the concept in the ancient world, see Riddle (1985, p. 20).

15. Various writings suggest its importance; see surveys like Stannard (1982), Court (1985).

16. Persistence of the doctrine is illustrated in a book (Harris, 1972) written by a pharmacist and "curator of economic botany" at the Worcester Museum of Natural History in Massachusetts. Harris, who employs the doctrine of signatures throughout, states: "I use the approach . . . derived directly from an ancient doctrine of signatures, and have found it an effective teaching device. . . . Instead of tedious memorization of the various uses of a plant, the doctrine of signatures offers in many (though not all) cases a reliable system of connecting the herb with its remedial use through symbolic association" (p. 39). Employment of the doctrine can still be found worldwide; examples appear in A. G. Morton (1981). See also J. F. Morton's article, "Caribbean and Latin American Folk Medicine" (1980). Bass sometimes refers to the concept; see "Walnut" and "Bloodroot" in volume 2.

17. For some background, see L. S. King (1963, pp. 111–26).

18. For instance, L. Gordon (1980).

19. For a sense of the aura of nonnatural beliefs, some found among Bass's visitors, see Hyatt (1970, vol. 1). Other plants well known to Bass for "superstitious use" include Adam-and-Eve, ginseng, and boarhog roots.

20. Various accounts exist on the introduction of British and European plants, many serving as food as well as medicines, into North America. See Leighton (1970), Favretti and Dewolf (1972). A helpful short review is Rea (1975). Most well-known food plants (including "greens," discussed below) and fruits were introduced in the seventeenth century. (An exception is broccoli, which became generally known around 1925.)

21. See Steele (1977).

22. Among much data for this opinion, a principal resource is the catalogue of Philadephia "chymist" John Day (1771). For general reviews, see Kraus (1940), Parascandola (1976); there is also much background information in Blanco (1979, esp. pp. 35–60), and Spiers (1977). Information about more extensive importation is available for later in the century (1750–70) from the records of such merchant houses as Robert Cary & Company, John Norton & Sons, Edward and Samuel Athowes, drug suppliers like Thomas Corbyn, and imports by American planters. (For specific information see Fitzpatrick [1931 onward].)

23. All the information on Sauer's *Herbal* is from C. M. M. Wells (1980, particular points on pp. 62, 250).

24. Ibid., p. 353.

25. For suggestions about medicines used widely in the nineteenth century, see Crellin (1979), Risse (1985).

26. For some factors at play in the evaluation not considered in the present account, see Crellin (ed.) (1982).

27. The heyday of distilling plants—a popular way of utilizing medicinal plants to obtain their "quintessences"—occurred during the late sixteenth and seventeenth centuries. For instance, calamus was included on a long list of plants used to prepare distilled waters in John French's *The Art of Distillation* (1653). As interest in distilled waters declined, relevant botanicals received less attention. Of the vegetable products listed in French's book, only mint, peppermint, dill, and cinnamon remained generally popular into the nineteenth century. (Compare with lists such as by Morson of London [1825, p. 11].)

28. Cullen (1775, p. 302).

29. W. Lewis (1791, p. 154).

30. W. P. C. Barton (1817–18, 2:71).

31. For instance, among American regular medical texts it was noted by Chapman, Eberle, and Wood and Bache (1870, p. 190), who said it was neglected by modern physicians "though well calculated to answer as a substitute for more costly aromatics." Among American botanic/domestic medical works, calamus received only spotty mention. A lack of enthusiasm for calamus also was seen in Britain. In 1874 it was reported that the plant was no longer gathered in the quantities of earlier years (mostly in Norfolk) and was only rarely employed in regular medicine (Flückiger and Hanbury, 1874, pp. 613–16).

32. Gerard (Johnson) (1636) pp. 1341 and 1274, respectively, describing oak astringency.

33. Teigen, "Taste and Quality in Late Galenic Pharmacology" (1983). Goldwater (1983, p. 48) notes the use of sensory properties in the past, but gives no indication whether it remains part of traditional medicine in Latin America.

34. It is appropriate to note that early classifications of taste (e.g., in the eighteenth century) were relatively complex. Linnaeus enumerated eleven categories. By fiat, it has been said, the basic list was reduced to four by Wundt (1893). For a review, see the introduction by Pfaffman to Pfaff (1985). Doubts are currently being raised

about the concept of four basic tastes; see, for example, Erikson (1985, pp. 129–50).

35. Other authors interested in sensory properties who were contemporaries of Floyer could be discussed; for example, influential Nehemiah Grew, who analyzed all plant tastes into ten basic elements in *The Anatomy of Plants* (1682), discussed by Arber (in Underwood, 1953). It also is appropriate to mention a work earlier than Floyer's with a similar title: *A Touchstone for Physick, Directing by Evident Marks and Characters to Such Medicines, as without Purgers, Vomiters, Bleedings, Issues, Mineral or Any Other Disturbers of Natures May Be Securely Trusted for Care in All Extreamities, and Be Easily Distinguished by Such as Are Hazardous or Dangerous* (1667). The preface is signed "W. W." but the author has not been identified.

36. Floyer added (p. 85) "I have not confin'd myself, in describing the Natures of plants to Hot, Cold, Dry or Moist; but have added all the compositions of tastes, and sensible effects of their modes; whereby I might particularly express the nature of each plant."

37. The quotation is taken from a long essay on medical education, advice to his son. Typescript kindly provided by Dr. W. W. Gibbs (pp. 40–41).

38. Floyer (1687, p. 90).

39. Cullen (1789, 1:139). The others probably included influential eighteenth-century physician Herman Boerhaave; the role of sensory properties is explicit in his *Materia Medica* (1741).

40. For example, Cullen (1775, p. 246).

41. Ibid., p. 161, and, for instance, Cullen (1812, 1:91–92).

42. Cullen (1775, p. 230).

43. G. M. Foster, "Concept" (1984).

44. See Schoepf ([1787] 1903, pp. xi–xii). Many writers like William Heberden encouraged change by stressing the need for careful assessment of therapeutic practices.

45. Murray (1815, 1:83–84).

46. For a sense of the impetus of interest in plant remedies following the isolation of alkaloids, see Magendie (1829).

47. Rafinesque (1828–30, 1:11).

48. Murray (1815, p. 83). It is of interest that certain classes of drugs were described based on sensory properties (e.g., astringents and aromatic stimulants) in some textbooks of the period.

49. Bass has been told about William Bryant, who collected herbs for Dr. Matthews. In the 1920s Bryant often identified the quality of plants by their smell; black snakeroot is especially remembered for its unpleasant odor. Bass has provided many examples of a plant new to him being "probably medical" because of sensory properties. He employed this widely during the 1960s when he collected plants from habitats new to him. He recognizes that most of his medicines are bitter and a few sweet. For some background to sweet medicines, see Farnsworth (1973).

50. Nine informants other than Bass recorded that some plants smell "medical." Rexrode (1980, p. 77) notes two informants who believed a medicine was effective after comparing its taste with one known to be good.

51. Comparatively few indigenous North American remedies acquired an established place in European medicine after the early "transfer" of sassafras, sarsaparilla, and senega into regular medicine. For the early story, see Cowen, "The British North American Colonies" (1966). In 1602 one of Raleigh's ships returned with a cargo of timber and sassafras, china root, benjamin, sarsaparilla, cassia lignea, and an unknown "strong bark." These had been obtained by trading with the Indians in the vicinity of Cape Fear. Cowen's article has much information on the early history of sassafras and the trade involving snakeroot, black snakeroot, dittany, turbith, mechoacon, Jamestown weed (jimsonweed), wild cherry bark, pokeroot, Jerusalem oak, and stickweed root. A few plants did become established in European home medicine, if only for short periods. The following are listed by Wheelwright (1974, pp. 136–37): *Podophyllum peltatum*, *Cimicifuga racemosa*, *Hamamelis virginiana*, *Grindelia squarrosa*, *Trillium pendulum* (bethroot), and *Phytolacca decandra*. The limited transfer of American plants to European medicine may have been because they merely replicated long-established, "well-tried" remedies. An interesting discussion with a useful outline of early authors on indigenous remedies is G. B. Wood (1838).

52. The literature on Amerindian concepts of disease is considerable. For recent information, see Wassén (1979), which includes Central America; also the thought-provoking work of Elferink (1984). The author concludes "there has been a relatively poor transfer of Aztec medicinal and pharmaceutical knowledge to Europe."

53. This statement, amplified below, is made notwithstanding Vogel's influential *American Indian Medicine*, (1970), which implies that Indians made substantial contributions to white medicine. Vogel indicates that over 170 plants entered the U.S. *Pharmacopoeia* through Indian influences. See also Vogel (1981, pp. 103–13). However, Vogel does note some reservations insofar as comparative studies between usages among Indians and whites have not been undertaken.

54. Writers like Vogel (1970), Ortiz de Montellano (1975), Chandler (1983), and many others may well overstate the case for empirical discoveries by Indians.

55. Josselyn (1672, p. 217), B. G. Hoffman (1964, p. 6). A helpful table of publications relevant to Indian influences in chronological order appears in Ford, "Ethnobotany: Historical Diversity and Synthesis" (1978, pp. 36–37). Studies of Indian medical practices indicate common uses, for instance, of astringent, cathartic, and bitter medicines. Sources for this statement include Mooney (1891, pp. 301–97), J. P. Evans (1859). The latter contribution suggests that reinforcement of knowledge held by white practitioners sometimes encouraged more intensive interest and investigation (e.g., *Apocynum cannabinum*). Also see W. H. Banks (1953). The Indian root-and-herb-doctor literature, such as Mahoney (1849), is generally eclectic and suggests (although the literature has not been subject to detailed study) that much exchange of information between Indians and whites had already taken place. Fogelson (1980) notes that Cherokee medical and conjuring practices were

once probably pragmatic and flexible and readily incorporated new information. Later, under duress, less flexibility existed. The dynamic aspect of all traditional medicine must always be remembered. Pertinent to this story of the employment of sensory characters and the doctrine of signatures in Cherokee Indian medicine are: personal communication, Cherokee physician Hawk Littlejohn; also, Mooney and Olbrechts (1932, p. 53), and Vogel (1970, p. 33).

56. Information on species found on both sides of the Atlantic is taken from Hultén (1958), who argues that toward the end of the Tertiary and during the Quaternary periods ice ages led to the fragmentation of circumpolar belts of formerly temperate and subtropical vegetation. Plants that withstood the changing conditions spread rapidly after the glacial periods and again occupied circumpolar ranges. Others are amphiatlantic, native to both sides of the Atlantic but no longer circumpolar. Of 5,523 eastern North America species listed in Fernald (1950), at least 1,100 (one-fifth) are introduced. About 320 European plants introduced and naturalized in eastern North America have amphiatlantic ranges, although those introduced are not strictly amphiatlantic in the sense of precolonial evolution. Another hundred European species are not established, but adventive (i.e., occur sporadically) in eastern North America. Many of the naturalized and adventive species are weeds in North America but occupy natural areas in Europe. Some European plants that are regarded as introduced to America are found only in the easternmost parts.

57. Petiver (1699). The possibility of independent discoveries noted above was not considered and has received little study, but see Otsuka (1986).

58. Letter in Controller Papers. In the region of the Carolinas earlier writings by Lawson and Brickell were sensitive to possible Indian contributions.

59. Cowen (1984). For details, see the monographs in volume 2, which note the early interest in Europe in, for example, sassafras, ginseng, and senega. Cowen's list is much smaller than Vogel's (1970). Many factors can be suggested to explain the lack of enthusiasm among whites, such as the hostility of Christian missionaries to Indian practices. A useful review, though somewhat condescending of medicine in the past, remains Duffy (1958), who stresses that much of the recording of Indian medical practice is judged in the light of white medical knowledge. Indians' acceptance of white men's medicines is also made clear, as is variation from one tribe to another associated with differences in flora.

60. For review of black contributions to botany, see Grimé (1976). Some physicians were attentive to black knowledge. Alexander Garden wrote from Charleston in 1753 about local doctors that, if it were not what they "learn from the Negro strollers and old women, I doubt much if they would know a common dock from a cabbage stock" (quoted in Berkeley and Berkeley, 1969, pp. 31–32).

61. It is not necessary to note the activities of John Josselyn, John Clayton, William Byrd, John Banister, John Lawson, John Brickell, John Curtis, and others, which can be best seen as contributions to a growing matrix of information, rather than, as often suggested, seminal influences in American medicine and botany. Although at least local usage of some plants occurred, perhaps only one indige-

nous American remedy (apart from the early introduction of sassafras, sarsaparilla, etc.) became widely accepted in colonial times, namely, senega. Colonial interest in natural history was perhaps not so widespread as sometimes imagined. Physician Alexander Garden, credited with generally introducing pinkroot to regular medicine, was critical when writing in 1753 to Charles Alston in Edinburgh about South Carolina doctors (see n. 60 above). Admittedly this may reflect a rather youthful, jaundiced view. For further background and beyond Garden, see Gifford (1975), Smallwood (1941).

62. For physicians' usage, see analysis of records of four eighteenth-century physicians in Estes (1980). The records indicate reliance on drugs well known to European physicians.

63. F. A. L. Bynum (1979). For background, see Fries (1922, 1:236–39), Long (1956). It can be added that the North Carolina newspapers of the 1770s were listing such imported items as rhubarb, cinchona bark, jalap, ipecacuanha, camphor, cinnamon, clove, and mineral substances (ibid.).

64. Thomas Jefferson's *Notes on the State of Virginia 1781* is known for the first comprehensive treatise on the topography, natural history, and natural resources of a state. Included were Virginia snakeroot, black snakeroot, senega snakeroot, and ginseng. A few years later (1787) German physician Johann David Schoepf, who had been a mercenary during the Revolutionary War, published summaries on indigenous plants which were quoted widely for fifty years or so. For some background on Schoepf and his publication, see Müller-Jahncke (1977, 1978). Schoepf also utilized earlier studies.

65. "American Medical Writers" (1832–33).

66. It is noteworthy that botany itself was a popular study encouraging interest in indigenous plants. See, for instance, "On the Utility of Botany," *Med. & Phys. J.* 11 (1804): 368–72, which mentions the not uncommon view that the stores of nature for the relief of her creatures are unbounded: "The disorders of the poor and those untainted with the corruptions of luxury, are, generally speaking, simple; and almost every field, every wood, every despised ditch, presents him with a variety of remedies for his sufferings, and palliatives for the consequences of his own folly."

67. Mease (1806) was only one of a growing number of practitioners in places like Boston, Charleston, and Philadelphia who were concerned with indigenous remedies. Many shared his views (for instance, in Philadelphia, *Medical Museum*, 1806, 2:157–63) that an "immense saving" could be made by using indigenous remedies. He listed *Ulmus americana*, *Sesamum orientale*, *Prinos verticillata*, *Sanguinaria canadensis*, *Asclepias decumbens* (pleurisy root), *Aralia spinosa* (a prickly ash), *Aralia nudicaulis* (can be substituted for sarsaparilla), *Arum triphyllum* (Indian turnip), *Chenopodium anthelminticum*, *Geranium maculatium*. Noteworthy, too, is the interesting collection of indigenous and some naturalized plants compiled by Benjamin Waterhouse for his course in natural history at Harvard in the late 1780s; it is perhaps the earliest American *hortus siccus herbarium* extant; a few plants have notes on medicinal uses. See Hawes (1974).

68. As an example of the eclectic approach of at least one eighteenth-century Philadelphia citizen: "Elizabeth Paschall's beliefs [in the middle of the eighteenth century]
were in line with the dominant and conservative medical tradition stretching back
to antiquity, but her activities showed that the system was a fluid one. Through
the integration of oral and written tradition, high and low culture concepts among
physicians and laymen, were constantly blending and changing to meet perceived
needs" (Gartrell, 1983).

69. Much information can be obtained from S. Thomson's autobiography, available
in *Bull. Lloyd Library* 11 (1909). A principal source of information for Thomson
was "an old lady by the name of Benton, whose sole practice was with roots and
herbs, applied to the patient, or given in hot drinks, to produce sweating." For a
recent review on Thomsonianism listing most earlier articles, see Wallace (1980).
It is generally felt that the success of Thomsonianism rested on providing milder
treatment than the mercury-calomel regimes of regular medicine, but basic treatments were not all mild (cf. Halstead, 1941). While Thomsonianism was in many
respects radical, much of its teaching on particular drugs, theory aside, differed
little from regular medicine.

70. For some review of the Indian doctor publications, see C. Meyer (1973). Other
interests in Indian remedies merit notice. For instance, scientific reports exemplified by Stacey (1873), who felt, as did many others, that relatively little was to be
learned. Most botanicals listed were already well known in regular and domestic
white medicine; for example, bethroot (*Trillium pendulum*), female complaints;
mulberry (*Morus rubra*), in human urine for fomentation in orchitis; wild cherry
bark (*Prunus virginiana*), tonic, dyspepsia, intermittents, and consumption; black
cohosh (*Cimicifuga racemosa*), rheumatism, coughs; blue cohosh (*Caulophyllum
thalictroides*), parturition; water avens (*Geum rivale*), debility; goldenrod (*Soli-
dago odora*), general sickness; masterwort (*Angelica atropurpurea*), flatulence and
colic; sweet clover (*Trifolium pratense*), sore eyes. Unfortunately, it is not clear
how the author determined the popularity of these medicines.

71. Earlier attempts to create standards for the United States, such as Coxe's *American
Dispensatory* (1806) did incorporate some information on indigenous remedies,
e.g., from B. S. Barton's *Collections for an Essay*.

72. *Pharmacopoeia of the United States of America* (1820, p. 21).

73. H. C. Wood (1874, pp. 5–6). Temkin (1964, p. 5) has described the scene around
1850 as chaotic. He also said the whole relationship between belief and disbelief
in drug therapy is difficult to disentangle because of, for instance, personal tem-
perament, social factors, and scientific considerations.

74. T. Hill (1894).

75. Minutes of Committees, Trent Collection, Duke University Medical Center.

76. Aside from certain naturopathic practices, Thomsonianism remains evident in
various facets of herbal medicine in the United States and Britain.

77. For example, Mattson (1841), which showed discrimination in assessing effectiveness of plants. Berman ("Striving," 1956; "Neo-Thomsonianism," 1956) refers
to the writings of Mattson and others. The original Thomsonian core of seventy

plant drugs was increased fivefold with the appearance of William Cook's *Physio-Medical Dispensatory* in 1869. Much emphasis was placed on "sanative" or "non-poisonous" medication, though in practice this was not always carried out. Wilder (1901, p. 761).

78. Numbers (1973).
79. Koch (1936, pp. 204, 205, and 207). Also in the *American Druggist* (February 1924).
80. J. U. Lloyd (1912).
81. Berman (1980). Many nineteenth-century pharmacists also encouraged interest in indigenous remedies. Pharmacy journals provided much space for medical botany. For a pertinent discussion of King's *American Eclectic Dispensatory*, see *Amer. J. Pharm.*, o.s. 26 (1854): 569–75. Typical of many articles are John M. Maisch's "Notes on Some Indigenous Remedies," *Amer. J. Pharm.* 61 (1889): 552–54, which drew attention, among other things, to southern reports on *Solanum carolinense* and *Chamaelirium luteum*.
82. Personal communication from James Massey about usage.
83. A. B. Miller (1976, p. 11).
84. Cowle Papers (1854–55), letter-press Book E, various letters in October.
85. Eli Lilly and Company, information from archivist.
86. Quotes from Mushet (1870), admittedly a British author but certainly relevant to the American scene.
87. Warner (1986).

3. Health Matters in a Changing Community

1. Bass remembers childhood illnesses and episodes of "numbness" and "rheumatism" lasting until his thirties. His accounts of pain and numbness in the leg and side, which he calls "strokes," were, so far as a detailed medical history suggests, episodes of cramps and exhaustion. This raises the issues of differences between lay and professional diagnoses and the "modernizing" of lay concepts noted later.
2. Bass's memories tend to be rosier than other accounts of isolated and generally more northerly parts of the Appalachians during the 1920s to 1940s. See, for example, Sherman and Henry (1923), Felterman (1967).
3. Raine (1924, pp. 209–10).
4. The idea that good sanitary conditions were necessary for health was bolstered by knowledge of the germ theory, which Bass says was "coming in" when he was growing up. But he has always known that "cleanliness is next to godliness." The historical significance of cleanliness in the health revolution is still debated. For a recent viewpoint, see Greene, 1984. See also n. 5 below.
5. Just how much preventive care has been pursued as part of traditional medicine is a question currently being asked; e.g., G. M. Foster, "How to Stay Well" (1984). Along with Foster, Bass's recollections (some noted below) imply that there is more to consider than public health issues long associated with nineteenth-century sanitary history. Within Western medicine, factors such as fresh air,

sleep, and exercise—called the nonnaturals—have a long cultural history which reached the twentieth century at conscious and unconscious levels. For a review of the concept, see Rather (1978). Close questioning of eleven elderly women over seventy years of age revealed no indication that the health reform movement of the early decades of the twentieth century had any memorable impact in Bass's area. On the other hand, the middle-class bias of the health reformers is well known; see Morantz-Sanchez (1985, pp. 28–46).

6. Information on asafetida, camphor, nutmeg, and turpentine (see "Pine", vol. 2) seemingly reached Bass by the oral tradition. He knows all the recommendations listed in R. B. Browne, *Popular Beliefs and Practices from Alabama* (1958). Relations between oral and written traditions are discussed later.

7. Lewis and Elvin-Lewis (1977, pp. 230–44), discuss chewing sticks at length, noting that the practice still exists in various parts of the United States, including Appalachia. They suggest that sticks were not used by the Indians and, quoting W. P. C. Barton (1817), imply that the practice was introduced into America by blacks. Sassafras, sweet gum, beech, wintergreen, dogwood, and species of *Populus* are characteristic of different regions of the United States. "The plants are very carefully selected for such properties as foaminess, hardness or bitterness and certain species are more popular than others." Elvin-Lewis (1979) extends earlier discussion; black gum, said to possess antibiotic activity, is noted as "still used among the 'Hill Folk' of eastern Tennessee and other areas of Southeast Appalachia, and perhaps also among the Eastern Band of Cherokee in North Carolina" (p. 444).

8. Bass tells many stories about teeth pulling. His account of the loss of his own teeth suggests the spread and genesis of certain beliefs about health:

> It happened about 1922 or 1923. We had good teeth—my family and me. But when we moved out on Lookout Mountain, we got cavities. We didn't know what in the world was happening.
>
> Now I was a guide . . . at a place they call Rock City. A bunch of ladies come up from Gadsden and wanted me and a Mackey boy to take them down to the spring . . . down below Rock City. . . . It's a beautiful spring—comes right out of a rock and runs down under ground so you don't see it no more.
>
> One of the ladies made a cup out of a grape leaf, and took a swallow of water, and said, "Lord to mercy—that's mineral water! That just eats up your teeth." It hit me that that was the matter with my teeth!
>
> Because our water was a whole lot more mineral than that was. The lady said we ought to drink it through a straw—a quill she called it. But anyway, that's how I found out that minerals would eat your teeth up. Had too much iron—that's one of the minerals, you know. They're using filters now, up on the mountain, to filter out the minerals.

The failure to replace teeth was something of a custom; see Sherman and Henry (1923, n. 2, p. 38).

9. A graphic vignette, "Fighting Filthy Flies," appears in R. G. Taylor (1984, pp. 137–38).

10. Eight informants gave similar accounts to that related by Taylor (1984, n. 9, pp. 46–48, "Coping with Itch and Lice"). Bass knows that the "itch" has started to come back among schoolchildren.

11. For accounts of pellagra, see Etheridge (1972), Roe (1981), Carpenter, "Effects of Different Methods" (1981), Carpenter, *Pellagra* (1981).

12. Sherman and Henry (1923, p. 38, n. 2).

13. For background to the emergence of vitamins, see A. D. Davis (1982).

14. For many references recorded in Alabama on medical uses of buttermilk, see Browne (1958). A discussion of "milk-cure" and "buttermilk cure" appears in Bartholow (1882, pp. 39–42).

15. Such plants, "wild greens," are described in many writings on edible wild plants, for example, in Hedrick (1919). Also of background interest to Bass's accounts is Ware (1937). It is noteworthy for the date (1937) that this work has a list of vitamins in vegetables to justify that "vegetables have long been valued for their health giving properties."

16. For Bass's recollections of food, see Crellin, ed. (1988).

17. Highlighting such problems and attempts to deal with them are Schoonover (1975), Stabler (1945). Much of the early story of public health deals with attempts to combat hookworm and the persistent but slow efforts to improve general health; the need was emphasized by the high percentage of rejections of recruits during the draft for World War I.

18. For general background, see Rosen (1975). Although such voluntary agencies as the National Safety Council for the Prevention of Blindness, the American Heart Association, the American Eugenics Society, and the American Social Hygiene Association reflect the emergence of ideological concerns in the early decades of the twentieth century, the practical effects of these organizations on the South need detailed study. It is widely believed that the South placed relatively little emphasis on social science compared with the North—in fact, regarded it with scorn and suspicion; see Peacock (1975, p. 201).

19. Compare the thought-provoking account of the slow emergence of public health regulations in another part of the Appalachians in Roemer and Foulkner (1951).

20. The issue of self-responsibility is underscored in much of the popular literature known to Bass and his generation. Bass thinks today's use of herbs is bringing people back to self-responsibility—currently much discussed—which was lost in the 1950s and 1960s.

21. Whether or not these medicines were the same ones now used by Bass is considered in detail elsewhere, but physicians in the Appalachians (and other places) had variable prescribing habits, and some relied on herbs more than others, either obtained locally, purchased, or in the form of manufactured medicines. For background pertinent to Bass's comments on doctors, see Stoeckle and White (1985), Crellin and Crellin (1988).

22. Local newspapers, a big part of Bass's life, have contributed much to his opinions.

Evidence of concern with the environment frequently emerges in his conversation. Popular magazines have been an important influence for him at the national level. See M. C. Smith (1983), who indicates that the press is often negative toward medicine.

23. Views on sexual mores were derived from discussions with sixteen men in the region over the age of sixty-five. See also comments on the new sexuality in H. A. Matthews (1980, pp. 120ff.), who suggests that the new morality might lead to more considerate behavior on the part of men.

24. Similar points are made by Stephenson (1968, esp. p. 192).

25. The answer and its accompanying comments result from twenty-three interviews with citizens over sixty years old in Bass's community.

26. Assessing the extent of nostalgia is not easy, but we consider it a real force. For a pertinent discussion, see Stekert (1970), including relevant comments by Pearsall.

27. Bass says a big change in local newspapers took place when the *Coosa River News* gave way to the *Cherokee County Herald* in 1958, which, says Bass, "tried to bring New York to Centre." Local interest in day-to-day events nevertheless continued, though not to Mr. Bass's satisfaction.

28. For an interesting discussion on a cluster of ideas about the simple life, see Shi (1985).

29. For an account of trends and relevant literature, at least in Britain, see Armstrong (1983).

4. Self-Treatment in the Community

1. Local surveys tend to overimply uniqueness, although regional characteristics exist, often relating to local availability of a remedy (e.g., yellowroot in the southern Appalachians), alongside nationally known remedies; see Messer (1978).

2. This implies, perhaps, as do other authors (e.g., Beier, 1981) a lack of public discrimination about an eclectic range of practitioners, but we believe that discrimination and eclecticism coexist. The influence of the vernacular literature —mediated primarily through the wealthy or middle class—in disseminating regular medical ideas and cementing existing lay ideas probably cannot be underestimated, but studies are needed. See Slack (1979).

3. For example, G. Harvey (1676, p. 4).

4. The "authority" of the recipes ranged widely from empirical, old wives' knowledge to a pedigree from the "establishment." For example, an eighteenth-century manuscript (private collection) contains a recipe entitled "King James the 2nd Receipt for the Cure of Dogs or Man or Any Creature." It included a celebrated panacea, Venice treacle, as well as astrological considerations.

5. For some background and printed version, see Berman (1960). A catalog of many such manuscripts appears in Brendle and Unger (1935, pp. 289–303). For relevant discussions, see Lacy and Harnell (1963), Sonnedecker (1972), McGrary (1975), L. S. King (1967), Dennie (1956).

6. For *Gentleman's Magazine*, see Porter (1985). Unfortunately, most early manu-

scripts are British or European, leaving the colonial scene open to much more interpretation in terms of relationships between printed sources and everyday practice.

7. Blake (1975). See also Lawrence (1975) for didactic role of many volumes, at least as represented by Buchan. Nineteenth-century inclusion of anatomy and physiology implies an increase in the level of educational sophistication. Blake notes this with such works as William Matthews's *Treatise on Domestic Medicine* (Indianapolis, 1848). Much of the literature described in Cowen (1985) seemingly belongs to the genre generally written without concern for educating the public. Cowen stresses the superstitious-magical nature of many formulas, though some of his examples contain tried-and-tested botanicals. He does note the gradual change in the hold of superstition and magic on folk medicine, which parallels an increasingly critical attitude toward materia medica within the framework of regular medicine. Blake (1975) provides another instance of parallels between domestic and regular medicine when noting the Americanization of Buchan's *Domestic Medicine* for "American diseases" and the decline in references to heroic therapy in later editions.

8. See Poynter and Bishop (1951, p. 20). The close relationship between physicians and patients has often been noted for early colonial times; see, for example, Rosenberg and Smith (1983). The authors suggest "medical care in seventeenth-century New England was a co-operative venture between patient and practitioner, each often adjusting theories or preferences on a case-by-case basis." Although we do not think this was always a conscious accommodation, many sources indicate a change in relations beginning in the nineteenth century (e.g., reflected in Thomas Percival, *Medical Ethics*, 1803.) For some aspects, see Porter (1985).

9. We are not implying that other writers have ignored coherency in traditional care, but investigations in Anglo-Saxon practices are limited in scope compared with, for example, Evans-Pritchard's 1937 account of practices among the Azande, which underscores how medical care fits into a society in which magic is a component part of religion and culture, a normal part of society, and a logical part of understanding nature and human behavior.

10. We cannot explore here the ethos, which was compounded of many factors. Sometimes it included practitioners treating ailments which were recognized to be within the province of self-treatment; see Loudon (1985) for the eighteenth century.

11. Some call this professionalization, but for cautions in interpretation, see Shortt (1983).

12. Rosenberg (1983), when discussing Buchan's *Domestic Medicine*, indicates that Buchan sought to delineate the roles of laypeople and medical practitioners. It is easy to overstate the case. All practitioners used "herbal remedies," and, in the case of dropsy, Buchan's suggestions for care and adjunct treatment included imported drugs—ipecacuanha, squill, seneca, jalap, camphor, and Virginia snakeroot—which cannot be said to be "implicitly or explicitly part of folk practice," at least when this is interpreted as having indigenous remedies as its core. The stress

placed on getting formal medical advice is illustrated in the booklets accompanying domestic medicine chests, a prominent feature of nineteenth-century self-care (Crellin, 1979).

13. Intensification of professional attitudes can be seen in such things as the expanding number of medical journals, as well as establishment comments often found in them; e.g., "slight catarrhs, headaches, and chronic eruptions induce millions at the present time to seek for medical advice." This merely echoed another opinion that, on reading popular advice, "the patient pines over his own image, and gathers fresh tortures at every page."

14. Amid much evidence for the continuing interest among rural folk is the interesting Gene Stratton Porter novel, *The Harvester*, published in 1911. It includes much on the collection of such plants as baneberry, blessed thistle, bloodroot, boneset, catnip, dandelion, jimsonweed, lobelia, mallow, sassafras, and sarsaparilla. See R. J. Mann (1975). Replacement of botanical remedies by chemicals at the time is clear: "In times of scarcity many of our people took to the woods and gathered commoner medicinal roots, such as blood root and wild ginger (there are scores of others growing in great profusion) but made only a pittance at it, as synthetic drugs have mostly taken the place of herbal simples in modern medicine" (Kephart, 1913, p. 41).

15. The following examples of labels on packaged items, dating mostly from the 1920s and 1930s, can be found in Patterson's Mill Country Store Museum, Durham, North Carolina, and so far as we can tell represent the more popular items: "American centaury," "bayberry bark," "black-haw," "blue cohosh," "blue flag," "blue vervain herb," "boneset leaves and stem," "buchu leaves-short," "catnip herb with stem," "chestnut leaves," "cleavers herb," "cransbill root," "culver's root or Leptandra," "Elecampane root," "elm bark (slippery elm)," "eucalyptus leaves," "foxglove," "goldthread herb," "hops," "horehound (white)," "Hungarian or German chamomile," "liverwort," "marigold flowers," "motherwort," "mullein leaves," "pennyroyal (American)," "peppermint leaves and tops," "pipsissewa," "pomegranate bark of root," "princes-pine," "Queen-of-the-meadow (or Joe-pye-weed or gravel-weed)," "rosemary leaves," "rosinweed," "senna," "senna pods," "spearmint root," "white poplar," "wintergreen," and "yarrow."

16. For reference to current usage, see Cook and Baisden (1986). For some pertinent background, R. B. Browne (1958) includes countless examples amid herbal remedies (e.g., alum, asafetida, borax, camphor, castor oil, goose grease, honey, kerosene with or without sugar, poultices, soda, tallow, turpentine); also see G. Wilson (1981). Noted are such items as alum, asafetida, axle grease (to treat piles), baking powder (for toothache), blueing (with milk for asthma and respiratory complaints and for burns), bluestone for croup, coal oil (kerosene), coffee (for indigestion), dynamite (chewed for toothache), Epsom salts, face powder (for chigger bites), gasoline (insect stings), glycerine, gunpowder (internally for boils, rubbed on for itch), lemon (for complexion), matches (moistened and applied to fever blisters), nail polish (for chigger bites), scorched whiskey, sulfur and molasses, sweet oil, turpentine. Interesting information on the use of store-bought family and pro-

prietary articles also appears in Rexrode's "Take Moonshine According to Age: Healing in Pendelton County, West Virginia, 1900–1940" (1980). Almost all are known to Bass and most are noted below. Surprisingly, in view of wide usage, no mention is made of alum and sugar as a cough remedy, pepper tea for cramps and indigestion, mixing asafetida and garlic, mullein leaves in alum water, and specific poultices such as flour, lard, turpentine, and onions for colds.

17. The story of family medicines is very much part of the social history of the general store. A few stores, like the old Mackey store, still exist, even if now oriented toward tourists and bric-a-brac. One in the Appalachians that has changed little is the Mast store in Valle Crucis, North Carolina. The store, which opened in 1883, still sells patent medicines, but not herbs collected locally.

18. See B. Kelly (1968, p. 15).

19. Hare (1909, p. 427).

20. Milk was considered to be of great value in sickness. "Milk was, along with rest, the major treatment in milksick and typhoid fever" (H. A. Matthews, 1980, p. 93).

21. Formulas appear in such works as Remington (1894). Despite contrary opinions, not all family medicines were totally safe; see Mack (1984).

22. G. Steele (1923, pp. 37–40). Raper (1936, p. 48) noted that in parts of Georgia, families that used midwives also generally employed patent medicines.

23. Of the many sources of information on such categories, we have used advertisements from eighteenth- and nineteenth-century newspapers. Many of the best-known medicines have at times been considered quack medicines. See also P. S. Brown (1976).

24. J. H. Young (1981).

25. A good example of successful radio advertising was Hadacol. "You couldn't go into a home that didn't have Hadacol. If they didn't have if they were going to get it the next day. It purified your blood."

26. Watkins's products are still sold by individual salesmen in the region and nationwide.

27. It should be noted that some tightening of legislation occurred after the Supreme Court decision already noted. For background, see J. H. Young (1967).

28. For an account of the use of glycerin, see Cowen and King (1966). These medicines reflected widespread interest in preparations containing the active constituents of plants in a palatable and standard form; for background, see Helfand and Cowen (1982, 1983). Bass notes that a good alternative to "Dr. Pierce's Favorite Prescriptions" was "Dr. Simmons Squaw Vine Compound." It was recommended "for the relief of diseases peculiar to women, and for derangements of female organs, as well as for general debility and a nerve tonic." Also firmly fixed in his mind is Lydia Pinkham's Vegetable Compound for Women, which he assumed contained squawvine. Less popular female remedies were "Dr. Kilgers Swamp Root," "Dr. Biggers Huckleberry Cordial Compound," "Southers Remedy" (this stressed the opium content and was recommended for children's teething and diarrhea, etc.).

29. Bass remembers opium (or at least paregoric) being used for children until the 1930s.

30. Risse (1973) discusses the story of Rush's involvement and the response by promoters of botanical remedies. He emphasizes that greenish stools after the ingestion of large amounts of calomel were considered to be due to increased secretion of bile.

31. Despite his grim recollections, calomel is described by Bass as "one of the most wonderful all-round remedies to remove bile and for stomach. We kept it as long as we can remember. It wasn't too bad to take—a whole lot pleasanter than Black Draught." Sources such as the London Fever Hospital casebooks (1824–25, Royal Free Hospital, London) indicate that the use of calomel (with rhubarb) and castor oil ("powder and oil") were then routine, and thus the long-standing nature of this practice. The iatrogenic effects of calomel have long been known. Indeed, in the nineteenth century, some spoke of creating another disease (recognized by salivation) to replace the original disease. See, for example, Warren (1813, p. ii). Warren was one who called calomel "the Sampson of the Materia Medica" (pp. 2, 39). Jalap was said not only to assist the cathartic effect of calomel, but also, in some instances, to increase its activity in promoting salivation.

32. See J. H. Young (1967, pp. 282–95).

33. Cf. "Mail-Order Health Frauds," in Consumers Union, *Health Quackery* (1980).

34. Even in the 1920s change was under way. In 1925 an authoritative commentator on pharmacy, J. G. Beard, in "Ethics in the Field of Drug Merchandising," noted that "a generation ago it was customary for retailers to buy drugs in the crude state and then build them into a form suitable for administration" (MS, School of Pharmacy, University of North Carolina, Chapel Hill). From then on, "traditional" practices for the pharmacist dwindled in the face of counting tablets from one bottle into another.

35. Helman (1978, p. 13).

36. These remedies are sold in at least one pharmacy in nearby Centre, Alabama. Dr. Pierce's Golden Medical Discovery is said to aid digestion and contains ("active ingredients"): gentian root, Oregon-grape root, blood-root, (and "other ingredients"), queen's root, and cascara bark. The formulas of many surviving old-time remedies have been revised and the names of others have been changed to avoid false therapeutic claims. Thus, Carter's Little Liver Pills are now marketed as Carter's Little Pills, but the association with the liver persists strongly in the minds of many, an association subtly encouraged by the arrangement of the lettering on the label. Cumarindine (for burns and indolent ulcers), though less of an herbal medicine, is, according to Bass, an old-timer with oil of peppermint. Bass's collection of old calendars advertising medicines also documents continuity; e.g., Black Draught and Cardui of the Chattanooga Medical Company for 1980.

37. Over-the-counter preparations unique to blacks, as implied in W. H. Watson (1984) have not been noted.

38. The main lines sold in local stores during 1983–84 were ginseng, goldenseal, bee pollen, aloe vera, chickweed, and yellowroot.

39. Some recent studies highlight continuing widespread usage. Kronenfeld and Wasner (1982) note that 94 percent of ninety-eight people interviewed reported a total of 366 cases of unorthodox remedies used. Topical medicines tend to be the most

popular. The total figure given is $1 billion of self-care remedies. The authors indicate that much of this is used in conjunction with regular therapy. Also see Snyder (1983). J. H. Young (1981, p. 385) gives a recent estimate of the number of individual proprietaries at around 350,000.

40. Papers on patients' expectations (e.g., Hartzema and Wertheimer, 1983) point up the relevance of antecedents but may imply a constancy of views among particular social groups. Structured conversations with Bass's visitors over a period of six years—albeit not a random sample—suggest that attitudes within a group can be very variable.

5. Acquiring Herbal Knowledge

1. Much has been written on the spectrum of practitioners in the past. For some of many contemporary comments on alternative practices during Bass's formative years, see L. S. Reed (1932); also of specific interest in the context of Bass are L. C. Jones (1949), a study based on a collection of folklore, and H. Cooper (1972, pp. 9–18). For general reviews, see Easthope (in R. K. Jones, 1985, pp. 52–71); Hand (1971).

2. One story about Molly Kirby told in 1983 by an informant (not Bass), merits recording since it reflects nineteenth-century anthropological attitudes now considered racist, but which still linger on: "She had better luck than all the doctors. You know what she did, she'd just get into bed and used her head for a battering ram, to push the baby out. You ever seen a nigger's skull? A white person's is about that thick on top, a nigger's is about that thick [demonstrated by the storyteller to be twice as thick]. If you want to show a nigger you hit him on the heel; you don't get him on the head; it's a battering ram." For other pertinent information, see "Voodoo Medicine," in Williams (1975, pp. 716–38).

3. A 1921 study of inhabitants in the North Carolina and Tennessee mountains showed that approximately one-third were Scotch-Irish in ancestry and another one-third were English. People of German ancestry constituted one-fifth of the population, and there were a few Welsh, French, and others (Campbell, 1921, p. 28). Studies are needed to show whether differences exist in various European influences. For discussion, see Hand (1981, introduction to Puckett Collection). One study (Brendle and Unger, 1935) considers information similar to Bass's. The literature on the early colonists lists many treatments embracing superstition and charms. The intertwining of superstition, theoretical notions, and empirical knowledge has been indicated by various authors.

4. Bass has other recollections of Nelson—a "lovable rogue." On one occasion "Doc" visited Bass and "brought a brand new woman—a wife—with him. He married about everytime the moon changed, the old man did." Doc seemingly fit the genre of the medicine-show doctor rather than more restrained practitioners like Bass.

5. This secular-experiential approach is often called empirical; we prefer experiential because it implies building up knowledge of herbs through constant use, rather than just observations.

6. Kern Kiser was featured in the film *Nature's Way*, by Appalshop. The quotations

here are from a transcript supplied with the film. Some additional notes are appropriate to appreciate something of the spectrum of practitioners in Bass's general region. One elderly "herb woman"—following in her parents' footsteps—practices out of Lewisville, North Carolina, and sells herbs at the farmers' market in Winston-Salem. In 1975 a high percentage (over 90 percent) of her customers were black (J. L. Fisher, 1975). By 1984, although her practice had not changed, the customers were no longer preponderantly black (personal observations; see also Strader, 1979).

The inherent dangers of trying to categorize diverse practitioners must be recognized. One example is Icy Plemon of Chatsworth, Georgia. In many ways she fits into a secular-experiential mold. Many of her recommendations for herbs—some remembered from childhood—(e.g., mullein, peppermint, yellowroot) are conventional and widespread, but she also has acquired certain enthusiasms difficult to rationalize on the basis of traditional uses or chemical constituents. For example, chickweed is a veritable panacea and is recommended for eyes, arthritis, and paralysis, and as a tonic and blood purifier. Furthermore, her views on the aetiology of many diseases (e.g., due to the presence of worms) are not common within the recent Anglo-Saxon tradition. (Basic information, though not interpretation, kindly supplied by Dr. Clive Kileff.) A well-known Appalachian person who defies precise classification is Clarence Frederick Gray ("Catfish") of Glenwood, West Virginia. Bass has Gray's mimeographed handouts (1982) but disagrees with the contents. Gray advertises visiting hours ("Thursday–Saturday, 8:00 A.M.–9:00 P.M."); his "handout" suggests he is a cross between an old-time medicine-show doctor (he prescribes his "special" bitters remedy for everything) and a modern health food faddist. He believes, for instance, that certain "poison" foods and drinks must be omitted from the diet: "pork, vinegar, cabbage, graham crackers, salt, saccharine, artificial sweeteners, grapefruit, cherries, plums, tomatoes, cranberries, fish that 'don't wear scales,' ducks and other web-footed fowl, round hoofed animals, and oysters." E. C. Green (1978) sees Gray as one of those who have adapted to changing conditions and have found or created a niche for themselves in modern America: a rare blend of traditionalist, modernist, fundamentalist Christian, populist, applied psychologist, exhibitionist, philosopher, and eccentric. Gray says that knowledge of herbs has been in his family for generations. Indian knowledge has been a big stimulus to his practice, as has media coverage.

For other practitioners difficult to categorize from the evidence available, see Smith and Young (1973), Wigginton (1968), and Miller (1969).

7. For one survey of the complex arena of recent health care practices, see Bauman et al., 1978.

8. Bass has heard of the role of curanderos through popular articles. For a recent review, see Trotter and Chavira (1981). While fundamental differences exist among curanderos (who cover a diversity of practices), there are similarities with Bass's practice.

9. His life and activities are described in Steedly (1979). Vernon Cooper is not to

be taken as necessarily representative of Indian practitioners, for Lumbees do not live on reservations.

10. Ibid., pp. 31–32. It is also not clear that his knowledge is unique to the Lumbees, as stated by Steedly (p. 54). Indeed, like many traditional practitioners he seems to have developed an eclectic practice.

11. Some commentators classify the diversity of black practitioners according to how their skills were acquired: ability conferred during an altered state of consciousness, at birth, or through learning (Snow, 1978). Yet other classifications rest on functions within a community (e.g., Baer, 1981, p. 150). Overlap in functions exists, often reflecting lack of an overarching theory; e.g., comments in B. Jackson (1973, pp. 259–72). A variety of review articles exist, many focusing on spiritual and faith-healing practices; see, for example, Ness and Wintrob (1981). Others highlight the practice of root work, some indicating interface with regular medicine; see Hillard and Rockwell (1978), Stitt (1983). While an increasing amount of discussion has taken place in recent years on the relevance of intracultural factors in regular medical care, the focus is largely on psychiatry. Apart from relevant journals, notably *Culture, Medicine, and Psychiatry*, many books provide introductions, e.g., Foulks et al. (1977).

12. Baer (1981, p. 151).

13. All writers on the practice of traditional medicine among blacks stress that a widespread belief in the teachings of the Bible exists among both healers and clients. See Snow (1978), and C. E. Hill (1976), an article which covers the attitudes of both blacks and whites in the lower socioeconomic groups. Snow argues that the scriptural explanations combine to form the symbols that give meaning to a system of folk medical belief.

14. Bass's concept of "hyssops" extends beyond the botanists' *Hyssopus* spp.

15. For relevant discussion on the recognition of natural groups of plants, see Berlin et al. (1966). For developments on this paper, see Berlin (1970), Berlin et al. (1973), Berlin (1977).

16. Berlin (1977, pp. 65, 98).

17. Hunn (1982) makes the point that a feature of folk classification is the large number of unclassified entities, "taxonomic space." This applies to Bass's limited knowledge, or at least appreciation, of many wild, nonmedical plants.

18. This view is based on an unpublished paper by Müller-Jahnke.

19. There is some debate over the relationship between oral and written sources of information. It has been said that for a long time after the introduction of printing, medical books challenged the oral culture and failed. We do not see the evidence for this, owing to the overlap between lay and professional practical knowledge, if not theoretical ideas. Some relevant comments are found in G. Smith (1985).

20. Gathering herbs for other than personal or family use is readily documented from the 1850s through the wholesale activities of C. J. Cowle of Elkville, North Carolina. This was almost certainly adding to Indian activities. Bartering also became a feature of Appalachian life. Reminiscences of the situation in the Appalachians in 1947–48 noted herbs as an integral part of the barter economy: "There was [a

country store] at Shell Creek, Tennessee. We would take roots and herbs to Shell Creek and sell them for goods. Only trade there was. White shirt buttons were twenty cents a dozen. We picked ellerbes, stagger balls, turkepee, angelico and ginseng. We never heard of galax then. I was a big boy of 12 or 13 before people picked any galax" (quoted in Harman, 1957, p. 54). For the importance of galax and other shrubs in the 1940s, see ibid., p. 88. Other insights into herb collecting in the Appalachians can be glimpsed in G. Peterson (1983). For most people collecting was a part-time seasonal business, but a few made it a year-round job. Items listed as being a major part of the business, past or present (though not all from all areas of the Appalachians), include goldenseal, catnip (sometimes stuffed into "toy-mice"), witch hazel, wild cherry, saw palmetto berries, comfrey, and passionflower. Four to six million pounds of botanicals a year are purchased currently. It is difficult to say how many people collect today in the Appalachians, but it probably runs into the thousands. (Personal communication from Kenneth Wilcox and Ray Bowkley, Wilcox Drug Company, November 1983.)

21. See Jacobs and Burlage (1958, p. 1 of introduction). The many companies collecting botanicals in the region in the late nineteenth and early twentieth centuries testify to the economic importance of botanicals for Appalachia. Jacobs and Burlage note that Wallace Brothers of Statesville, North Carolina, was the first (1879) important commercial establishment. Not mentioned is the sizable activity of C. J. Cowle of Elkville for many years from the 1840s onward. In 1908 the well-known S. B. Penick and Company opened an office at Marion and subsequently in Asheville. A helpful list of six hundred plants and names of other herb companies appears in Simpson (1894). Core (1967) aims to give a sense of tradition, but much of the medical information is culled from modern sources and precise references are, unfortunately, not provided.

22. These figures are provisional. They are based on a review of information, especially distribution maps, in Radford et al. (1968). Justice and Bell (1979, p. xiv), note that of 2,915 North Carolina species, 1,716 are to be found in the mountains. To these were added other assessments such as Mohr (1901), Strausbaugh and Core (1978), Small (1933), Massey (1961). For medicinal plants we have used a variety of sources in hand with Jacobs and Burlage (1958), who list 1,443 plants found in North Carolina, but not all growing in the mountains.

23. These figures were derived from field studies and from recent published studies such as Bolyard (1981), Krochmal et al. (1971). The phrase "living force" is used to stress the belief that Appalachian traditional medicine is much more than a quaint curiosity. See also Evans et al. (1982). Aikman (1977) gives only a little space to the Appalachians in her worldwide survey, but noted "no-where, I found, is folk medicine more popular than in the Appalachian Mountains—one of America's leading herb-using and distributing regions" (p. 40). The well-known *Foxfire* books (ed. Wigginton) include a variety of information. See *The Foxfire Book* (1972, pp. 230–48, 346–68, on faith healing, primarily for burns, bleeding, and "thrash" or thrush); *Foxfire 2* (1973, pp. 31, 49–53, 69, 274–303, 381–85), *Foxfire 3* (1975, pp. 245–73, 331–42), and incidental references indexed for *Foxfires 1–3*, in *Foxfire 3*;

Foxfire 4 (1977, pp. 445–48). Not all of the information, it should be added, indicates that the tradition is alive today (except in the form of memories), but taken with the considerable literature on folk medicine a striking continuum is evident, though frequently modified.

24. About the rheumatism medicine: "My daddy, he made an awful good rheumatism medicine. He'd take so much Espom salt, so much cream of tartar, and yellow sulfur, and saltpeter—put it all in a jar and add so much sugar. Of course, Mother would generally make it. You take a teaspoonful three times a day."

25. Raine (1924, p. 229).

26. Visitors sent to Bass by Molly Kirby commonly asked him for cedar weed, burdock, yellow dock, Sampson snakeroot, and butterfly weed. Mrs. Kirby generally made these up in whiskey, a popular method in the region.

27. Bass has a large collection of almanacs from the 1930s to 1970s; he rarely throws anything away.

28. For instance, *Health from Field and Forest*, published in 1917.

29. A 1915 edition is still owned by Bass. Though he had not looked at it for many years, he remembers information from it. See chapter 7 for his views on the liver.

30. Quoted in J. H. Young (1967, p. 321). Young discusses fully the fascinating saga of Dudley J. Leblanc and Hadacol during the years 1943–51. The product contained 12 percent alcohol, B vitamins, iron, calcium, phosphorus, and honey. Young bemoans "the millions needlessly expended, or spent for Hadacol instead of proper medical care" (p. 332). Although this is a conventional comment, the testimonies to Hadacol noted by Young and those of Bass and his neighbors indicate that, at the time, many people felt better after taking the preparation.

31. See discussion in Fellman and Fellman (1981). At the same time, it must be stressed that the volume was clearly promotional literature for Pierce's products; Stoeckle (1984).

32. James (1969, p. 11).

33. For an account, see Whorton (1982, pp. 331–39). For eulogy on Rodale, see "J. I. Rodale [1891–1971] in Memoriam," *Prevention* 23, no. 8 (1971): 14–18, which indicates the emphasis Rodale placed on promoting organic living and natural health ideas.

34. The role of the mineral springs in Bass's region has not been told. For an introduction to this once very popular form of health care, see Sigerest (1946).

35. This attitude to vitamins is noted many times; e.g. National Analysts, Inc. (1972, p. 9). The implication of much of the report is that this rests on empiricism, but it is an example of where a cultural stock of knowledge is at play.

36. Bass has acquired a lot of information because of the countless people he has met. Some were particularly influential, such as Dr. Cross, physician and druggist of Gadsden in the 1920s. "Dr. Cross taught me quite a bit. He used lots of herbs." Cross's influence extended well beyond Gadsden in many ways. One was through supplying local general stores with medicines on a sale-or-return basis.

37. Bass has many thoughts about the economics of herb collecting, which we do not pursue here. Typical is the remark: "They didn't get much for them in the

old days. One man dug herbs for a Doc Carver in Flintstone for $5 per hundred pounds. But then dealer Mr. Campbell came along and paid him $1 a pound for Solomon's seal."

38. For some other information on Sanders, see E. Lawrence (1987, p. 137).

39. Other local newspapers carried reports at the time; e.g., "Leesburg Man Knows Plants' Secrets," *Anniston Star*, 15 April 1971.

40. There has been much discussion on the differences between the shaman (primarily a mediator between the supernatural powers and man) and the medicine man (primarily the curer of diseases through traditional techniques). See, for example, Hultkrantz (1985), who says: "There is in my mind no doubt that the 'wise old men' [of folk societies in advanced cultures] and folk healers of both sexes are carriers of many of the qualities that distinguish the shaman." Omitted from many such discussions is the importance of the "eye of the beholder" in categorizing practitioners. Certainly different views are identifiable among visitors to Bass.

41. See Hammer (1983) for recent review.

6. The Practice: Setting and Visitors

1. Bass's premises are a reminder that for many years herbalists' establishments commonly have had a distinctive character and often an apparent state of chaos. Budge (1928, pp. 5–7) describes in picturesque terms a London establishment of the 1860s and 1870s. References to dustiness, bowls of seeds, berries, and dried herbs, sarsaparilla wine, lavender, rosemary, mint, chamomile, dandelion, and sorrel, although vastly removed in time, place, and circumstances, evoke an atmosphere reminiscent of Bass's shacks.

   Listed here are dried herbs—using Bass's names—stored throughout the various shacks as of February 1983. Seventy-three items are included, but others are available at times: anise seed, apple tree bark, bamboo root, bay leaves, bearsfoot root, bethroot, blackberry root, black cohosh root, black-haw bark, bloodroot, blueberry, blue lobelia, blue vervain, boneset, butterfly weed, button snakeroot, calamus root, catnip, chickweed, clover bloom, comfrey, corn silk, devil's shoestring, dogwood bark, elder blooms, gall-of-the-Earth root, garden sage, ginseng, goldenrod, goldenseal, goosegrass, ground-ivy, horsemint, Jerusalem oak, mayapple root, maypop, mistletoe, mullein, peach tree leaves, pennyroyal herb, peppermint, plantain leaves, poplar bark, Queen Anne's lace, queen-of-the-meadow root, rabbit-tobacco, raspberry leaves, ratsvein, red maple bark, red oak bark, redroot, red sage, red sassafras root, red sumac berries, red sumac root, willow tree bark, sarsaparilla root, skullcap, slippery elm bark, smartweed, sourwood bark, star-root, strawberry leaves, sweet gum bark, tag-alder bark, yellowroot, white oak bark, wild alumroot, wild cherry bark, wild ginger, wild hydrangea, wild yam.

2. The mail-order business has prospered through extensive advertising, including "wants," in the widely read *Alabama Farmers' Bulletin*. For background information, see E. Lawrence (1987).

3. Since 1980 or so, newspaper publicity has been increasingly extensive. Many of Bass's local talks have been reported in full in the *Cherokee County Herald*. An example, "Bass Speaks to Dist. II Garden Club Members" (4 May 1983, p. 9), includes a long list of medicines. Articles like this one bring many visitors and queries to Bass.

4. Store run by Mrs. Woodall, who provided much insight into the extent of usage.

5. For an account of the medicine show, see McNamara (1976). This and other medicine-show literature was shown to and discussed with Bass. His affinity with the mix of entertainment and salesmanship is obvious.

6. See Dorson (1983, pp. 57ff.).

7. There are various ways of understanding Bass's attitudes toward God and nature. One is to see them in the pattern of certain nineteenth-century views on natural theology—as expressed in influential works like William Paley's *Natural Theology* (first published London: Fauldner, 1802)—that an appreciation of God's wisdom can be seen through nature.

8. Bass's sensitivity to Indian ideas has been observed many times, especially after meetings between him and an Indian medicine man, Hawk Littlejohn. However, nature and supernature in southern Appalachia are closely intertwined; see Pearsall (1966). Bass's observation on the popular beliefs and practices recorded in Alabama by R. B. Browne (1958) is that "witchery" and knowledge based on experience are indiscriminately mixed, but that only a few herbs are used according to superstition.

9. There are problems with asking questions which require answers resting on graded responses such as "strongly agree, agree, uncertain, disagree, strongly disagree," a common format for data collection. Difficulties arise because respondents often supply socially acceptable answers, and a quantitative attitudinal score for each respondent is not readily obtainable. For discussion on attitudes toward medicine, see Hulka et al. (1975), who indicate that the public is more willing to criticize the system rather than particular doctors, especially in a community where 95 percent of the populace professed to have a regular physician of their choice. Blacks were more critical than whites.

10. The lack of clear answers is noted in other studies; for example, National Analysts Inc. (1972) concluded that this indicates a lack of a generalized, systematic set of beliefs. This, we believe, is correct, but not the implication that sets of beliefs cannot be uncovered. For an instance of consideration of psychological factors, see Holland (1981).

11. A detailed discussion of the various opinions including stereotypes about Appalachian people appears in Friedl (1978, pp. 13–19). Looff (1973) is of special relevance by showing how poverty affects attitudes.

12. Coles (1971).

13. These figures and those below are as accurate an estimation as possible. They are derived from our assessments of numbers visiting Bass daily and figures furnished for a nine-month period by Bass in the form of tape-recorded daily reports. The number two thousand includes many groups of two, three, and sometimes four. Not everyone arrives with a medical problem; but, on the other hand, most leave

with advice. One suspects that they intended to ask about their own problem from the start.

The ratio of blacks to whites in the area is low, and this is complicated by many black visitors arriving from Gadsden and Birmingham. The fact that a large proportion of Bass's visitors are elderly reflects a high incidence of ailments in the elderly. For a recent overview of patterns among those seeking medical care, see Cockerham (1982, pp. 68 ff.). Evidence has been gathered to support the generally held view that the elderly are more likely to visit a physician than younger people, except for those under five (e.g., National Center for Health Statistics, Washington, D.C.: Department of Health, Education, and Welfare, 1979). It also has been shown that parochial groups tend to subscribe more readily than cosmopolitan groups to popular rather than strictly scientific beliefs about medicine. Similarly, low-income blacks tend to seek the services of nonphysician practitioners much more than whites (Cockerham, 1982, p. 72). This has been correlated with the lower number of visits to regular physicians compared with whites, but, among Bass's visitors, shopping around for medical care is as common among blacks as among whites. We have been unable to confirm among Bass's visitors the view that patterns of medical-care-seeking behavior by blacks in American society is influenced less by ethnicity than by conditions of poverty. Undoubtedly economics is a factor for many, but its extent is unclear.

14. Koos (1954, esp. chap. 1). For supplementary remarks on the study, see Kunitz and Sorensen (1975).

15. See, for example, Kunitz and Sorensen (1975).

16. For introduction to this, see R. A. Jones et al. (1981). The decision to seek medical care is affected by whether a symptom is new or not, but this cannot be differentiated clearly in Bass's practice.

17. Many accounts are available on people's reasons for seeking care. In addition to other references given above, difficulties in fully understanding the factors affecting the seeking of medical care are underscored by Mechanic (1979, 1981), who shows that in the United States the main factors in decisions to seek medical care are social network influence and beliefs, rather than demographic or structure-of-care variables. See also Levin (1981), and Naisbitt (1982) for "megatrends" toward self-care.

18. Employing both a regular practitioner and alternative medicine has been noted many times; see, for example, G. G. Meyer (1974, 1981).

19. For some pertinent background comments, see Sankar (1984).

20. Such episodes highlight some of the issues, widely debated during the 1970s, involved in establishing health plans for ambulatory care. Bass's treatment with an astringent lotion might, in this case, be compared favorably with the lysine tablets from the chiropractor, or even the painkillers from the regular physician, who, most important, determined that no known underlying pathology existed.

21. He is also asked about Adam-and-Eve root, probably *Aplectrum hyemale*, but he has no experience with it.

22. For discussion of nonnatural beliefs among blacks, see Snow (1978); and for an account of the use of animal blood, etc., see Hand (1980, pp. 187–200).

23. Bass knows a wealth of popular sayings and beliefs. Those linking zodiacal signs with planting crops serve as one reminder of diverse elements in his rural culture. Discussions with him and visitors suggest a present-day pervasiveness of folk beliefs as commented on by Hand in his introduction to Hand et al. (1981, vol. 1). Bass says one of the commonest is: "If anyone has a child with asthma, cut a sourwood stick and put it under the bed. Or cut a sourwood stick two inches taller than the child. When the child is grown as tall as the stick the asthma will have disappeared."

24. Assessing the extent of black influence on white medicine is not easy. A number of studies imply substantial influence, e.g., Grimé (1976); less infuence is recorded in Sea Islands and low country populations; see F. Mitchell (1978), and J. F. Morton (1974), though the latter makes no clear distinction between black and white knowledge. Both works rely heavily on publications by Porcher, especially his *Resources of the Southern Fields and Forests* (1863), which is based on many of his earlier writings. Porcher, while summarizing a great deal of published information, included some firsthand observations of usage on plantations. Much of this, however, implies at least some influence by whites treating slaves. See, for example, *Aralia spinosa* (rattlesnake master), p. 50, *Aristolochia serpentaria* (snakeroot), p. 356; *Cynara scolymus* (Jerusalem artichoke), p. 428; *Eupatorium perfoliatum* (boneset), p. 411; *Liriodendron tulipifera* (tulip tree), p. 40; *Podophyllum peltatum* (mayapple), p. 123; *Quercus rubra* (red oak) p. 262. Although it is difficult to determine with confidence the overall black contribution to white medicine, many incidental episodes are recorded. Savitt (1978, p. 174) discusses information reported in the regular medical literature (*Mon. Steth.*, 2 (1857): 7–14), although he focuses more on the part played by conjure doctors within black medicine. Conjure doctoring, in the form of root work, is active today (see, for instance, Jordan, 1975), but the influence in disseminating herbal knowledge is unclear. Jordan notes a number of plants used by voodoo doctors for purposes known to Bass; e.g., corn silk (congestive heart failure), catnip (anxiety and hives), asafetida (anxiety), persimmon bark (external bleeding), peppermint tea (colic), kerosene (cough), and pomegranate (worms). Puckett (1926, pp. 358–91), despite emphasizing the concept of evil spirits, includes many sayings and beliefs well known to Bass and probably empirically based; for instance, the use of liniments, tonics of red or black snakeroot, and febrifuges. Many examples of the latter, however—smartweed, mullein, life-everlasting, dog fennel, Jerusalem oak, and bitterweed (p. 367)—are, according to Bass, only effective when teas prepared from them are taken hot. Also mentioned are kerosene for sore throats, sweet gum, mullein, or pine straw (p. 369) for colds and respiratory disorders, and poultices for boils.

    One facet of the story of black influence is the possible impact of ideas and information that arrived with slaves. McClure (1982) considers this in relation to *Citrus aurantifolia*, *Ricinus communis*, and *Abrus precatorius*. See also Sheridan (1985), although he gives few precise details on drug usage.

25. Bass's attitudes toward Indians are complex. Few non-Indian visitors seem to agree with his frequent comment: "We're ashamed of the way the white man done

them, the Indians. This was their home and we come in and took it away from them. If we had come in and made peace and paid for it, it would be another thing. Someday the white race will suffer for the way they treated the Indian."

26. Much has been written on issues relating to consumer attitudes. Pertinent to the region are Richardson and Scutchfield (1973), and Stekert (1970), who indicates a general background of suspicion of doctors. We have not found this to be widespread, though certainly a reluctance to visit a doctor is commonplace. Stekert's interesting article lists other sources of conflict such as self-diagnosis and use of traditional remedies.

27. A vast literature exists on criticisms of medicine by physicians, some written for the public. Chodoff (1983) is advertised as written by a "respected surgeon" who "rips the lid off the medical profession as no book has done since *Intern* by Dr. X—junior doctors." And in this case the author, Dr. Richard Chodoff, is not "hiding behind a pseudonym." Much criticism published in professional journals is aired in public, especially when it comes from leaders of the profession. See, for example, Pickering (1978), who echoes much that we have found in our study: "Service and integrity were the watchwords. . . . Now medicine seems to be in danger of ceasing to value or respect learning. What would have been regarded as unprofessional behaviour is not only tolerated but encouraged."

28. Many studies on attitudes to alternative medicine have found entrenched views arguing for freedom of choice in medical care "as a right"; for example, Cassileth et al. (1984).

29. J. H. Young (1983), and Young (1983, in Parascandola and Whorton) discuss the well-known sulfanilamid case. The latter explains many of the sequelae of the episode, and provides some interesting insights into medical practices in the north Georgia mountains not far from Bass.

30. For some discussion on this aspect of traditional care, which has important considerations for health education, see A. Young (1981).

31. This complex issue cannot be elaborated here; however, it seems clear that it is linked to the richness of feelings and images that are invariably part of an illness; see Viney (1983). Much of this relates to the role of metaphors and symbols in medicine in contributing to a feeling of unwellness. For an introduction for serious illnesses, see Sontag (1977).

32. As an example amid a growing literature, see Furstenberg and Davis (1984). No doubt exists that lay consultation is the means whereby, in the past, most people have learned about Bass.

33. Finkler (1984) raises questions about various aspects of shared beliefs and their significance; also see Cassileth et al. (1984). Much discussion has appeared on patients' attitudes in the medical sociological literature; for example, Armstrong, *An Outline of Sociology* (1983, esp. chap. 2).

We have not explored fully attitudes among blacks. Snow (1974) has interpreted many features of folk medicine and attitudes among blacks as follows: (1) the world is viewed as a hostile and dangerous place; the individual is liable to attack from external sources and is helpless, with no internal resources to combat such attack, having to depend on outside aid; (2) basic to the folk medical system are happenings described as "natural" or "unnatural" (or supernatural) (for the latter with respect to Southern whites, see Pearsall, 1959, pp. 106, 119–20, 114–57); (3) supernatural and magical elements are widespread; (4) there is a tendency to see events in terms of opposites: natural (having to do with the world as God made it and as he intended it to be) and unnatural. This is seen in such expressions as "for every birth there is a death," "every illness has its cure," "every poison has an antidote," "every herb has a healing purpose." This belief is largely responsible for the view that all illnesses are curable. Our semistructured discussions with black visitors revealed a widespread acceptance of the fourth point.

34. It is difficult to overstress the emphasis placed on cleanses for removing "toxins." The following set of directions is an example of a cleanse, quoted verbatim from a widely circulated leaflet.

> One Day Cleanse
> Start your cleansing with 12 oz. of prune juice. Use the full 12 oz. After the evening meal start drinking your prune juice. You can drink it during the evening as long as you drink all of it before retiring. Next morning start the program. Take the following [capsules]:
>
> 4 LBS [lower bowel system]
> 4 Special Formula
> 4 Black Walnut
> 8 Psyllium or 1 tablesp. Psyllium hulls if you prefer (in juice)
>
> You choose the juice you intend to drink on your cleanse. Do not mix juices, drink one of a kind throughout the program. No orange or grapefruit. You may have all the juice you wish. Anytime you're hungry, take a glass of juice. You may add as much psyllium as you like.
> Take these cleansing herbs 4 times during one day. Morning, Noon, Evening and at bedtime. DO NOT EAT. Drink lots of juice.
> You may feel discomfort in the stomach or even in the muscles of the arms and legs or other large muscles of the body. This is cleansing. The herbs are drawing toxins out of the body. THIS IS GOOD. Do not be alarmed. You may feel as if you have a slight case of flu. You will pass much mucus through the bowels. After the cleanse you need to replenish the calcium and potassium in the body. The day after the cleanse you should go back to eating very gently. Start with some potato peeling soup and then a very light bland diet for the following day. It is good to do this once weekly. You do your herbal health building in between cleansings. If you have had bowel problems, try Cascara Sagrada for a week before your cleanse.

35. Bass has apparently heard of reported differences in the incidences of many serious diseases between Mormons and non-Mormons (see Lyon et al., 1976). No serious suggestion that this is associated with herbs has been made.

36. This has led to concerns from many quarters about suggestions for treatment given in health food stores. See Stoffer et al. (1980).

37. J. H. Young (1978) describes as mythical the notion of America being analogous to

the original Garden of Eden. This is correct, but for many people the myth is an ideological reality, which we believe can still be discerned today. Cooter (1981) is helpful.

38. We cannot even mention all the complexities of the health food movement. Some background is found in the following. For Graham, see Nissenbaum (1980). Conspicuous among visitors is interest in organic gardening; a key feature—the view that "what is natural is good"—is pervasive. See Hufford (1971), Kandel and Pelto (1980). Ideological unity (including revitalization and the role of communication-distribution centers) and diversity are features highlighted (as is health food use) in alternative medical systems.

39. The literature, fact and fiction, on hypoglycemia is vast. Much is considered misleading and the extent of the problem overstated; see Consumers Union (1980, pp. 70–81).

40. Anomymous contribution.

41. We cannot discuss the many social roles and influences of the rural church, but they have been studied since the 1920s. The potential role of the church in health matters today is being increasingly appreciated.

42. For some introduction to these concepts, see Wallis (1985).

7. Treating Ailments and Symptoms

1. Some students of folk life recognize the need for interpretive studies on published lists of uses (e.g., M. O. Jones, 1967, based on reflections on volume 6 of Brown, *Collection of North Carolina Folklore*, 1961.) Many other lists of traditional remedies are published but, unfortunately, often poorly documented.

2. The literature on ethnomedicine is growing rapidly, but a still-helpful perspective on its scope is Fabrega (1975).

3. For discussion on ethnomedical concepts in another part of Appalachia, see Nations et al. (1985).

4. Some commentators imply that all diagnoses should be considered to have a meaning (cf. Good and Good, 1981), but it is often difficult to discern specific cultural factors at play in visitors' accounts of their symptoms.

5. We say this while recognizing the widespread place of anxiety in society (discussed later) and the subtleties of somatization of psychosocial factors. A well-known example is couvade; see, for example, Lipkin and Lamb (1982). Biochemical explanations for the physiological impact of stress, which are attracting more and more interest (e.g., Gruckow, 1979), may have special relevance to events within traditional practice. For an introduction to varied literature discussing directly or indirectly the psychological troubles of Appalachian people, see Coles (1971, pp. 632–33).

6. The link between herbal practice and the drugstore of the past has been made by others: "There's something in the woods good for everything that ails you. When you goes to the drugstore that's all you gets—some kind of herb something that's

diluted and weakened down. It just costs you more that's all" (quoted in H. Lewis, 1955, p. 75).

7. Debate continues over the role of pharmacists, offering advice pertinent to our later discussion on the plurality of health care. For example, Edwards and Stillman (1983) reflect pharmacists' involvement in self-treatment, albeit from an establishment position.

8. See Modell (1961, p. 38). The suggestion that assessing symptoms stands apart from the cornerstone of medicine may seem misleading because, contrary to much public opinion, understanding symptomatology remains as important for many physicians as the results of laboratory and other tests, especially in general practice. Much is written on the significance of symptoms; see Morrell (1972), who notes variations in patients' thresholds, which determine seeking advice, and suggests that, in part, concern with symptoms relates to patients' expectations of their health, expectations higher in age groups 45–64 than over the age of 65. R. A. Jones et al. (1981) concluded from studies on young adults that symptoms are pursued primarily when perceived as threatening, disruptive, and painful; many symptoms are generally not pursued—at least not taken to a physician— but many Bass visitors are pleased to be able to be able to "drop in" to see Bass about their symptoms.

9. We are not implying that other writers have ignored coherency in traditional care, but investigations in Anglo-Saxon practices are limited in scope compared with, for example, Evans-Pritchard's 1937 account of practices among the Azande, which underscores how medical care fits into a society in which magic is a component part of religion and culture, a normal part of society, and a logical part of understanding nature and human behavior.

10. We feel that a helpful designation for such theories is "hot-cold *balance* theory" or "sweet-bitter *balance* theory," rather than merely "hot-cold" and "sweet-bitter," if only because Bass and others are primarily concerned with balance in the body.

11. Keill (1738, p. x).

12. Ames (1770, in "An Essay on Physick").

13. Beard (1875).

14. Sir Arthur Keith's *The Engines of the Human Body*, which reached many editions (e.g., 1926), was but one popular book with a similar title. A quick glance at almost any medical or physiological text can reinforce a mechanical view. From the viewpoint of the present account—attitudes among laypeople—such college texts as Carlson and Johnson, *The Machinery of the Body* (1946) are perhaps especially significant. Physicians often recognize that in communicating with patients they sometimes simplify accounts of a disease and pathology; omitting, for instance, discussions on biochemistry, they describe processes in purely mechanical terms.

15. The Hadacol jingle is from F. M. Clay (1973, p. 167), through the courtesy of W. H. Helfand. For an indication of the persuasiveness of popular literature where mechanical analogies appear, see Frost and Frost (1985, p. 62).

16. For some introduction to autointoxication, see Lambert (1978), and for details, Bouchard (1898).

17. One recent discussion illustrating the pervasiveness of past ideas is in Helman (1978), who provides an example of a physical or at least sensory orientation which helps sustain long-standing ideas about the roles of hot and cold. Helman also makes the interesting point that "in some respects the 'operational model' used on a day-to-day basis by the general medical practitioners is closer to that of the lay model than to the official biomedical model of disease."

18. Comments on classification are appropriate. John Gerard, in his celebrated *Herball* (1597), defined medicines according to traditional Galenic qualities (hot, cold, dry, and moist) but grouped plants by growth forms (e.g., grasses and grass-like plants, herbs, shrubs, etc.). Such botanical arrangements for herbal remedies as well as alphabetical listings have remained popular to the present time, but neither are ideal for medical education and clinical practice. In consequence, numerous authors have organized drugs according to therapeutic properties. Acceptable classifications are difficult since almost every substance has more than one action, sometimes dependent on dose; some botanicals, therefore, are confusingly classified variously among emetics, cathartics, anthelmintics, antacids, tonics, astringents, narcotics, stimulants, diaphoretics, etc. Notwithstanding confusion, arranging medicines according to therapeutic properties highlighted the relative ineffectiveness of many, thus encouraging the revision of the materia medica already noted.

19. Tournefort (1708, preface, pp. A2–A3).

20. For an early definition mentioning blood impurities, see James (1743–45, vol. 1, under "blood"). By the early nineteenth century definitions were generally more limiting; for instance, as "altering and amending the animal fluids without any immediately sensible operation" (Coxe, 1817, p. 30).

21. Paine (1857, pp. 156–57).

22. Hare (1909, p. 37).

23. It is difficult to say when alteratives, or any medicine, completely disappeared from regular practice. In 1918 a textbook for pharmacy students defined alteratives as drugs modifying nutrition and restoring to normal various functions of the body. The term still appears in much modern herbal literature in the context of improving the condition of the system.

24. For example, Motherby (1785), who described alteratives as a type of medicine "making changes in the blood for the better without any manifest operation or evacuation." See also Buchan (1772, p. 452).

25. If regular medical books did not mention blood purifiers, they at least made clear that good health depended on well-functioning blood (e.g., G. Moore, 1850, p. 54). Some works, such as Stevens (1832), did not specifically mention the term blood purifier, although it recommended them in treatment (e.g., sarsaparilla and wild cherry bark).

26. It should be added that the term "purificantia" was sometimes used in regular medicine for "drugs that purify the blood" (*New Sydenham Society Lexicon*, 1899).

27. The list of items used occasionally as spring tonics, not just in Appalachia, is

extensive. Others noted variously are sweet gum, spicewood, witch hazel, winter-green, or powdered sulfur in molasses (2 tablespoons taken over a week). The popularity of some of these depended on availability.

28. Local persistence of knowledge of the use of plants for a condition such as malaria, once commonplace, is frequent.

29. For a wide-ranging account dealing generally with nonbotanical remedies, in fact the more unusual kinds of inhalants, see Hand (1968). Attention is given to change of air (including that near gasworks), animal odors, fumes from tar, and a wide range of household remedies.

30. More detailed practical information can be gathered from specialist articles and books, e.g., Dobell (1872). A few specific articles appeared in the medical press, e.g., J. Fothergill (1875), which focused attention on restoring balance "betwixt the two heat-producing and heat-losing areas" (p. 38).

31. Tonics often were given in the context of supportive care.

32. Among many relevant quotes: "Such an obstructed perspiration, therefore, as is sufficient to produce the disease most commonly called a cold" (J. Chandler, 1761, p. 31).

33. For reference to this and a general account of expectorants, see Dobell (1872, pp. 186–98), Hatcher and Wilbert (1907, pp. 219–36; p. 233 for hydrocyanic acid). Others listed as used at the time were ammonium chloride, apomorphine, balsam of Peru, balsam of tolu, benzoin, codeine, ipecacuanha, licorice, pine tar, senega, squill, and tartar emetic.

34. However, some still recognized in 1944 were: benzoin, bryony, coccillana, ele-campane, eriodictyon, euphorbia, grindelia, poppy, sanguinaria, and white hore-hound.

35. The literature on folk medicine lists countless remedies for colds.

36. Bass has a comprehensive knowledge of other plants which have been used in the form of hot teas to produce sweats, or "warmth and comfort" for chills; examples include yarrow, pennyroyal, chamomile, and ginger, all mentioned in J. Meyer (1979). He also recognizes many remedies listed in R. B. Browne (1958), all of which tended to be used more in home medicines. Regular physicians commonly used the time-honored antimonial wine.

37. Bass does not have a specific recommendation for dry, irritating coughs that keep many people awake at night. However, he does say that passionflower or some-thing else for the nerves might help.

38. Bass has noted that a laxative can be used for colds; this may be a recollection of old proprietary preparations like De Witt's Laxative Cold Tablets. One type of ingredient in old proprietary medicines which Bass does not use is anodynes. Opium or morphine were old favorites; Bass would not use anything as strong as narcotics, even if he could.

39. Woodard Papers, North Carolina State Archives.

40. By folk remedies Bass means those that he does not believe have been collected commercially or employed by regular physicians.

41. For discussion on feed a cold, etc., see Helman (1978). Incidental references illus-

trating and reinforcing the idea that the environment is an important factor in connection with catching colds and rheumatism are commonplace today. For example, the *Manchester Guardian Weekly* reported 23 January 1983 (p. 23) a sailor's prediction about those who surf in the winter sea: it will "produce a generation of rheumatic old surfriders."

42. See Crellin and Nowell-Smith (forthcoming).

43. Potter (1913, p. 494).

44. Goth (1981, pp. 513–14). It is of interest that a health-care review panel for the FDA reported recently that in over-the-counter medicines there are no ingredients as safe and effective as expectorants to help remove thick secretions from the mouth and throat. They said potassium iodide is not safe and effective, and ammonium chloride, horehound, and tolu balsam need further testing (*FDA Consumer*, 12 September 1982).

45. Paine (1847, p. 317).

46. For remarks on "muscles swellin' up"—admittedly as pain and tension in the stomach and neck and without it being made clear whether the subjects had "diagnoses"—see Nations et al. (1985).

47. No comprehensive history of rheumatism has appeared. For information, see Rodnan (1977), and Copeman (1964). The view about causation differs somewhat from other recorded lay beliefs, e.g., Gray (1983).

48. This is clear from many texts and manuscripts, e.g., Fuller (1814, fn. 13).

49. "Camphorated oil" products are no longer available, primarily because of reported cases of poisoning by ingestion (accidental or deliberate) and occasional toxic effects when applied with frequency to the chests of infants: "Any benefits from having camphorated oil available are insignificant when compared to the risk" (see Thompson, 1983). For regulation, see *Federal Register*, 21 September 1982.

50. For example, R. B. Browne (1958), and Brown, *Collection of North Carolina Folklore* (1957–64, 6:254–69).

51. Some of the issues are raised by Ring and Trotman (1983).

52. See references in n. 50 above.

53. This can be seen by comparing twentieth-century textbooks with, for instance, Erasmus Wilson's prestigious and influential *Diseases of the Skin*, 1st ed. (1852), which is the basis for the following comments on nineteenth-century practices. For a general account of dermatology, see Pusey (1933). This does not replace earlier reference accounts such as Frik et al. (1928).

54. For background to Vaseline, see Vaseline (1884).

55. Mentioned in countless writings, e.g., Kaposi (1895, p. 83).

56. SSS tonic, not discussed in the account of patent medicines (chap. 4), is well entrenched in Bass's memory. Still marketed from Atlanta, it contains iron, vitamins, and alcohol, but in the past the preparation has contained many botanical drugs. For instance, in 1914 it included chionanthus root (*Chionanthus virginicus*) as the principal ingredient, with smaller amounts of swamp sumac (*Rhus vernix*) and sumac (*Rhus glabra*). Later, three additional botanicals were added: queen's delight (*Stillingia sylvatica*), prickly ash (*Zanthoxylum* spp.), and pokeroot (*Phytolacca americana*). Information from Tyler (1984).

57. Bass further modifies the formula on occasion, depending on the availability of ingredients. If hog lard, for instance, is difficult to obtain, it is supplemented by paraffin.

58. Many visitors hold similar views about "all sores being the same" and keep an "all-purpose" salve in the home.

59. Requests for help with prickly heat have declined in recent years, reflecting that it causes less concern than formerly. Renbourn (1958) gives a review but little discussion on therapy.

60. Typical "sores" brought to Bass are healing or slowly healing wounds, abscesses, carbuncles, and cold sores. Surprisingly, since they are so common, he is rarely asked about varicose veins.

61. Few visitors appear to have any real comprehension of the pathology of a hiatus hernia; namely, a portion of stomach slipping through the diaphragm.

62. Bass is familiar with such other demulcents—still well known—as gelatin and glycerin. See, for instance, *FDA Consumer*, 12 September 1982. Alternative plants he recommends for sore mouths include five-finger grass, black gum, spicebush, tag-alder, and persimmon, recommendations seemingly based primarily on astringent properties.

63. The literature recording folk medicine includes innumerable references to such poultices as Irish potato, house leek, alder bark, and bread and milk.

64. Countless suggestions have been made for treating poison ivy and poison oak. A helpful account appears in McNair (1923, pp. 147–71). Soap and nonbotanical remedies are mentioned prominently. More recent information can be found in Whitener (1981, pp. 29, 55). This also notes the use of Octagon soap. The use of milk rather than water is noted, but using milkweed rather than plantain. Jewelweed (snapweed in the Appalachians) also is highly recommended. See also Hand, et al. (1981, 1:426–29).

65. The idea of eating a small portion of the root in the spring to build up resistance during the year is well established as a popular concept. See F. C. Brown (1961–62, 6:251).

66. Walnut is recorded among folk treatments in Alabama. Other listed plant remedies known to Bass include green fig leaves, milkweed, and yellow dock. He has no recollection of cocklebur or some of the "magical" treatments listed in R. B. Browne (1958, pp. 90–91).

67. Ibid., pp. 101–2.

68. W. N. B. Watson (1971).

69. R. B. Browne (1958) lists seventeen Alabama popular sayings on treating itch, including six for poke.

70. The introduction of ice for treating burns is a complex story. For general issues of its use for treating burns, see Aurness (1906).

71. Rook and Savin (1980, pp. 288–90); letter subsequent to article by Burton (1984).

72. Despite the widespread interest in warts, no comprehensive account has yet appeared. For some review of selected facets, see T. Browne (1970). "Removal of Warts," *New Eng. J. Med.* 255 (1956): 625, provides some interesting comments on methods such as wart charming. Wart cures galore are recorded in Brown (1961–

62, 6:309–50). Especially relevant to Bass's practice is evidence of the popularity of milkweed juice.

73. For variations on use of the potato; e.g., cutting it into halves, see Brown (1961–62, 6:329–30).

74. Latex is widely distributed in the plant kingdom. Metcalf (1967) indicates its presence in 12,500 species. An interesting discussion, "Milkweeds and Wartworts," appears in Clute (1939, pp. 91–102). Clute notes what a number of later writers have reported; namely, that celandine (Chelidonium majus) with an abundance of orange-colored, alkaloid-rich juice was one of the more reputable cures. See also Lassek and McCarthy (1983, p. 124). Plants known as wart-worts (wort-spurge, wart-weed, wart-grass, etc.) include Euphorbia heliscopia, Gnaphalium uliginosum, and Coronopus procumbens.

75. Quoted in Dagnall (1964).

76. Brown (1961–62, 6:160–61).

77. The presumed use of salicin—or at least the use of a paste made from the ash of a willow bark—is often said to have a long historical pedigree (e.g., reference to Pliny by Dagnall, 1964), while salicylic acid generally is recognized as safe and effective for hard corns and calluses (e.g., FDA Consumer, 22 March 1982). Salicylic acid presumably is more potent than aspirin.

78. R. B. Browne (1958, pp. 84–85) lists a number of astringent medicines for the same purpose, such as red oak, alum water, peach tree leaves in lard.

79. C. T. Johnson (1811, p. 95).

80. Banister (1622, sig. 2).

81. For background, Shapiro (1959).

82. As is well known, much interest exists in the possible value of "traditional remedies" for cancer; see, for example, Hartwell (1982); for another discussion, see Duke, "Folk Anticancer Plants Containing Antitumor Compounds" (in Etkin, 1986, pp. 70–90); Cassileth et al. (1984); B. R. Smithe (1980), and the voluminous literature on Laetrile. Overall, however, much skepticism exists within the scientific community. In particular, such remedies as "resolving" poultices and plasters are dismissed; see Moulin (1983, p. 43).

83. For agave, see Davidson and Ortiz de Montellano (1983). This paper is noteworthy for testing formulated preparations as generally available, rather than merely considering the action of active ingredients. As noted later, there has been much interest in antibiotic activity in higher plants. For recent discussions on sugar, see Chirife et al. (1982), which notes that "natural substances such as honey and molasses have been used throughout history for the treatment of infection." Certain bacterial pathogens were shown to be affected. For comments, negative and positive, see R. D. Forrest (1982); B. Bose (1982; a note favoring honey); Chirife and Herszage (1982). A brief review by Bush (1974) notes references to bed sores and traditional treatments for internal use.

84. For some suggestions see Benoit et al. (1976); Gábor (1979), though most suggestions are not concerned with external applications.

85. For example, A. A. Fisher (1977).

86. Instances of counterirritation can be found in Hartwell (1967).
87. For influence of podophyllum, see Hartwell (1967, p. 379); and for periwinkle, Farnsworth and Kaas (1981).
88. For background, see Rather (1978).
89. Spjut and Perdue (1976) suggest that greater emphasis be given to bioassays that detect toxicity. For comments on this, see Farnsworth and Kass (1981), who point out the limited sources of information used and that differences between in vitro and in vivo assays were not distinguished.
90. Bass promotes and sells a booklet summarizing much of his knowledge; see D. C. Meyer (1978).
91. Scarpa and Guerci (1987).
92. Describing nerves in biological terms is less of a stigma than explanations in terms of mental illness. See Ludwig and Forrester (1981, 1982); Ludwig (1982). A significant paper by Barlett and Low (1980) nevertheless indicated a common view that "nervios is an illness of the nerve endings or of the brain." For provocative discussion in reifying pathogenic emotions, see Helman (1985).
93. It is accepted widely that in Western countries more females than males have depressive illnesses.
94. The book was perhaps prompted by the high incidence of hypochondriasis in Cheyne's medical practice. Cf. p. 11 (quoted in Fischer-Homburger, 1972). The figure includes female hysteria. See also helpful background in Veith (1968). For a selective overview, see Hofling (1977). For some account of secularization, see MacDonald (1982).
95. William Cullen (quoted from Spillane, 1981, p. 163). For other pertinent background, see Bowman (1975). It is not always easy to be sure that changing theoretical concepts altered everyday therapy. S. W. Jackson (1983) suggests that changing theories had little impact.
96. Cullen (1812, 2:154ff.).
97. Cullen also included *Cicuta*, but wrote a critical account of its reputation (p. 189): "As it has manifestly strong powers in affecting the human system, I conclude, that, like all other substances possessed of such powers, it may be a very efficacious medicine. This, we believe, will be allowed; but it may still be a question in what diseases."
98. Cullen (1812, 2:94–95).
99. Quoted from Buchan (1807, Philadelphia edition, p. 277). In emphasizing non-drug treatment, Buchan was echoing such influential writers as George Cheyne already noted.
100. Rippere (1980, 1981). Among the various factors, the role of the atmosphere was considered especially important in the etiology of disease. It may be viewed as part of a constitutional "wholistic" approach to medicine. For just one example, see J. Johnson (1818). Rapid changes in temperature were considered to be especially dangerous for some people.
101. For example, Cullen (1812, 2:95) noted that tonics and stimulants (acting on the nervous system) should be distinguished, but admitted, perhaps confusingly: "we

cannot clearly explain wherein the difference consists." Much discussion exists on a common feature of bitterness among tonics; e.g., Lassek and McCarthy (1983, pp. 75–77). The authors note (p. 75) that some of the "most popular" tonics were prepared from two small gentianaceous herbs, *Centaurium spicatum* and *Sebea ovata*, as well as from the bark of the apocynaceous tree *Alstonia constricta*. Also mentioned (p. 76) is *Smilax glyciphylla*, commonly known as "native sarsaparilla," once extensively used as a tonic and antiscorbutic.

102. Fischer-Homberger (1972, p. 396), notes that Beard's work reduced a Babel-like diversity of terminology to a single term.

103. For symptoms and background, see Sicherman (1977, p. 37).

104. Beard (1875, p. iv).

105. For documentation, see Crellin, "From Tonics to Vitamins" (in preparation).

106. Burdock Blood Bitters Almanac, Foster, Milburn & Co. (1893, p. 7).

107. Another formula is a teacup of peach, bay, passionflower, and catnip, respectively, and one-half teacup of skullcap.

108. Flint (1879, p. 650).

109. The argument that tonics prolong life appears to rest on loose interpretations of a range of papers discussing the effects of drugs on plasma cholesterol; for instance, Shanmugasundaram et al. (1983).

110. Quotations from Greenblatt et al. (1984). For a recent survey of many aphrodisiacs, but far from complete on botanicals, see Taberner (1985). For recent comments: *Federal Register*, 1 October 1982; "Natural Aphrodisiacs," *Lawrence Rev. Nat. Prod.* 15 (1982): 57–59. This classifies them as myth and folklore, centrally acting agents (e.g., yohimbine, strychnine), urogenital irritants, nitrites, pheromones, and other hormones.

111. Cf. J. Johnson (1826); we have found many references to torpid and sluggish livers in nineteenth-century medical correspondence. A "burning sensation" is less common, but see letter from Desmarest in Snyder Correspondence, Illinois State Archives, 26 August 1892. For some background to lithemia or torpid liver, see Chen and Chen (1984, pp. 173–74).

112. Poynter and Bishop (1951, p. 25).

113. J. Johnson (1818, p. 100).

114. For example, ibid.; Johnson said that the dandelion had lately come into use for "biliary obstructions."

115. Fantus (1920, p. 27).

116. Personal communication from Dr. D. V. Kuang.

117. R. B. Browne (1958, p. 77); and Brown (1957–64, 6:228); both give examples of the use of mayapple. Another popular, less-drastic laxative, senna, was used. Bass also remembers that many foods were considered good for the liver, such as oranges, sauerkraut, and tomatoes (Browne, p. 77).

118. For milk thistle, at least for the flavanolignans present as antihepatotoxic agents, see G. Vogel (1977). For other examples, see "Garlic", in volume 2.

119. Capron and Slack (1848, p. 58). Bass no longer receives queries about Bright's disease: "I understand it's not so bad as it was. But back in 1961 when my sister was in the hospital, I helped the nurse with a young boy who had Bright's disease."

120. Digitalis should perhaps be added to the list but its action is on the heart, not the kidney. The improved action of the heart rather than the kidney is behind the elimination of edema.
121. For an example of a clear statement of being "powerfully diuretic, and hence antisyphilitic," see Lindley (1838, p. 450).
122. A list of seventy-three items assembled from lay publications, old materia medica herbals, and in some few cases, the scientific literature, appears in "Herbal Obstetrics," *Lawrence Rev. Nat. Prod.*, 1984. It is said that no scientific evidence exists to justify the use of most of the plants as diuretics.
123. Quoted in Rolleston (1942).
124. Boric acid has lost favor in the medical profession.
125. For a reminder of the importance of knowing whether the juice is administered in the form of drops, see Gentry and Cook (1984).
126. Lewis and Elvin-Lewis (1977, p. 224) have singled out *Achillea* spp., and for ears *Asarum canadense* (which they suggest is due to the antimicrobial properties of aristolochic acid), and *Polygala senega*, for anti-inflammatory properties. The authors also mention, from "folk medicine," other plants used as eyewashes or poultices to treat sore or bruised eyes: *Achillea* spp., *Argemone intermedia*, *Maclura pomifera*, *Salix* spp., *Hydrastis canadensis*, *Linum* spp., *Monotropa uniflora* (juice), *Prosopis* spp. (leaves applied directly). Decoctions of *Saponaria officinalis*, *Hydrastis canadensis*, and *Hyssopus officinalis* were noted for bruises around the eye. We have found no evidence that these were commonly used.
127. For general background to treatment of ear complaints, see Kennedy (1713), J. H. Curtis (1819; this accepted the notion of the importance of the stomach for the sound functioning of the body as a whole), W. Kramer (1838, esp. p. 40), R. H. Lewis (1886), Milligan and Wingrave (1911).
128. R. B. Browne (1958) and other lists of folk remedies.
129. Of the various nonbotanical remedies listed in the folk medicine literature, bessbug blood is commonplace; e.g., see Waller and Killian (1972).
130. Hooper's Female Pills obtained British patent no. 592 in 1743, but unfortunately the patent did not divulge the constituents, merely stating they were the "best purging stomacick and antihysterick ingredients." The latter reflected a long-standing belief that female problems have a nervous component. Various nineteenth-century formularies published recipes for Hooper's pills.
131. Quoted in Stage (1979, p. 69). Much discussion has taken place on attitudes to women; see Morantz-Sanchez (1985, pp. 203–31).
132. A useful "obstetric materia medica" (also gynecological) is included in J. King (1871, pp. 684–743).
133. Some indication of the large number of plants is given in N. R. Farnsworth et al. (1975). Knowledge of only a small proportion of these has reached Bass; in fact, Bass has not heard of the emmenagogue/abortifacient properties of even many that do grow in his area, and when questioned about them discounts the reputation (e.g., of calamus, beet root, and chamomile). For a list pertinent to Bass's practice see Kost (1859, pp. 445–57). This excludes ergot, often listed as an emmenagogue; see Ellis (1849, pp. 101–2). For emmenagogues still attracting a little

interest in 1944, see Allport (1944, pp. 149–50): aletris rhizome, apiol, black-haw, black hellebore, calendula, canella, caulophyllum, cimicifuga, cotton-root bark, pulsatille, rue, savin. Generally, remedies for female complaints were not discussed widely in the medical literature (except those for childbirth).

Current interest exists in various parts of the world on abortifacient emmena-gogues and potential contraceptives. A recent publication that references earlier articles and underscores different concepts is Browner and Ortiz de Montellano (1986, pp. 32–47). Also see Conway and Slocumb (1980).

134. L. F. Newman (1979) notes some warnings against abortion (e.g., from Andrew Boordes, *Breviary of Health*, 1547); Jochle (1972).

135. Meigs (1848, pp. 406–23).

136. Farnsworth et al. (1975, pp. 582–83).

137. Plantain has been noted by Conway and Slocumb (1980).

138. For examples of the hypothesis of action mediated through prostaglandin synthe-sis, see Kong (1981).

139. Exercise was another factor; for remarks within the context of general practice, see Alexander (1897). An interesting handwritten note on the flyleaf of Mundé (1895, Country Doctor Museum Library) underscores the interest in one of a num-ber of chemical emmenagogues: "In amenorrhoea or suppressed mensium give biniodide manganese in 2 gr. dose (gelatin-coated pills) 3 times per day. Be careful that pregnancy does not exist lest this should produce an abortion."

140. A noteworthy plant with a strong reputation as a galactogogue over which there is recent conflicting clinical evidence has been discussed in detail by Rosen-garten (1982). Feiz and Moattar (1985) presented evidence for galactogogue actions in *Pimpinella anisum, Carum corde, Foeniculum vulgare, Anethum graveolens, Trigonella foenum-graecum,* and *Petroselinum sativum.*

141. Of interest is a recent note on *Oxytropis* spp: "to increase milk flow of nursing mothers or to make the mother's milk more agreeable to the infant" (in Hort, 1981).

142. For discussion of this concept as a folk belief, see Blumhagen (1980).

143. Singer et al. (1984).

144. A large number of plants (over two hundred) are reputed by Lewis and Elvin-Lewis (1977, pp. 218–19) to have a hypoglycemic action. Others noted by them and also known to Bass include Jerusalem artichoke, Solomon's seal, black co-hosh, and goldenseal. For examples, see Karawya et al. (1984).

145. Hare (1909, p. 265).

146. For recommendations on the two alum roots, see J. King (1878, pp. 624–54).

147. For example, D. R. Stevenson (1986).

148. Cf. Burland et al. (1974). Bass recognizes that some people lose water, but says that the herbs "eat up calories." Herbal teas, he says, have to be taken over a long period of time. Unfortunately, in follow-up studies the authors have not met any-one who has taken the tea for more than a month. Short-term weight losses are clear, but not long-term results. At least, for those trying, in turn, the long list of commercially marketed preparations (commonly with no long-term success), Bass's suggestions are inexpensive.

149. Cowle Papers.

150. In the home, "dish" rags cut from fertilizer or feed sacks often were used as toilet paper. Such general-purpose sacks also were fashioned into underwear or clothes. Toilet paper became commonplace in the Mackey-Leesburg area during the 1930s. Bass recognizes that many over-the-counter medicines still contain natural products; e.g., Carter's Little Pills (aloe, podophyllum); Metamucil and Seratan (psyllium); Nature's Remedy (aloe, cascara).

151. The notion that taking an excessive amount of laxatives caused constipation was often stressed in the early twentieth century. See Fantus (1920, p. 9).

152. Bass adds that a substantial amount of peanuts produces a mild action. The cathartic action of some of the items listed is not mainline. For instance, black Indian hemp was regarded primarily as a cardiac stimulant. In fact, its one-time recognition as a cathartic is not mentioned in most twentieth-century texts on materia medica.

153. Capron and Slack (1848, p. 209).

154. Some confusion exists over the difference between carminatives and antispasmodics. The latter substances—to relieve spasms, cramps, and convulsions—were not used only for gastrointestinal upsets. Well-known ones were ammonia, asafetida, belladonna, camphor, castor, cicuta, ether, musk, opium, and valerian. See Capron and Slack (1848, p. 33).

155. The long-standing, widespread use of bitters is readily appreciated from, say, many seventeenth- and eighteenth-century writings indicating that the infusion of common bitters are useful to support the stomach, open the liver, and move the bowels.

156. These are included in the *Brown Collection of North Carolina Folklore* (1957–64, 6:212ff.) along with many others.

157. Ibid., pp. 212–19.

158. Crellin and Nowell-Smith, forthcoming.

159. Publications such as J. de Baïracli Levy's *The Complete Herbal Book for the Dog* (1983) have helped to stimulate interest in herbs for dogs. Comparatively little is written on traditional veterinary care, but see Brookman (1978, pp. 67–74), which underscores the limited amount of published information.

8. Reflections on the Region and Beyond

1. The comments rest on twenty-six interviews with people aged sixty-five and over. At least a few elderly Appalachian women who practice herbal medicine on what can be best described as an extended family basis use more drugs. An example, perhaps, is Etta Banks, who in 1973, when aged eighty-three, discussed her homemade salve and its lineage (she claimed the formula was well over one hundred years old):

> Call it homemade salve; didn't have any name, only that. Well, my mother-in-law learned me. Just when I watched her make it, then I got to makin' it

myself and that's been . . . sixty-four years ago, and I've made it all along through my life when I'd need it. I kept it all the time . . . for the children when they was, when I was araisin' the children. That's what I used for their sores and their burns and things. It'd take two days not for me to make it 'cause I work some two days. But used to be, I could have done that in half a day; got the bark, scraped it, and made it. Have to have, uh, tree resin, tree turpentine, and mutton's "taller" [tallow] and lard . . . hog's lard. And . . . of all these four barks and the buds off of the . . . balm of Gilead. It's good for all kinds of sores, you know, after they get infected. People don't have sores like they used to, the little children would have. And burns, it's good for burns.

I don't remember ever havin' a doctor when I was growin' up, never takin' any doctor medicine; and I hain't much since. I never have been in the hospital, only just go to visit. (From published transcript of film *Nature's Way*, Appalachian Film Workshop)

2. The expression "living force" is used in Evans et al. (1982). The vigorous and persistent nature of "alternative health systems," already noted, is emphasized by Hufford (1984, esp. pp. 4–5).

3. The hot-cold concept in present-day cultures has attracted much recent discussion; a useful introduction which indicates some sound medical practices under the rubric of hot-cold theory is Logan (1977). Other recent contributions especially pertinent to the present account highlight how the hot-cold concept can shape aspects of Western health care. They include Harwood (1971), which provides interesting examples of the classification of such new substances as penicillin as hot because it can cause hot-classified symptoms such as a rash or diarrhea. Much accepted treatment rests on treating with opposites. Some studies also indicate how the concept leads to treatment approaches similar to those of Bass. For Bolivia, Bastien (1983, p. 98) stresses the focus on symptomatic treatment: "make a person sweat (sudorific), reduce fever (febrifuge), remove mucous (expectorant), calm pain (analgesic), regulate bile (biliary regulant), cause menstruation (emmenagogue)," etc. Many herbs are also listed as blood purifiers. "Andeans are very concerned about their blood." Problems with the liver are another focus of attention. Earlier publications by Bastien analyze the function of Qollahuaya diviners in ritual curing. See also G. M. Foster (1979). Many examples given deal more with lay concepts, such as "feed a cold, starve a fever." Additionally, G. M. Foster (1984) emphasizes the role of "thermal temperature," though does not show that many of the notions have been generally prominent in Western medicine within recent centuries. For series of articles: *Soc. Sci. Med.* 25 (1987): 329–41.

4. From knowledge of incompatibilities and interactions in compounded medicines employed in regular medical practice, it is reasonable to assume similar phenomena occur in herbal preparations. Unfortunately, little concrete data is available, but see, for example, Kimata et al. (1985).

5. Many authors talk optimistically of natural plant remedies in the context of potential new drugs for Western medicine. Two of many examples are Huxtable (1980),

and Etkin (1981). For reference to plant products in prescriptions, see Farnsworth (1983). Figures also in Farnsworth and Bingel (1977, n. 6).

6. For responses, explicit and implicit, to the view that results emerging from a vast amount of chemical screening are disappointing, see Moerman (1979). Another article by Moerman, "Symbols and Selectivity" (1979), describes regression analyses of plants used by native Americans and argues that, while much of medicine (ethno- or otherwise) is symbolic—based on meaning—substantial selectivity in medical usage by native Americans can be shown. Much recent discussion has appeared on improving methods of evaluation of plants. For a helpful discussion, see Farnsworth and Bingel (1977, pp. 1–22), which highlights some of the problems of using animal models. The authors discuss studies that indicate the chance of finding a clinically useful natural product is on the order of one in four hundred. Among various points stressed in terms of pharmacological screening are the need for careful identification of specimens and variation within samples from the same lot of plant material. Various suggestions have been made for brief assays to encourage more widespread testing of plants. See Trotter et al. (1983), who describe a simple method using brine shrimp.

7. Issues about research have been sharpened in recent years, partly as a result of attacks on alternative medicine. Many "defensive" studies incorporating standard scientific methodology are intended to answer the question whether or not alternative practices really alter the natural history of disease and, if so, to see if it is the result of providing more than time and kindness. Double-blind clinical trials on homeopathic medicines published in non-homeopathic scientific journals are one expression of this. But for discussions raising questions about the applicability of scientific methodology in other areas, see G. M. Foster (1987).

Specific issues relevant to the discussion include debate on the value of whole-plant extracts compared with employing the active constituents; few scientists and physicians support the use of extracts, but see Scarpa (1981), who repeats the view that infusions prevent accumulation of digitalis glycosides and hence toxic effects; and Burch (1972): "with elegant and proper administration, digitalis leaf is superior, though subtle at times, for the management of patients with cardiac disease." Somewhat different attitudes are implied in a recent study, which does not address the issue directly: Aronson (1985), who discusses variability of action and bioavailablity. Also relevant are Weil (1981, pp. 287–312), and Izaddoost and Robinson (1987).

8. It seems appropriate to stress that some consider practices like homeopathy, with its use of infinitesimally small doses not explicable in terms of modern physiology, to rest primarily on effects other than placebo responses. For insights into the problem of definition, see B. L. White et al. (1985, pt. 2).

9. Much discussion on the origin of the idea of placebo action has appeared, resting largely on dictionary definitions. The concept was, however, appreciated by many authors—without being specifically defined—during the eighteenth century, if not long before. Attempts to understand the placebo quickened in the 1950s (Shapiro, 1959). For other discussion on background, see S. White (1985).

10. For recent reviews, see W. R. Phillips (1981); Gowdey (1983); Berg (1983).

11. For discussion, see Gowdey (1983, p. 924), Shapiro and Morris (1978). An often-cited statistic in the placebo literature is that placebo effects occur in 30–40 percent of treated patients.

12. For pertinent comments and different views on the placebo effects of over-the-counter medicines, see J. K. Jones (in Lasagne, 1980, pp. 26–39).

13. The role, for instance, of endorphins in explaining analgesia as a placebo phenomenon is producing much speculation; see "Shamans and Endorphins" (1982).

14. J. K. Jones (1980, p. 30). For criticisms of much of the literature on placebos, see Shapiro et al. (1980). Shapiro (1978) has said that anxiety is the only consistent factor.

15. See Jospe (1978, p. 104, quoting Shapiro).

16. Ibid.

17. See also Gowdey (1983).

18. For example, Jospe (1978, p. 3).

19. Discussions on placebo theories are commonplace; e.g., B. L. White et al. (1985). For introductions: Brody (1980, esp. pp. 18–24), Byerly (1975–76), Adler and Hammett (1973—a discussion stressing the importance of the cognitive world), Twemlow and Gabbard (1985). For reference to biological view of placebo action, see Kleinman and Sung (1970). This paper includes the results of Kleinman's study of medicine in Taiwan. Kleinman's ideas are developed fully in his *Patients and Healers in the Context of Culture* (1980, esp. pp. 311–44). Emphasis is placed on cross-cultural comparisons, the considerable amount of somatization, the need for follow-up studies on patients and, as other authors have indicated, that patients' perceptions of improvement may differ from the perceptions of their practitioners.

20. Kleinman (1980, p. 72).

21. Ibid., p. 361.

22. Shapiro and Shapiro (1982).

23. Cf. Zabrowski (1952), Wolff and Langley (1968).

24. The literature on the subject of stress is vast—over 200,000 papers on the subject since Hans Selye's embryonic description of the concept of stress in 1936. For background, see Selye (1984, pp. 1–20). Selye deals mostly with biological factors. He considers that stress plays some role in the development of every disease. See also Kasl (1984, pp. 79–102). Some argue that despite the large number of studies, links between general effects of stress and subsequent organic disease have not been proved definitively. The question of how much stress may be considered a "social disease" remains a controversial issue. It is appropriate to note that even where personality factors seem to be primarily at play behind stress (for instance, the association of type A personalities with a high incidence of heart disease), cultural factors, as in a goal-oriented society, can do much to accentuate personality traits. See Chesney and Rosenman (1984).

25. Such thoughts are prompted by questions that challenge conventional thinking about the role of placebos; e.g., Moerman, "General Medical Effectiveness and Human Biology" (1979).

26. Many commentators state that the doctor-patient relationship plays an important role—probably an essential role—in positive placebo responses. Countless discussions focus on facets of this; e.g., C. V. Ford (1983, p. 224). It is the thrust of Agich (1983, pp. 233–50) that a full analysis of the scope of the therapeutic relationship will necessarily indicate how rights and duties are woven into the concept of the relationship within the practice of medicine. He argues that values and beliefs also need to be made clear.

27. For some background, see "The Epidemiology of Well-Being" (in Hine et al., 1983, pp. 165–76).

28. The relevance of symbolism is commonly suggested in the context of faith and spiritual healing; e.g., Ness and Wintrob (1981). Some commentators argue that symbolic communication forms a pathway of sorts between social and cultural events and psychophysiological reactions. E.g., Kleinman (1973). See also Moerman, "Anthropology of Symbolic Healing" (1979). Moerman argues that a variety of biological mechanisms suggest that "metaphorical concepts or performances [can] affect human physiology." For an interesting discussion from a different vantage point, see Atkinson (1978). Some studies emphasize that shamans, who may on occasion be strikingly successful in responding to patients' personal troubles, do not systematically recognize or attempt to relieve the psychosocial burden of illness; see Eisenberg and Kleinman (1981, p. 10). The authors also indicate that romanticism in anthropology and sociology can lead to an overevaluation of the skills of traditional healers. Difficulty in evaluation is made clear by studies indicating that discrepancies exist between rates of ulcer healing and rates of symptom improvement. Some patients with healed ulcers continued to have symptoms, whereas others whose ulcer persisted had no complaints of pain (Peterson et al., 1977).

29. MacDonald (1981, p. 183), for instance, suggests that in the seventeenth century physicians placed greater emphasis on the curative powers of the imagination than we do today.

30. Multiple factors were at play in the genesis of the movement in the 1960s. Berliner and Salmon (1980) state that the "holistic health movement arose as the creation of a large and colorful cast of characters, ranging from established medical professionals to psychic healers and Indian Shamans. Like most American experiential movements, it is centered on the West Coast, though its practitioners are scattered around the nation." Many people, however, give special credit to the influence of Granger E. Westberg (see his Theological Roots of Wholistic Health Care, 1979). Berliner and Salmon highlight positive features of wholistic medicine in giving people a sense of caring for themselves.

31. Fabrega (1982, p. 34) states "at least diagnosis and treatment of illness in modern societies constitute enterprises that have, relatively speaking, [few] immediate religious and political overtones."

32. It is difficult to summarize the literature criticizing the medical profession because it is written from multiple positions. For some discussion, see Fox and Willis (1983).

33. See Vanderpoof (1984). For an instance of blanket condemnation, see Glymour

and Stalker (1983), who point out some of the banal rhetoric of wholistic medicine, its attempt to substitute a magical for an engineering conception of the physician, and its attack on scientific understanding and reasoning. The authors state emphatically: "Holistic medicine is a pablum of common-sense and nonsense offered by cranks and quacks and failed pedants who share an attachment to magic and an animosity toward reason." The literature on wholistic medicine is vast, but little of it provides a balanced account. See Allender (1984, pp. 215–23).

34. G. M. Foster (1983, pp. 17–24) considers some stereotype views, including wholism, which he believes can be overrated in the context of traditional medicine.

35. This point is often made; e.g., by Saegert and Young (1983), considering the extent of nutrition and health knowledge. Also see Bruch (1974), Herbert (1980), Barrett and Barrett (1981).

36. For discussion on Germany, with some comparison to the United States, see Maretzki and Seidler (1985). In the United States not everyone would agree that practices are changing toward increased sensitivity to wholistic concepts. Armstrong (1984) notes that despite the widespread endorsement of an extended patients' view in the medical literature, most clinical practice today—particularly hospital-based—probably relies on older approaches to eliciting information.

37. For an introduction from a considerable range of literature, see Rosenblatt and Moscovice (1982). Much of the discussion is on inadequacy of health care due to lack of availability and accessibility of services. For a general review, see Parker and Sorenson (1978), who indicate that while a number of factors are at play —economic, social, and professional—unsatisfactory professional situations are probably the major factor. However, the authors note a study of reasons why physicians left rural Appalachian practices. They stressed lack of educational opportunities for children and lack of cultural activities for spouses (p. 156). The vast amount of discussion on rural sociology, much of which has been published in the journal *Rural Sociology*, cannot be summarized here.

38. Quotations from videotape prepared by Brian Alf. In 1978 a new group of people evolved who are interested in working on health issues outside clinics. Special attention is being paid to lay health advocacy programs. Many articles have appeared indicating problems of communication; e.g., King-ming New and Hessler (1972), which emphasizes the trend to hospital ambulatory care.

   Numerous interpretations have been put forward to account for patterns of behavior among Appalachian people. Many have described it as irrational recalcitrance. Some have said it is an institutionalized, nonrational response to frustration, which has been called an "analgesic subculture" (Ball, 1968). Among the informants we met, we rarely found views that can be interpreted as obstinate traditionalism. It is more a profound faith in experience and fundamental religious views and kinship amid a culture among which commercial pressures to change have been relatively limited owing to comparative isolation.

39. Arguments in the general medical literature for a basic knowledge of folk medicine by physicians are not commonplace, but see views in Saunders and Hewes (1953), which have been repeated from time to time. For some relevant comments on a rather limited comprehension of health care by many physicians, see Ben-

net (1974). The reductionist approach has often been questioned; e.g., Pellegrino (1983, pp. 153–72). For a discussion of this approach to defining medicine in terms of its goals, see Kass (1975). For one of many articles underscoring the value of understanding symbolism associated with drugs and treatment, see Helman (1981).

40. Vogel (1970, p. 129) quoting an 1894 publication.

41. It is appropriate to stress again that the promotion of old remedies is both obvious and subtle in, for instance, repeated newspaper articles, some with the imprimatur of regular practice. For example, Francis Head Tripp, writing a feature in the *Chapel Hill Newspaper* (19 June 1983, p. 6A) on "Home Remedies Worked Sometimes," concluded: "Imagine my surprise recently when I discovered from a pharmacist that these remedies actually had a scientific basis." Examples noted in the article include castor oil, Black Draught, senna-leaf tea, Carter's Little Liver Pills, Epsom salts, 666 tonic, "the dangerous calomel," and kerosene. On the other hand, it also is appropriate to note the long lists of quite extraordinary remedies used nowadays for such problems as arthritis and herpes; they tend to cast doubt on any rationality in home medicine—for herpes, from carburetor fluid to peanut butter have been used (*Time*, 2 August 1984, p. 69). For a view that 90 percent of medical problems are managed by self-care, see Dean (1981).

42. Limited compliance has been shown to be common among persons of all social and demographic types. For a review, see Podell (1975), which stresses that patient noncompliance cannot be explained by any single factor; it is multifactorial, with the physician-patient relationship playing a key role. Reviews prior to 1974 indicate that of patients with symptomatic disease, about 20 percent do not keep their appointments and about 50 percent do not take their medicines as directed. Noncompliance was higher with symptomless problems, 50 percent and 60 percent, respectively. Such figures apply to hospital clinic situations and also probably private practice. Physicians often underestimate the extent of noncompliance. While health education generally is thought to be of considerable value in improving compliance, the pitfalls of health education—at least health education "programs"—must not be underestimated. See, for example, B. T. Williams (1984).

43. Such topics might facilitate communications between pharmacists and customers. For suggestions on the need for this, see Dickson and Rodowskas (1975).

44. Brody (1980, p. 103).

45. Gowdey (1983, p. 924).

46. Helman (1978, p. 133). It is appropriate to add that the number of failures in communication over prescription products is high. See R. W. Miller (1983).

47. *British National Formulary*, no. 6 (1983): 120.

48. Cf. "The European Region," in Bannerman et al. (1983, p. 240).

49. Omitted is reference to analogies to other traditional practices found in America and elsewhere; for example, witchcraft, sorcery, spirit or demon intrusion, susto, evil eye. A number of comparative studies are especially pertinent; for example, W. I. Jones (1976) indicates that common features can be found among matrices of ideas reflecting traditional patterns of thinking or preconceptions: static/dynamic, continuity/discreteness, abstract/concrete, and immediacy/medications.

Jones indicates that such concepts serve to explain differences and common threads between Western and Chinese science. For bibliographies providing other key references, see Harrison and Cosminsky (1976).

50. For some background discussion, see McQueen (1985). The rise and fall of interest is documented, mainly in professional medicine. It seems clear to us that, in herbal medicine, word-of-mouth testimonials about Chinese herbs have been very important. Nevertheless, Bass recollected for us one such article found in *Prevention* 28 (1976): 23–30 ("Looking for Chinese Health Secrets"). For discussion on bicentric patterns, see H. Li (1952).

51. Bass and the author reviewed in detail *A Barefoot Doctor's Manual* (1977).

52. Personal communication, Dr. K. Y. Kuang.

53. Ibid.

54. Ibid. At the same time belief in the presence of active constituents exists; see Brekhman et al. (1981), Brekhman and Grinevitch (1981).

55. Bibeau (1985) discusses trends in traditional Chinese medicine, except for information on the new integrated medicine, which was obtained from Dr. Kuang.

56. The title of an article by Akerele (*World Health*, 1983). Akerele discusses the activities of WHO's promotional efforts and highlights dangers of exploitation. Various directions include consideration of plants for fertility control, various diseases, and safety.

57. Quick (1982, p. 247), from which our summary of major directions is taken. For other perspectives, likewise somewhat critical, see Vuori (1982).

58. This point has been made for many cultures by G. M. Foster (1984). Factors affecting a mix of "modern" and traditional medicine are considered by Elling (1981).

59. A paper that prompts thought on this issue is A. Young (1981).

60. G. M. Foster (1984, p. 849) highlights the declining numbers of traditional practitioners. From different perspectives, we follow views by Mechanic and many others who argue that the ability to exercise alternatives—to choose—is basic. Admittedly he mentions this in the context of regular medicine, but we believe the ability to choose extends beyond this. See also Relman (1980).

61. Pertinent background appears in such articles as Baer (1984).

62. A paraphrased quote from Robert Coles is used by R. B. Browne (1983–84). This is one of many recent discussions arguing for a better understanding of popular culture. Much discussion exists on the social roles of folklore, but still very useful is Bascom (1954).

Annotated Bibliography

Aakster, C. W. "Concepts in Alternative Medicine." *Soc. Sci. Med.* 22 (1986): 265–73.

Abel-Smith, B. "Global Perspective on Health Service Financing." *Soc. Sci. Med.* 21 (1985): 957–63. Background for consideration of cost of traditional practices.

Ackerknecht, E. H. *Medicine and Ethnology, Selected Essays*, edited by H. H. Walser and H. M. Koelbing. Bern: Huber, 1971. Emphasis on health care shaped by culture, though many papers focus on medical practices.

————. *Therapeutics from the Primitives to the 20th Century.* New York: Hafner, 1973.

————. "Zur Geschichte der Krebsbehandlung." *Gesnerus* 37 (1980): 189–97.

————. *A Short History of Medicine.* Baltimore: Johns Hopkins University Press, 1982.

Adams, C. F. *Nutritive Value of American Food, in Common Units.* Washington, D.C.: Agricultural Research Service, U.S. Department of Agriculture, 1975.

Adler, H. M., and V. B. Hammett. "The Doctor-Patient Relationship Re-visited, An Analysis of the Placebo Effect." *Ann. Int. Med.* 78 (1973): 595–98.

Agich, G. J. "Scope of the Therapeutic Relationship." In *The Clinical Encounter, The Moral Fabric of the Physician-Patient Relationship*, edited by E. A. Shelp, 233–50. Dordrecht, Netherlands: Reidel, 1983.

Ahmed, P. I., and G. V. Coelho, eds. *Toward a New Definition of Health, Psychosocial Dimensions.* New York: Plenum Press, 1979.

Aikman, L. *Nature's Healing Arts. From Folk Medicine to Modern Drugs.* Washington, D.C.: National Geographic Society, 1977. Overview of herbal and other practices in various parts of the world. Documentary photographs.

Akerele, O. "Which Way for Traditional Medicine?" *World Health* June (1983): 3–4.

————. "The WHO Traditional Medicine Program: Policy and Implementations." *Int. Trad. Med. Newsletter* 1, no. 1 (1985): 1–3.

Albert-Puleo, M. "Fennel and Anise as Estrogenic Agents." *J. Ethnopharmacol.* 2 (1980): 337–44.

————. "Physiological Effects of Cabbage with Reference to Its Potential as a Dietary Cancer-Inhibitor and Its Use in Ancient Medicine." *J. Ethnopharmacol.* 9 (1983): 261–72.

Alcorn, J. B. *Huastec Mayan Ethnobotany*. Austin: University of Texas Press, 1984.

Alexander, A. L. "Menstrual Disorders." *Trans. Med. Soc. North Carolina* 44 (1897): 83–88.

Allen, H. B. *The Useful Companion and Artificer's Assistant*. New York: N.p., 1893.

Allender, E. "Holistic Medicine as a Method of Causal Explanation, Treatment, and Prevention in Clinical Work: Obstacle or Opportunity for Development?" In *Health, Disease, and Causal Explanations in Medicine*, edited by L. Nordenfelt and B. I. B. Lindahl, 215–23. Boston: Reidel, 1984. A critique of thinking within wholistic medicine.

Allport, N. L. *The Chemistry and Pharmacy of Vegetable Drugs*. Brooklyn: Chemical Publishing, 1944.

"American Medical Writers." *Boston Med. Surg. J.* 6 (1832–33): 142–44.

Ames, N. *An Astronomical Diary or Almanack, for the Year of Our Lord Christ 1770*. Boston: N.p., 1770.

Anderson, F. J. *An Illustrated History of the Herbals*. New York: Columbia University Press, 1977.

Anderson, L. A., and J. D. Phillipson. "Herbal Medicine, Education, and the Pharmacist." *Pharm. J.* 236 (1986): 303–5, 311.

Andrews, T., with W. L. Corya and D. A. Stickel, Jr. *A Bibliography on Herbs, Herbal Medicine, "Natural" Foods, and Unconventional Medical Treatment*. Littleton, Colo.: Libraries Unlimited, 1982. An invaluable bibliography with 749 extensively annotated entries.

Arber, A. "Analogy in the History of Science." In *Studies and Essays in the History of Science and Learning*, edited by M. F. Ashley-Montagu, 221–33. New York: Schuman, 1944.

————. "From Medieval Herbalism to the Birth of Modern Botany." In *Science, Medicine and History. Essays in Honor of Charles Singer*, edited by E. A. Underwood, 317–36. London: Oxford University Press, 1953.

————. *Herbals, Their Origin and Evolution*. Cambridge: Cambridge University Press, 1953.

Armstrong, D. *An Outline of Sociology as Applied to Medicine*. Bristol: Wright, 1983. Short textbook with many sections relevant to present account.

————. *Political Anatomy of the Body. Medical Knowledge in Britain in the Twentieth Century*. Cambridge: Cambridge University Press, 1983.

————. "The Patient's View." *Soc. Sci. Med.* 18 (1984): 739–44.

Aronson, J. K. *An Account of the Foxglove and Its Medical Uses, 1785–1985*. London: Oxford University Press, 1985.

Ataudo, E. S. "Traditional Medicine and Biopsychosocial Fulfillment in African Health." *Soc. Sci. Med.* 21 (1985): 1345–47. The positive conclusion that traditional medicine can be used as "psychological" opium prompts questions relevant to the present study.

Atkinson, P. "From Honey to Vinegar: Levi-Strauss in Vermont." In *Culture and Curing. Anthropological Perspectives in Traditional Medical Beliefs and Practices*, edited by P. Morley and L. Wallis, 168–88. London: Owen, 1978.

Aurand, A. M., Jr. *The "Pow-Wow" Book*. Harrisburg: Aurand Press, 1929.

Badura, B. "Life-style and Health: Some Remarks on Different Viewpoints." *Soc. Sci. Med.* 19 (1984): 341–47. Emphasizes personal attitudes, many of which are prominent among Bass's visitors.

Baer, H. A. "Prophets and Advisors in Black Spiritual Churches: Therapy, Palliative, or Opiate?" *Culture, Medicine, and Psychiatry* 5 (1981): 145–70.

———. "A Comparative View of a Heterodox Health System: Chiropractic in America and Britain." *Med. Anthropol.* 8 (1984): 151–68. Raises questions about narrow functions and legitimization, and broadening of functions.

Bailey, L. H. *How Plants Get Their Names.* New York: Macmillan, 1933.

Baillon, H. "Botanique Médicale." In *Dictionnaire Encyclopédique des Sciences Medicales.* Paris: Asselin, 1869, 10:109–62. A helpful review with historical perspective.

Ball, R. A. "A Poverty Case: The Analgesic Subculture of the Southern Appalachians." *Amer. Soc. Rev.* 33 (1968): 885–95.

Balon, A. D. J. "Response to Symptoms." *Pharm. J.* 234 (1985): 532–36, 235:752–55. Reflects trends within modern pharmacy toward a more clinical practice. Raises questions about errors in interpreting symptoms without tests, a key problem for herbal practitioners.

Banister, R. *A Treatise on One Hundred and Thirteen Diseases of the Eyes and Eye-Liddes.* London: Kyngston, 1622.

Banks, A., ed. *First-Person America.* New York: Knopf, 1980.

Banks, W. H. "Ethnobotany of the Cherokee Indians," Master's thesis, University of Tennessee, 1953. Valuable for firsthand data collected.

Bannerman, R. H., et al., eds. *Traditional Medicine and Health Care Coverage.* Geneva: World Health Organization, 1983.

A Barefoot Doctor's Manual. Rev. and enl. ed. Seattle: Revolutionary Health Community of Hunan Province, 1977.

Barlett, P. F., and S. M. Low. "Nervios in Rural Costa Rica." *Med. Anthropol.* 4 (1980): 523–64.

Barrett, V. H., and S. Barrett. *Vitamins and "Health" Foods. The Great American Hustle.* Philadelphia: Stickley, 1981.

Bartholow, R. *A Practical Treatise on Materia Medica and Therapeutics.* 1876. Reprint. New York: Appleton, 1882.

Barton, B. S. *Collections for an Essay towards a Materia Medica of the United-States.* 3d ed. 1798. Reprint of 1810 edition. *Bull. Lloyd Library,* no. 1, series 1. Cincinnati: Lloyd, 1900.

———, ed. *Professor Cullen's Treatise of the Materia Medica.* Philadelphia: Parker, 1812. Contains interesting annotations to *Treatise;* see Cullen, 1789.

Barton, W. P. C. *Vegetable Materia Medica of the United States, or, Medical Botany.* 2 vols. Philadelphia: Cary, 1817–18.

Bartram, W. *The Travels of William Bartram.* Edited by F. Harper. New Haven: Yale University Press, Naturalist's ed. 1958.

Bascom, W. R. "Four Functions of Folklore." *J. Amer. Folklore* 67 (1954): 333–49. A seminal paper on the role of beliefs, many considered in our account.

Bastien, J. W. "Pharmacopoeia of Qollahuaya Andeans." *J. Ethnopharmacol.* 8 (1983): 97–111.

Bauman, E., et al. *The Holistic Health Handbook. A Tool for Attaining Wholeness of Body, Mind, and Spirit*, compiled by Berkeley Holistic Health Center. Berkeley: And/Or Press, 1978.

Baumann, E. D. "Historische Betrachtungen über die vis medicatrix naturae." *Janus* 40 (1936): 148–70.

Beach, W. *The American Practice Condensed, or the Family Physician: Being the Scientific System of Medicine: On Vegetable Principles, Designed for All Classes.* New York: M'Allister, 1848. Influential in the development of Eclectic botanical medicine.

Bean, W. B. "The Natural History of Error." *Trans. Assoc. Amer. Physicians* 72 (1959): 40–55.

Beard, G. M. *Our Home Physician: A New and Popular Guide to the Art of Preserving Health and Treating Disease.* New York: Trect, 1875. Gives a sense of keeping lay public up-to-date on medical developments.

Beckett, S. *Herbs for Rheumatism and Arthritis and Herbs for Prostate and Bladder Troubles.* Boulder: Shambhala, 1980. One of many advocacy books, widely known but with little historical or scientific basis for most of the claims made.

———. *Herbs to Soothe Your Nerves.* Boulder: Shambhala, 1981. An advocacy book uncritically employing historical sources.

Beier, L. M. "The Creation of the Medical Fringe, 1500–1700." *Society Social Hist. Med. Bull.* 29 (1981): 29–32.

Bell, J. *A Practical Dictionary of Materia Medica.* Philadelphia: Haswell, 1841. Adds articles on indigenous plants to English edition.

Bell, J. W. *The Colonial Physician and Other Essays.* New York: Science History Publications, 1975.

Benezra, C., et al. *Plant Contact Dermatitis.* Toronto: Decker, 1985.

Bennet, G. "Scientific Medicine?" *Lancet* 2 (1974): 453–56. "Just how scientific can we claim to be?"

Benoit, P. S., et al. "Biological and Phytochemical Evaluation of Plants. 14. Anti-inflammatory Evaluation of 163 Species of Plants." *Lloydia* 39 (1976): 160–71.

Benson, A. B., ed. *Peter Kalm's Travels in North America. The English Version of 1770.* New York: Wilson-Erickson, 1937.

Berg, A. O. "The Placebo Effect Reconsidered." *J. Fam. Pract.* 17 (1983): 647–50.

Bergen, F. D. "Popular American Plant Names." *J. Amer. Folklore* 6 (1893): 135–42; 7 (1894): 89–104; 8 (1896): 179–93; 10 (1897): 49–54.

———, ed. *Animal and Plant Lore.* Boston: American Folk-Lore Society, 1899. An interesting list of beliefs "collected from the oral tradition of English speaking folk." Most are known to Bass.

Berger, P. L., and T. Luckmann. *The Social Construction of Reality, A Treatise in the Sociology of Knowledge.* New York: Doubleday, 1966. A seminal study relevant to the present account by reminding readers of the complexity of factors that mold knowledge.

Berkanovic, E., et al. "Structural and Social Psychological Factors in the Decision to Seek Medical Care for Symptoms." *Med. Care* 19 (1981): 693–709. Raises questions regarding ability to understand decisions to use health services.

Berkeley, E., and D. S. Berkeley. *Dr. Alexander Garden of Charles Town.* Chapel Hill: University of North Carolina Press, 1969.

——. *The Life and Travels of John Bartram: From Lake Ontario to the River St. John.* Tallahassee: University Presses of Florida, 1982.

Berlin, B. "A Universalist-Revolutionary Approach to Ethnographic Semantics." *Bull. Amer. Anth. Assoc.* 3 (1970): 1–18.

——. "Speculations on the Growth of Ethnobotanical Nomenclature." In *Sociocultural Dimensions of Language Change*, edited by B. E. Blount and M. Sanches, 63–101. New York: Academic Press, 1977.

Berlin, B., et al. "Folk Taxonomies and Biological Classification." *Science* 154 (1966): 273–75. One of a number of papers raising questions about present-day herbalists' understanding of plants.

——, et al. "General Principles of Classification and Nomenclature in Folk Biology." *Amer. Anthropol.* 75 (1973): 214–41.

Berliner, H. S., and J. W. Salmon. "The Holistic Alternative to Scientific Medicine: History and Analysis." *Int. J. Health Services* 10 (1980): 133–47.

Berman, A. "Neo-Thomsonianism in the United States." *J. Hist. Med. All. Sci.* 11 (1956): 133–55.

——. "A Striving for Scientific Respectibility: Some American Botanics and the Nineteenth Century Plant Materia Medica." *Bull. Hist. Med.* 30 (1956): 7–31.

——. "A Confederate Recipe Book." *Amer. J. Hosp. Pharm.* 17 (1960): 169–71.

——. "The Eclectic 'Concentrations' and American Pharmacy (1847–1861)." *Pharm. Hist.* 22 (1980): 91–103.

Betts, L. "Folk Medicine in North Carolina." *North Carolina Med. J.* 35 (1974): 156–58.

Bhardwaj, S. M. "Medical Pluralism and Homoeopathy: A Geographic Perspective." *Soc. Sci. Med.* 14B (1980): 209–16.

Bhopal, R. S. "The Inter-Relationship of Folk, Traditional, and Western Medicine within an Asian Community in Britain." *Soc. Sci. Med.* 22 (1986): 99–105. Highlights culinary ingredients employed as medicinals.

Bianchini, F., and F. Corbetta. *Health Plants of the World. Atlas of Medicinal Plants.* New York: Newsweek Books, 1977.

Bibeau, G. "From China to Africa: The Same Impossible Synthesis between Traditional and Western Medicines." *Soc. Sci. Med.* 21 (1985): 937–943.

Bigelow, J. *American Medical Botany.* 3 vols. Boston: Cummings and Hilliard, 1817–21. A milestone in the publication of botanical books (see R. J. Wolfe below).

Bingham, S. *The Everyman Companion to Food and Nutrition.* London: Dent, 1987.

Black, W. G. *Folk-Medicine: A Chapter in the History of Culture.* New York: Folk-Lore Society, 1883. Still a valuable reference book.

Blake, J. B. "The Compleat Housewife." *Bull. Hist. Med.* 49 (1975): 30–42.

Blanco, L. *Physicians of the American Revolution.* New York and London: Garland STPM Press, 1979.

Blatherwick, N. R. "The Specific Role of Foods in Relation to the Composition of Urine." *Arch. Int. Med.* 14 (1914): 409–50.

Blumhagen, D. "Hyper-tension: A Folk Illness with a Medical Name." *Cult. Med. Psychiat.* 4 (1980): 197–227.

Blunt, W., and S. Raphael. *The Illustrated Herbal.* New York: Thames and Hudson, in association with the Metropolitan Museum of Art, 1979.

Boatright, M. C., et al. *Mesquite and Willow.* Dallas: Southern Methodist University Press, 1957. Various essays on Texas folklore, including medical practices.

Boerhaave, H. *Materia Medica; or, A Series of Prescriptions Adapted to the Sections of His Practical Aphorisms.* London: Innys and Manby, 1741. One of a number of Boerhaave's writings influential in establishing various treatments. Lists of drugs in pharmacological classification.

Bohm, H. "The Biochemical Genetics of Alkaloids." In *Biochemistry of Alkaloids,* edited by K. Mothes et al., 25–75. Weinheim: VCH, 1985.

Bolsterli, M. J., ed. *Vinegar Pie and Chicken Bread: A Woman's Diary of Life in the Rural South 1890–1891.* Fayetteville: University of Arkansas Press, 1982. Helpful for community-oriented values.

Bolyard, J. L. *Medicinal Plants and Home Remedies of Appalachia.* Springfield: Thomas, 1981. Records similarities to Mr. Bass's practices. Differences due to many factors, including regional, and probably to idiosyncracies of many informants.

Bordley, J., et al. *Two Centuries of American Medicine, 1776–1976.* Philadelphia: Saunders, 1976.

Borell, M. "Brown-Séquard's Organotherapy and Its Appearance in America at the End of the Nineteenth Century." *Bull. Hist. Med.* 50 (1976): 309–20.

Bose, B. "Honey or Sugar in Treatment of Infected Wounds." *Lancet* 1 (1982): 963.

Bouchard, C. *Lectures on Auto-Intoxication in Disease.* Philadelphia: Davis, 1898.

Bowers, J. Z., and E. F. Purcell. *Advances in American Medicine: Essays at the Bicentennial.* 2 vols. New York: Josiah Macy, 1972.

Bowman, I. A. "William Cullen (1710–1790) and the Primacy of the Nervous System," Ph.D. diss., Indiana University, 1975.

Boyer, L. B. "Folklore, Anthropology, and Psychoanalysis." *J. Psychoanalytic Anthropol.* 3 (1980): 259–79.

Boyle, C. M. "Difference between Patients' and Doctors' Interpretation of Some Common Medical Terms." *Brit. Med. J.* 2 (1970): 286–89. Significant differences shown between the "majority doctors' definition" and the number of patients agreeing with that definition.

Bradon, W. W. *The Oral Tradition in the South.* Baton Rouge: Louisiana State University Press, 1983. Considers southern oratory to be a genre all its own.

Brekhman, I. I. *Man and Biologically Active Substances. The Effects of Drugs, Diet, and Pollution on Health.* Translated by J. H. Appleby. Oxford: Pergamon Press, 1980. The view of an influential Russian author on the effects on health of a wide range of biologically active substances.

Brekhman, I. I., and I. V. Dardymov. "New Substances of Plant Origin which Increase Nonspecific Resistance." *Ann. Rev. Pharmacol.* 9 (1969): 419–30.

Brekhman, I. I., and M. A. Grinevitch. "Oriental Medicine: A Computerized Study of Complex Recipes and Their Components: Analysis of Recipes Intended to Cure Certain Diseases." *Amer. J. Chinese Med.* 9 (1981): 34–38.

Brekhman, I. I., et al. "Oriental Medicine. A Computerized Study of Complex Recipes and Their Components: Herbs Most Frequently Used in Traditional Japanese and Korean Medicine." *Amer. J. Chinese Med.* 9 (1981): 134–43.

Brendle, T. R., and C. W. Unger. *Folk Medicine of the Pennsylvania Germans: The Non-Occult Cures.* Norristown: Pennsylvania German Society, 1935.

Brieger, G. H. "History of Medicine." In *A Guide to the Culture of Science, Technology, and Medicine,* edited by P. T. Durbin, 121–94. New York: Free Press, 1980. Helpful bibliographic essay.

——— , ed. *Medical America in the Nineteenth Century: Readings from the Literature.* Baltimore: Johns Hopkins University Press, 1972.

Brockman, J., et al. "Facts or Artifacts? Changing Public Attitudes toward the Mentally Ill." *Soc. Sci. Med.* 13A (1979): 673–82.

Brody, H. "Persons and Placebos: Philosophical Dimensions of the Placebo Effect," Ph.D. diss., Michigan State University, 1977.

——— . *Placebos and the Philosophy of Medicine: Clinical, Conceptual, and Ethical Issues.* Chicago: University of Chicago Press, 1980.

Brookman, R., "Folk Veterinary Medicine in Southern Appalachia." In *Glimpses of Southern Appalachian Folk Culture,* edited by C. H. Faulkner and C. K. Buckles, 67–74. Tennessee Anthropological Association, Miscellaneous Paper, no. 3, 1978.

Brown, F. C. *The Frank C. Brown Collection of North Carolina Folklore.* 7 vols. Durham: Duke University Press, 1957–64. Vols. 6 and 7.

Brown, P. S. "The Vendors of Medicines Advertised in Eighteenth-Century Bath Newspapers." *Med. Hist.* 19 (1975): 352–69.

——— . "Medicines Advertised in Eighteenth-Century Bath Newspapers." *Med. Hist.* 20 (1976): 152–68. A review, primarily of commercialism behind the marketing of 302 proprietary medicines.

——— . "Herbalists and Medical Botanists in Mid-Nineteenth Century Britain with Special Reference to Bristol." *Med. Hist.* 26 (1982): 405–20.

——— . "The Vicissitudes of Herbalism in Late Nineteenth- and Early Twentieth-Century Britain." *Med. Hist.* 29 (1985): 71–92. Emphasizes diversity of herbalists.

Browne, R. B. *Popular Beliefs and Practices from Alabama.* Berkeley: University of California Press, 1958. Bass has heard of over 80 percent of the beliefs recorded. Most of those unfamiliar to him are, he believes, from black sources.

——— . "Popular Culture as the New Humanities." *J. Popular Culture* 17 (1983–84): 1–8.

Browne, T. *The Works of Sir Thomas Browne.* Vol. 4, *Letters.* Edited by G. Keynes. London: Faber and Faber, 1964.

——— . "Charming in Devon." *Folklore* 81 (1970): 37–47.

Browner, C. H., and B. R. Ortiz de Montellano. "Herbal Emmenagogues Used by Women in Colombia and Mexico." In *Plants in Indigenous Medicine and Diet. Biobehavioral Approaches,* edited by N. L. Etkin, 32–47. Bedford Hills, N. Y.: Redgrave, 1986.

Bruch, H. "The Allure of Food Cults and Nutrition Quackery." *Nutr. Rev.* 32 (supplement) (1974): 62–66. Deals with exploitation of scientific nutrition, etc.

Buchan, W. *Domestic Medicine.* London: Stahon, 1769, 1772.

Budge, E. A. T. W. *The Divine Origin of the Craft of the Herbalist.* London: Society of Herbalists, 1928.

Bulloch, V. L. *Sex, Society and History.* New York: Science History Publications, 1976.

Burch, G. E. "Experiments of Nature: Whole Leaf and Purified Alkaloids." *Am. Heart J.* 83 (1972): 845. Discussion on merits of extracts and purified active principles.

Burke, P. *Popular Culture in Early Modern Europe.* New York: Harper and Row, 1978.

Burland, W. L., et al., eds. *Obesity Symposium.* Edinburgh: Churchill Livingstone, 1974.

Burns, J. J., and P. J. Tsuchitani, eds. *United States–China Pharmacology Symposium Proceedings.* Papers presented by the delegation from the Chinese Academy of Medical Sciences and by American participants. Committee on Scholarly Communications with the People's Republic of China. Washington, D.C.: National Academy of Sciences, 1980.

Burton, C. S. "Warts and All." *North Carolina Med. J.* 45 (1984): 344. A letter recording a variety of cures.

Bush, A. "The Sweetest Cures." *Econ. Bot.* 28 (1974): 175–78. Sugar as a panacea.

Byerly, H. "Explaining and Exploiting Placebo Effects." *Perspect. Biol. Med.* 19 (1975–76): 423–36.

Bynum, F. A. L. *Cultivated Plants of the Wachovia Tract in North Carolina 1759–1764.* Winston-Salem, N.C.: N.p., 1979. Christian Gottlieb Reuter's list of plants grown at Bethabara, in the vegetable garden, the medical garden, and in fields. Pamphlet available from Old Salem, North Carolina.

Bynum, W. F. "Cullen and the Study of Fevers in Britain, 1760–1820." In *Theories of Fever from Antiquity to the Enlightenment,* edited by W. F. Bynum and V. Nutton, 135–47. *Med. Hist.,* supplement no. 1, London: Wellcome Institute, 1981.

Caliendo, M. A. "Factors Influencing the Dietary Status of Participants in the National Nutrition Program of the Elderly. Part 1: Population Characteristics & Nutritional Intakes." *J. Nutr. Elderly* 1 (1980): 23–39.

Calixto, J. B., et al. "Pharmacological Actions of Tannic Acid. I. Effects on Isolated Smooth and Cardiac Muscles and on Blood." *Planta Med.* 52 (1986): 32–35. Suggests there may be pharmacological action due to tannins in tannin-rich herbs.

Campbell, C. M. *The Lazy Colon.* New York: Blue Ribbon Books, 1924.

Campbell, J. C. *The Southern Highlander and His Homeland.* New York: Russel Sage Foundation, 1921.

Caplan, A. L., et al., eds. *Concepts of Health and Disease, Interdisciplinary Perspective.* London: Addison-Wesley, 1981. Some background on the way people handle illness.

Capp, N. *English Almanacs 1500–1800. Astrology and the Popular Press.* Ithaca: Cornell University Press, 1979.

Capron, G., and D. B. Slack. *New England Popular Medicine.* Boston: Curtis, 1848.

Carawan, G., and C. Carawan. *Ain't You Got a Right to the Tree of Life!* New York: Simon and Schuster, 1966.

Carlson, A. J., and V. Johnson. *The Machinery of the Body*. Chicago: University of Chicago Press, 1946.

Carmer, C. *Stars Fell on Alabama*. New York: Farrar and Rinehart, 1934. Includes list of "mountain superstitions" from Alabama mountain country.

Carpenter, K. J. "Effects of Different Methods of Processing Maize on Its Pellagragenic Activity." *Fed. Proc.* 40 (1981): 1531–35.

———, ed. *Pellagra. Benchmark Papers in the History of Biochemistry*. Stroudsbury: Hutchinson Ross, 1981.

Carroll, A., and E. de P. Vona. *The Health Food Dictionary and Recipes*. New York: Weathervane, 1973.

Carroll, M. P. "On the Psychological Origin of the Evil Eye: A Kleinian View." *J. Psychoanalytic Anthropol.* 7 (1984): 171–87. One of a number of works influenced by Alan Dundes's belief that folk traditions would die out if they were not constantly revivified with each succeeding generation. Discussions with Mr. Bass and other informants reinforce this interpretation.

Cartwright, A. *Health Surveys in Practice and in Potential: A Critical Review of Their Scope and Methods*. London: King Edward's Hospital Fund for London, 1983. Much pertinent information on gathering data, including memory errors, sampling errors.

Cartwright, F. F. *A Social History of Medicine*. London: Longman, 1977. A collection of essays.

Carver, J. *Travels through the Interior Part of North America in the Years 1766, 1767, and 1768*. Toronto: Coles, 1774. Reprint. *Bull. Lloyd Library*, no. 9. Reproduction Series, no. 5, 1907. Includes comments on general economic uses and incidental medical references.

Cassileth, B. R., et al. "Contemporary Unorthodox Treatments in Cancer Medicine. A Study of Patients, Treatments, and Practitioners." *Ann. Int. Med.* 101 (1984): 105–12. Shows wide range of treatments, including "detoxification and restoration," diet therapies, megavitamins, mental imagery, spritual faith healing, and "immune" therapy.

Castiglioni, A. *A History of Medicine*. Translated by E. B. Krumbhaar. New York: Knopf, 1941.

Castillo-Salgado, C. "Assessing Recent Developments and Opportunities in the Promotion of Health in the American Workplace." *Soc. Sci. Med.* 19 (1984): 349–58. Argues that health promotion goes beyond individual concerns, considering it in the setting of an environmental-social approach.

Cato, M. P. *On Farming*. Translated by E. Brehaut. New York: Columbia University Press, 1933.

———. *On Agriculture*. Translated by W. D. Hooper and H. B. Ash. Cambridge: Harvard University Press, 1934.

Chambers, C. D.; J. A. Inciardi; and H. A. Siegal. *Chemical Coping. A Report of Legal Drug Use in the United States*. New York: Spectrum, 1975. Estimated that nine million people are "currently or regularly coping chemically" on over-the-counter sleep inducers, stimulants, and tranquilizers.

Chandler, J. *A Treatise of the Disease Called a Cold*. London: Millar, 1761.

Chandler, R. F. "Vindication of Maritime Indian Herbal Remedies." *J. Ethnopharmacol.* 9 (1983): 323–27.

Chandler, R. F., et al. "Controversial Laetrile." *Pharm. J.* 233 (1984): 330–32.

Chapman, A. "Astrological Medicine." In *Health, Medicine, and Mortality in the Sixteenth Century*, edited by C. Webster, 275–300. Cambridge: Cambridge University Press, 1979.

Chapman, N. *Discourses on the Elements of Therapeutics and Materia Medica*. Philadelphia: Webster, 1817–19. A useful volume containing many evidently firsthand observations. One of a number of books that implies much Indian usage.

———. *Elements of Therapeutics and Materia Medica*. 2 vols. Philadelphia: Carey, 1821–22 and 1831. An edition of Chapman's *Discourses* which included further critical thoughts and indicated differences between domestic and regular medicine.

Chappelle, M. L. "The Language of Food." *Am. J. Nursing* 72 (1972): 1294–95.

Chaudhury, R. R. "Folklore Herbal Contraceptives and Remedies." *Trends Pharmacol. Sci.* 7 (1986): 121–23. Includes interesting suggestions for testing folklore remedies.

Chen, T. S., and P. S. Chen. *Understanding the Liver. A History*. Westport: Greenwood, 1984.

Chesney, M. A., and R. H. Rosenman. "Specificity in Stress Models: Examples Drawn from Type A Behaviour." In *Stress Research. Issues for the Eighties*, edited by C. L. Cooper, 21–34. Chichester: Wiley, 1984.

Cheyne, G. *The English Malady: Or a Treatise of Nervous Diseases of All Kinds as Spleen, Vapours, Lowness of Spirits, Hypochondrial, and Hysterical Distempers*. London: Strahan and Leake, 1733.

Chirife, J., and L. Herszage. "Sugar for Infected Wounds." *Lancet* 2 (1982): 157.

Chirife, J., et al. "Scientific Basis for Use of Granulated Sugar in Treatment of Infected Wounds." *Lancet* 1 (1982): 560–61.

Chodoff, R. *Doctor for the Prosecution, A Fighting Surgeon Takes the Stand*. New York: Putnam, 1983.

Chowan College Creative Writing Group. *Southern Home Remedies*. Murfreesboro: Johnson Publishing, 1968. A useful collection reflecting commonplace and idiosyncratic remedies.

Christison, R. *The Life of Sir Robert Christison Bart, Edited by Sons*. 2 vols. Edinburgh: Blackwood, 1886. Includes much on promotion of plant remedies.

Clark, J. D. "Folk Medicine in Colonial North Carolina as Found in Dr. John Brickell's *Natural History*." *North Carolina Folklore J.* 17 (1969): 100–124. Useful compilation.

Clarkson, R. E. *The Golden Age of Herbs and Herbalists*. (Formerly *Green Enchantment*.) New York: Dover, 1972. An overview of generally well-known herbal literature.

Clay, F. M. *Coozen Dudley Le Blanc*. Gretna, La.: Pelican, 1973.

Claypole, E. W. "The Migration of Plants from Europe to America, with an Attempt to Explain Certain Phenomena Therewith." *Canad. Pharm. J.* 13 (1879–80): 172–79, 215–20, 252–55.

Clayton, J. "Medicinal Practices of the Virginia Indians." 1687. See B. G. Hoffman (1964) below.

Cleng, E. W., and W. Burroughs. "Estrogenic Substance in Forages." *Publ. Amer. Assoc. Adv. Sci.* 53 (1959): 195. Reflective of many papers of the time.

Clowes, W. *Treatise for the Artificiall Cure of Struma.* London, 1602. Reprint. New York: Da Capo Press, 1970.

Clute, W. N. *A Dictionary of American Plant Names.* Joliet: W. N. Clute, 1923. "Designed to bring together in a single list, all the vernacular names by which the plants of northeastern America are known." Invaluable list, though no indication of sources or which are the commonest names.

————. *A Second Book of Plant Names and Their Meanings.* Indianapolis: Clute, 1939.

————. *The Common Names of Plants and Their Meanings.* Indianapolis: Clute, 1942.

Cockerham, W. C. *Medical Sociology.* Englewood Cliffs: Prentice-Hall, 1982.

Colden, J. *Botanic Manuscript of Jane Colden 1724–1766.* New York: Garden Club of Orange and Dutchess Counties, 1963.

Coles, R. *Migrants, Sharecroppers, Mountaineers.* Vol. 2 of *Children of Crisis.* Boston: Little, Brown, 1971. Much background on the region.

"Complementary Medicine: Exploring the Effectiveness of Healing," *Lancet* 2 (1985): 1177–78.

Comstock, G. W., and K. B. Partridge. "Church Attendance and Health." *J. Chron. Dis.* 25 (1972): 665–72.

Conrow, R., and A. Hecksel. *Herbal Pathfinders.* Santa Barbara: Woodbridge Press, 1983. Brief portraits of a diverse range of practitioners promoting herbal remedies, including Tommie Bass.

Consumers Union. *Health Quackery. Consumers Union Report of False Health Claims, Worthless Remedies, and Unproved Theories.* New York: Holt, Rhinehart, and Winston, 1980. One of many combative publications, but providing judicious warnings.

Controller Papers. Southern Historical Collections. University of North Carolina, Chapel Hill.

Conway, G. A., and J. C. Slocumb. "Plants Used as Abortifacients and Emmenagogues by Spanish New Mexicans." *J. Ethnopharmacol.* 1 (1979–80): 241–61.

Cook, C., and D. Baisden. "Ancillary Use of Folk Medicine by Patients in Primary Care Clinics in Southwestern West Virginia." *Southern Med. J.* 79 (1986): 1098–1101. Seventy-three percent of the respondents used one or more remedies during twelve months. Many botanicals listed.

Cook, W. H. *The Physio-Medical Dispensatory.* Cincinnati: Cook, 1869.

Cooper, C. L., ed. *Stress Research Issues for the Eighties.* Chichester: Wiley, 1984.

Cooper, H. *North Carolina Mountain Folklore and Miscellany.* Murfreesboro: Johnson Publishing, 1972.

Cooter, R. "Interpreting the Fringe." *Society Social Hist. Med. Bull.* 29 (1981): 33–36.

Copeman, W. S. C. *A Short History of the Gout and the Rheumatic Diseases.* Berkeley: University of California Press, 1964. Much information on specific treatments and moderate regimens.

Core, E. L. "Ethnobotany of the Southern Appalachian Aborigines." *Econ. Bot.* 21 (1967): 199–214.

Corlett, W. *The Medicine Man of the American Indian and His Cultural Background.* Springfield: Thomas, 1935.

Cornut, J.-P. *Canadensium Plantarum.* 1635. Reprint. Murphreesboro: Johnson, 1966. The first book devoted entirely to North American plants. J. Stannard's introduction to reprint edition includes a list of probable modern identifications.

Corsi, P., and P. Weindling. *Information Sources in the History of Science and Medicine.* London: Butterworth Scientific, 1983. Useful surveys and bibliographies.

Cosminsky, S., and I. E. Harrison. *Traditional Medicine: Implications for Ethnomedicine, Ethnopharmacology, Maternal and Child Health, Mental Health, and Public Health. An Annotated Bibliography of Africa, Latin America, and the Caribbean.* Vol. 1. New York: Garland, 1976.

———. *Traditional Medicine. Current Research with Implications for Ethnomedicine, Ethnopharmacology, Maternal and Child Health, Mental Health, and Public Health. An Annotated Bibliography of Africa, Latin America, and the Caribbean.* Vol. 2, *1976–1981.* New York: Garland, 1984.

"Coste's Compendium Pharmaceuticum." Reprinted in *Badger Pharmacist,* nos. 27–30 (1940). Coste's *Compendium* (1780) indicated a basis of European drugs, though many items (e.g., couch grass, roots, yellow dock roots) could be obtained locally.

Coulter, H. L. "Divided Legacy: A History of the Schism in Medical Thought." In *Science and Ethics in American Medicine, 1800–1914.* Vol. 3. Washington, D.C.: McGrath, 1973.

Court, W. E. "The Doctrine of Signatures or Similitudes." *Trends Pharmacol. Sci.* 6 (1985): 225–27.

———. "Squill—Energetic Diuretic." *Pharm. J.* 235 (1985): 194–97.

Coury, C. "The Basic Principles of Medicine in the Primitive Mind." *Med. Hist.* 11 (1967): 111–27.

Cowen, D. L. "The British North American Colonies as a Source of Drugs." *Veröff Int. Gesell. Gesch. Pharm.* 28 (1966): 47–59.

———. "The Impact of the Materia Medica of the North American Indians on Professional Practice." *Veröff Int. Gesell. Gesch. Pharm.* 53 (1984): 51–63.

———. "Zum Dienst des germeinen Mannes, insonderheit für die Landleute" (The domestic and veterinary medicine books printed in colonial North America and the United States in the German language). In *Orbis Pictus: Kultur- und pharmaziehistorische Studien,* edited by W. Dressendörfer and W. D. Müller-Jahnke, 43–66. Frankfurt: Govi-Verlag, 1985.

———. "The Nineteenth Century German Immigrants and American Pharmacy." In *Perspektiven der Pharmaziegeschichte. Festschrift für Rudolf Schmitz,* edited by P. Dilg et al., 13–28. Graz: Akademische Druck in Verlagsenstalt, 1983. For reference to Charles Theodore Mohr (1824–1901), author of *Plant Life of Alabama.*

Cowen, D. L., and L. D. King. "George Beringer and Fluid-glycerites." *J. Amer. Pharm. Assoc.,* n.s. 6 (1966): 435–40.

Cowen, D. L., et al. "Nineteenth Century Drug Therapy: Computer Analysis of the 1854 Prescription File of a Burlington Pharmacy." *J. Med. Soc. New Jersey* 78 (1981):

758–61. Raises questions about everyday prescribing and common vegetable remedies such as opium, camphor, squill, cinchona, and rhubarb.

Cowle, C. J. Manuscript collections and North Carolina State Archives, Raleigh and
Southern Collections, University of North Carolina, Chapel Hill. Unless otherwise
noted, material quoted is in N.C. State Archives.

Cowle's Catalogue of Roots, Herbs, Seeds, &c. Leaflet. [1850s]. Southern Collection,
University of North Carolina, Chapel Hill.

Coxe, J. R. American Dispensatory. 1806. Reprint. Philadelphia: Dobson, 1814 and
1827. Based upon Duncan's Edinburgh New Dispensatory. It subsequently went
through nine editions. The third edition (1814) included much of the influential
dispensatory of James Thacher.

———. The Philadelphia Medical Dictionary. Philadelphia: Dobson, 1817.

Craker, L. E., and J. E. Simon, eds. Herbs, Spices, and Medicinal Plants: Recent Advances in Botany, Horticulture, and Pharmacology. Phoenix: Oryx Press, 1986.

Crellin, J. K. "Domestic Medicine Chests: Microcosms of 18th and 19th Century Medical Practice." Pharm. in Hist. 21 (1979): 122–31.

———, ed. Plants in Medicine: From Yesterday to Today. Durham: Medical History
Program and Trent Collection, 1982.

———, ed. Plain Southern Eating from the Reminiscences of A. L. Tommie Bass,
Herbalist. Durham: Duke University Press, 1988.

Crellin, J. K., and F. Nowell-Smith. "Popular Health Care. Historical Perspectives Based
on the Drake Collection." MS.

Crellin, J. K., and J. R. Scott. "Pharmaceutical History and Its Sources in the Wellcome
Collections. III. Fluid Medicines, Prescription Reform and Posology, 1700–1900."
Med. Hist. 14 (1970): 132–53.

Crellin, P. I., and J. K. Crellin. From Blackberries to Fishing Worms: Glimpses of Herbal
Medicine toward the End of the Nineteenth Century. A Manuscript, Written by
Willie Jordan Batts Around 1880, Illustrating the Persistence of Thomsonian Medi-
cine. Bailey, N.C.: Country Doctor Museum, 1987.

———. By the Patient and Not by the Book. Constancy and Change in Small Town
Doctoring. Durham: Acorn Press, 1988.

Crum, M. Gullah Negro Life in the Carolina Sea Islands. Durham: Duke University
Press, 1940.

Cullen, W. Lectures on the Materia Medica. Philadelphia: Bell, 1775; and Dublin, 1781.
An influential publication though unauthorized by the author.

———. A Treatise of the Materia Medica. 2 vols. Edinburgh: Elliot, 1789. An elaborated
version of the Lectures.

———. Professor Cullen's Treatise of Materia Medica . . . Including Many New Articles
Wholly Omitted in the Original. Edited by B. S. Barton. Philadelphia: Parker, 1812.

Culpeper, N. Complete Herbal and English Physician. Manchester: Gleave, 1826.

Cumston, C. G. An Introduction to the History of Medicine from the Time of the Pha-
raohs to the End of the XVIII Century. London: Kegan Paul, 1926. Reprint. London:
Dawsons, 1968.

Cunningham, J. J., and R. J. Cote. Common Plants, Botanical and Colloquial Nomenclature. New York: Garland, 1977.

Currie, W. *An Historical Account of the Climates and Remedies and Methods of Treatment which Have Been Found Most Useful and Efficacious Particularly in Those Diseases which Depend upon Climate and Situation.* Philadelphia: Dobson, 1792.

Curtis, J. H. *A Treatise on the Physiology and Diseases of the Ear.* London: Anderson, 1819.

Cutler, M. *An Account of Some of the Vegetable Productions Naturally Growing in this Part of America, Botanically Arranged.* 1785. Reprint. Bull. Lloyd Library, no 7. Reproduction Series, 1903. A useful list of plants with annotations, medical and nonmedical.

Czajka, P., et al. "Accidental Aphrodisiac Ingestion." *J. Tenn. Med. Assoc.* 10 (1978): 747–50. Indicates difficulty in ascertaining ingredients in over-the-counter preparations. A number contain red pepper amid various nontoxic products.

Daems, W. F. "Terminologische Probleme Mittelalterliche Pharmakobotanik." *Ber. Physico-Medica* (Würzburg) 88 (1981–83): 97–110.

Dagnall, J. C. "History of Corn Treatments." *Brit. J. Chiropody* 29 (1964): 249–52.

Darling, Dr. "Indian Diseases and Remedies." *Boston Med. Surg. J.* 34 (1846): 9–10.

Daugneaux, C. B. *Appalachia: A Separate Place, A Unique People.* Parsons: McClain, 1981. Innumerable facets of Appalachian life discussed.

Davenport, E., comp., "Plants, Other Remedies for Diseases, Superstitions, and Signs of Early Illinois Settlers." MS. 1914. Illinois Historical Survey, University of Illinois.

Davidson, J. R., and B. R. Ortiz de Montellano. "The Antibacterial Properties of an Aztec Wound Remedy." *J. Ethnopharmacol.* 8 (1983): 149–61.

Davis, A. D. "The Rise of the Vitamin-Medicinal as Illustrated by Vitamin D." *Pharm. Hist.* 24 (1982): 59–72.

Davis, R. B. *Intellectual Life in the Colonial South, 1585–1763.* Knoxville: University of Tennessee Press, 1978.

Dawkins, R. M. "The Semantics of Greek Names for Plants." *J. Hellenic Stud.* 56 (1936): 1–11.

Day, J. *Catalogue of Drugs, Chymical and Galenical Preparations, Shop Furniture, Patent Medicines, and Surgeon Instruments.* Philadelphia: Dunlap, 1771.

Dean, K. "Self-Care Responses to Illness: A Selected Review." *Soc. Sci. Med.* 15A (1981): 673–87.

———. "Lay Care in Illness." *Soc. Sci. Med.* 22 (1986): 275–84. Mostly covers Danish studies.

de Baïracli Levy, J. *Herbal Book for the Dog.* New York: Arco, 1983.

Debus, A. "Scientific Truth and Occult Tradition: The Medical World of Ebenezer Sibly (1751–1799)." *Med. Hist.* 26 (1982): 259–78. Debus sees Sibly as someone concerned with the severely mechanical approach to interpreting nature. Many who develop interests in alternative systems of medicine share similar concerns.

de Gorine, I. "The Socio-Cultural Aspects of Nutrition." *Ecology, Food, and Nutrition* 1 (1972): 143–63.

de Laszlo, H. G. *Library of Medicinal Plants.* Cambridge: Heffer and Son, 1958. Includes a useful bibliography.

Demling, L. "Volksmedizin, Erfahrungstherapie Ein Bestandteil moderner Behandlung?" *Fortschr. Med.* 94 (1976): 1193–1204, 1242–44. Like many writers, the author sees folk medicine as "empirical medicine," which we feel is an oversimplification.

Demlo, L. K. "Assuring Quality of Health Care. An Overview." *Eval. Health Prof.* 6 (1983): 161–96.

Dennie, C. C. "Old Doc." *Virginia Med. Man.* 83 (1956): 278–84. Various other references quoted.

Dickson, W. M., and C. A. Rodowskas, Jr. "Verbal Communications of Community Pharmacists." *Med. Care* 13 (1975): 486–98. Raises issues about communication in self-treatment.

Diethelm, O. "The Medical Teaching of Demonology in the 17th and 18th Centuries." *J. Hist. Behav. Sci.* 6 (1970): 3–24.

Doane, N. L. *Indian Doctor Book.* Privately published, Charlotte, N.C., n.d. Grandmothers' recipes, the type of small book that encourages Bass's faith in Indian medicines.

Dobell, H. *On Winter Cough, Catarrh, Bronchitis, Emphysema, Asthma.* Philadelphia: Lindsay and Blakiston, 1872.

Dodds, E. C., et al. "Oestrogenic Activity of Certain Synthetic Compounds." *Nature* 141 (1938): 247–48.

"Does Self-Medication Have a Role in Our Society?" *Food, Drug, Cosmetic J.* 36 (1981): 604–21.

Donnelly, W. J., et al. "Are Patients Who Use Alternative Medicine Dissatisfied with Orthodox Medicine?" *Med. J. Australia* 142 (1985): 539–41. Shows that 76.4 percent were satisfied with both orthodox and alternative medicines.

Dorson, R. M., ed. *Folklore in the Modern World, and Traditional History.* The Hague: Mouton, 1973.

———, ed. *Handbook of American Folklore.* Bloomington: Indiana University Press, 1983.

Dossie, R. *Theory and Practice of Chirurgical Pharmacy Comprehending a Complete Dispensatory for the Use of Surgeons.* London: J. Nourse, 1761. Notes a preposterous multiplicity of ingredients jumbled together in the manner of the ancients.

Dowling, H. F. "Comparisons and Contrasts between the Early Arsphenamine and Early Antibiotic Periods." *Bull. Hist. Med.* 47 (1974): 236–49. Issues about excessive unnecessary use.

Dragendorff, G. *Die Heilpflanzen.* Stuttgart: Enhe, 1898.

Driver, H. C. *Indians of North America.* Chicago: University of Chicago Press, 1969. Pp. 397–430.

Duffy, J. "Medicine and Medical Practices among Aboriginal American Indians." *Inter. Rec. Med.* 171 (1958): 331–49.

———. *The Healers: The Rise of the Medical Establishment.* New York: McGraw-Hill, 1976.

Dundas, R. *Interpreting Folklore.* Bloomington: Indiana University Press, 1950.

Dunglison, R. *New Remedies: The Method of Preparing and Administering Them; Their Effects on the Healthy and Diseased Economy.* Philadelphia: Waldie, 1839, 1843. Shows surge of interest in therapy following isolation of alkaloids.

———. *General Therapeutics and Materia Medica.* 2 vols. 1843. Reprint. Philadelphia: Lea and Blanchard, 1853 and 1857.

———. *A Dictionary of Medical Science.* 7th ed. Philadelphia: Lea and Blanchard, 1848.

Durant, M. *Who Named the Daisy? Who Named the Rose?* New York: Cogdon and Weed, 1976. More than a book on names; contains a potpourri of information.

Durkin-Longley, M. "Multiple Therapeutic Use in Urban Nepal." *Soc. Sci. Med.* 19 (1984): 867–72. A salutary reminder that questionnaire data do not always reflect actual practice.

Durodola, J. "Contribution of Traditional Medicine to the Chemotherapy of Cancer." *Nigerian J. Med.* 9, no. 5 (1979): 613–18. Review of treatments from many countries.

Dymock, W. *Pharmacographia Indica. A History of the Principal Drugs of Vegetable Origin Met with in British India.* 3 vols. London: Kegan Paul, 1890–93.

Earles, M. P. "Early Theories of the Mode of Action of Drugs and Poisons." *Ann. Sci.* 17 (1961): 97–110.

———. "The Pharmacopoeia Londinensis 1618: A New Look at an Old Problem." *Pharm. Hist.* 12, no. 2 (1982): 4–5. Relevant to the question of how much textbooks reflect everyday practice.

Eaton, A. H. *Handicrafts of the Southern Highlands.* New York: Russell Sage Foundation, 1937. Lists dyes and herbs.

Eberle, J. *A Treatise of the Materia Medica and Therapeutics.* Baltimore: Meeteer, 1824. A book of special interest for American viewpoints and firsthand observations.

Edwards, C., and P. Stilman. "Responding to Symptoms, Case Studies in Community Pharmacy." *Pharm. J.* 230 (1983): 110. The first of a series reflecting a trend within pharmacy.

Eidinger, R. N., and D. V. Schapira. "Cancer Patients' Insight into Their Treatment, Progress, and Unconventional Therapies." *Cancer* 53 (1984): 2736–40.

Eisenberg, L. "Disease and Illness. Distinctions between Professional and Popular Ideas of Sickness." *Culture, Medicine, and Psychiatry* 1 (1977): 9–23.

———. "The Subjective in Medicine." *Perspect. Biol. Med.* 27 (1983–84): 48–61.

Eisenberg, L., and A. Kleinman. "Clinical Social Science." In *The Relevance of Social Science for Medicine,* edited by L. Eisenberg and A. Kleinman. Dordrecht, Netherlands: Reidel, 1981.

Elferink, J. G. R. "Pharmacy and the Pharmaceutical Profession in the Aztec Culture." *Janus* 71 (1984): 41–62.

Ellers, R. *Miners, Millhands, and Mountaineers. Industrialization of the Appalachian South, 1880–1930.* Knoxville: University of Tennessee Press, 1982.

Elling, R. H. "Political Economy, Cultural Hegemony, and Mixes of Traditional and Modern Medicine." *Soc. Sci. Med.* 15A (1981): 89–99.

Ellingwood, F. "*Echinacea angustifolia.*" *Therapeutic Gazette* 29 (1905): 298–300.

———. *American Materia Medica, Therapeutics, and Pharmacognosy.* Evanston: Ellingwood's Therapeutist, 1915.

Elliott-Binns, C. P. "An Analysis of Lay Medicine." *J. Royal Coll. Gen. Pract.* 23 (1973): 255–64. Stresses importance of home medical care.

Ellis, B. *The Medical Formulary.* Philadelphia: Lea and Blanchard, 1849.

Ellis, H. *A History of Bladder Stone*. Oxford: Blackwell Scientific, 1969.

Elvin-Lewis, M. "Empirical Rationale for Teeth Cleaning Plant Selection." *Med. Anthropol.* 3 (1979): 431–58.

Elyot, T. *The Castel of Helth*. London: Berthelet, 1539.

Emboden, W. A. *Narcotic Plants, Hallucinogens, Stimulants, Lubricants, and Hypnotics, Their Origins and Uses*. New York: Macmillan, 1979.

Encyclopaedia Britannica. 18 vols. in 20. Edinburgh: Bell and Macfarquhar, 1797. Sections on medicine and on pharmacy.

Endecott, Z. *Synopsis Medicinae, or a Compendium of Galenical and Chymical Physick*. Salem: N and G, 1914. Publication of collection of seventeenth-century colonial recipes compiled by a practitioner. No clear influence of indigenous remedies, but at least references to readily available strawberry, plantain, sumac, and wild mallow.

Engs, R. C. "Health Concerns Over Time: The Apparent Stability." *Health Ed.* 16 (1985): 3–6.

Ephraim, J. W. *Take Care of Yourself*. New York: Simon and Schuster, 1937.

Erasmus, C. J. *Man Takes Control: Cultural Development and American Aid*. Minneapolis: University of Minnesota Press, 1961.

Ergood, B., and B. F. Kuhre. *Appalachia: Social Context Past and Present*. Dubuque: Kundull/Hunt, 1983.

Erikson, R. P. "Definitions: A Matter of Taste." In *Taste, Olfaction, and the Central Nervous System*, edited by D. W. Pfaff, 129–50. New York: Rockefeller University Press, 1985.

Estes, J. W. "Therapeutic Practice in Colonial New England." In *Medicine in Colonial Massachusetts 1620–1820*, 289–383. Boston: Publications of the Colonial Society of Massachusetts, 1980.

Etheridge, E. W. *The Butterfly Caste: A Social History of Pellagra in the South*. Westport: Greenwood, 1972.

Etkin, N. L. "Biomedical Evaluation of Indigenous Medical Practices." *Med. Anthropol.* 3 (1979): 393–400. Call for consideration of cultural context in the study of medicinal plants.

———. "A Hausa Herbal Pharmacopoeia: Biomedical Evaluation of Commonly Used Plant Medicines." *J. Ethnopharmacol.* 4 (1981): 75–98.

———, ed. *Plants in Indigenous Medicine and Diet. Biobehavioral Approaches*. Bedford Hills: Redgrave, 1986.

Evans, E. R., et al. *That Was All We Ever Knew. Herbal Medicine: A Living Force in the Appalachians*. Durham: Medical History Program and Trent Collection, Duke University Medical Center, 1982.

Evans, J. P. "Medicinal Plants of the Cherokees." *Proc. Amer. Pharm. Assoc.* 8 (1859): 390–97.

Evans-Pritchard, E. E. *The Azande. History and Political Institutions*. 1937. Reprint. Oxford: Oxford University Press, 1971.

Ewan, J. "Plant Collectors in America: Background for Linnaeus." In *Essays in Biohistory*, edited by P. Smit and R. J. Laage. Utrecht: International Association for Plant Taxonomy, 1970.

————. "Five Pupils of Benjamin Smith Barton: The Men and Their Minds." *Trans. Stud. Coll. Physicians Philadelphia* 5, ser. 5 (1983): 309–20. Their influence on and attitudes about popular remedies.

————, ed. *A Short History of Botany in the United States.* New York: Hafner, 1969.

Ewan, J., and N. Ewan. *John Banister and His Natural History of Virginia 1678–1692.* Urbana: University of Illinois Press, 1970.

"Exploring the Effectiveness of Healing." *Lancet* 2 (1985): 1177–78.

Fabrega, H., Jr. "The Need for an Ethnomedical Science." *Science* 189 (1975): 969–75. An oft-quoted call for new perspectives in medicine.

————. "The Idea of Medicalization: An Anthropological Perspective." In *The Use and Abuse of Medicine,* edited by M. W. De Vries et al., 19–35. New York: Praeger, 1982.

————. "The Scope of Ethnomedical Science." *Culture, Medicine, and Psychiatry* 1 (1977): 201–28.

Fantus, B. *Useful Cathartics.* Chicago: American Medical Association, 1920.

Farnsworth, N. R. "Current Status of Sugar Substitutes." *Cosmetics and Perfumery* 88 (1973): 27–35.

————. "The Development of Pharmacological and Chemical Research for Application to Traditional Medicine in Developing Countries." *J. Ethnopharmacol.* 2 (1980): 173–81. Notes how studies can contribute to safety.

————. "A Treasure House of Herbs." *World Health* (June 1983): 16–17.

Farnsworth, N. R., and A. S. Bingel. "Problems and Prospects of Discovering New Drugs from Higher Plants by Pharmacological Screening." In *New Natural Products and Plant Drugs with Pharmacological, Biological, or Therapeutical Activity,* edited by H. Wagner and P. Wolff, 1–22. Berlin: Springer-Verlag, 1977. Salutary review of practical problems.

Farnsworth, N. R., and C. J. Kass. "An Approach Utilizing Information from Traditional Medicine to Identify Tumor-Inhibiting Plants." *J. Ethnopharmacol.* 3 (1981): 85–99.

Farnsworth, N. R., and D. D. Soejarto. "Potential Consequence of Plant Extinction in the United States on the Current and Future Availability of Prescription Drugs." *Econ. Bot.* 39 (1985): 231–40. Of special interest for its lists of plants employed within the framework of regular medicine in the United States during 1980. Also, at least nine useful drugs derived from higher plants were developed and/or discovered during the thirty-one years from 1950 through 1981.

Farnsworth, N. R., et al. "Potential Value of Plants as Sources of New Antifertility Agents." *J. Pharm. Sci.* 64 (1975): 535–98, 717–54.

Farnsworth, N. R., et al. "Oncogenic and Tumor-Promoting Spermatophytes and Pteridophytes and Their Active Principles." *Cancer Treatment Rep.* 60 (1976): 1171–1206.

Farr, S. S. *More than Moonshine. Appalachian Recipes and Recollections.* Pittsburgh: University of Pittsburgh Press, 1983. Basically a cookbook, but contains some family remedies.

Faulkner, C. H., and C. K. Buckles. *Glimpses of Southern Appalachian Folk Culture.*

Tennessee Anthropological Association, Miscellaneous Paper, no. 3. 1978. Much background information.

Favretti, R. F., and G. P. Dewolf. *Colonial Gardens*. Barre: Barre Publishers, 1972.

Feiz, J., and P. Moattar. "Formulation; Preparation and Evaluation of Medicinal Plants on Quantity and Quality of Human Milk." Paper presented to International Research Congress on Natural Products, July 1985, Chapel Hill, North Carolina.

Fellman, A. C., and M. Fellman. *Making Sense of Self: Medical Advice Literature in Late Nineteenth-Century America*. Philadelphia: University of Pennsylvania Press, 1981.

Felter, H. W. "Biographies of John King, M.D., Andrew Jackson Howe A.B. M.D., and John Milton Scudde M.D." *Bull. Lloyd Library* 19. Pharmacy Series, no. 5, 1912.

————. "Genesis of American Materia Medica, Including a Biographical Sketch of John Josselyn and His Two Voyages." *Bull. Lloyd Library* 26 (1927).

Felterman, J. *Stinking Creek*. New York: Dutton, 1967.

Fenton, W. N. "Contacts between Iroquois Herbalism and Colonial Medicine." *Ann. Rep. Smithsonian Inst.* (1941): 503–26.

Fernald, M. L. *Gray's Manual of Botany*. 8th ed. New York: American Book Company, 1950.

Finkler, K. "The Nonsharing of Medical Knowledge among Spiritualist Healers and Their Patients: A Contribution to the Study of Intra-Cultural Diversity and Practitioner-Patient Relationship." *Med. Anthropol.* 8 (1984): 195–209. Raises the question whether cultural sharing is necessary between sacred healer and patient. Authority and other factors at play.

Fischer-Homberger, E. "Hypochondriasis of the Eighteenth Century—Neurosis of the Present Century." *Bull. Hist. Med.* 46 (1972): 391–401.

Fisher, A. A. "The Notorious Poison Ivy Family of Anacardiaceae Plants." *Cutis* 20 (1977): 570–91.

Fisher, J. L. "Development of Ethnobotanical Medicine and Its Prevalence among Afro-Americans in Winston-Salem, North Carolina." Unpublished MS, Bowman Gray School of Medicine, Wake Forest University, Winston-Salem, N.C., 1975.

Fisher, J. T. *A Familiar Treatise of Asthma, Difficulty of Breathing, Wheezing, Winter Cough, and Consumption of the Lungs with Other Information, and Explicit Directions for the Use of Stramonium Herb*. London: Sherwood and Jones, 1811.

Fisher, P. "Aims and Priorities for Research in Complementary Medicine: A Proposal for an Adverse Effect Reporting Scheme." *Complementary Med. Res.* 2 (1987): 35–44.

Fitzpatrick, J. C., ed. *The Writings of George Washington from the Original Manuscript Sources*. Washington, D.C.: Government Printing Office, 1931–44.

Flannery, E. J. "Should It Be Easier or Harder to Use Unapproved Drugs and Devices?" *Hastings Center Report* 16 (1986): 17–23. Individual choice versus government protection.

Flint, A. *Clinical Medicine*. Philadelphia: Lea, 1879.

Floyer, J. *Touchstones of Medicines. Discovering the Virtues of Vegetables, Minerals, and Animals by Their Tastes and Smells*. London: Johnson, 1687–91.

Flückiger, F. A., and D. Hanbury. *Pharmacographia: A History of the Principal Drugs of Vegetable Origin Met with in Great Britain and British India.* London: Macmillan, 1874, 1879.

Fogelson, R. D. "The Conjuror in Eastern Cherokee Society." *J. Cherokee Stud.* 5 (1980): 60–87.

"Folk Beliefs, Understanding of Health, Illness and Treatment." In *The Health of a Rural County: Perspectives and Problems*, edited by R. C. Reynolds et al., 111–19. Gainesville: University of Florida Press, 1976.

"Folk-lore Scrap Book." *J. Amer. Folk-lore* 9 (1896): 143–47. Information on Afro-American witchcraft.

Ford, C. V. *The Somatizing Disorders: Illness as a Way of Life.* New York: Elsevier Biomedical, 1983.

Ford, R. I., ed. *Nature and Status of Ethnobotany.* Anthropology Papers, no. 67. Ann Arbor: Museum of Anthropology, University of Michigan, 1978.

Forrest, R. D. "Sugar in the Wound." *Lancet* 1 (1982): 861.

Foster, G. M. Preface to *Modern Medicine and Medical Anthropology in the United States–Mexico Border Population*, edited by B. Velimirovic, 3–9. Washington, D.C.: Pan American Health Organization, 1978.

———. "Humoral Traces in United States Folk Medicine." *Med. Anthropol. Newsletter* 10, no. 2 (1979): 17–20.

———. "Introduction to Ethnomedicine." In *Traditional Medicine and Health Care Coverage*, edited by R. H. Bannerman et al., 103–13. Geneva: World Health Organization, 1983.

———. "Anthropological Research Perspectives on Health Problems in Developing Countries." *Soc. Sci. Med.* 18 (1984): 847–54.

———. "The Concept of 'Neutral' in Humoral Medical Systems." *Med. Anthropol.* 8 (1984): 180–94.

———. "How to Stay Well in Tzintzuntzan." *Soc. Sci. Med.* 19 (1984): 523–33.

———. "World Health Organization Behavioral Science Research: Problems and Prospects." *Soc. Sci. Med.* 24 (1987): 709–17.

Foster, G. M., and B. G. Anderson. *Medical Anthropology.* New York: Wiley and Sons, 1978.

Foster, S. *East-West Botanicals: Comparisons of Medicinal Plants Adjunct between Eastern Asia and Eastern North America.* 1986.

Fothergill, J. "Remarks on that Complaint Commonly Known under the Name of the Sick Headach." *Med. Obs. & Inquir.* 6 (1777–84): 103–37.

Fothergill, J. M. "On the Treatment of a Common Cold." *Practitioner* 15 (1975): 37–40.

Foulks, E. F., et al., eds. *Current Perspectives in Cultural Psychiatry.* New York: Spectrum, 1977.

Fox, R. C., and D. P. Willis. "Personhood, Medicine, and American Society." *Milbank Memorial Fund Quarterly Health and Society* 61 (1983): 127–47.

Francis, F. J. "Witchcraft, the Shaman and Active Pharmacopoeia." Paper 0549, presented at the Ninth International Congress of Anthropological and Ethnographical Sciences, Chicago, 1973.

Frank, R. G. "The John Ward Diaries. Mirror of Seventeenth Century Science and Medicine." *J. Hist. Med. All. Sci.* 29 (1974): 147–79.

Fraser, J. L. *The Medicine Men. A Guide to Natural Medicine.* London: Thames, 1981.

Frazier, K., ed. *Science Confronts the Paranormal.* New York: Prometheus Books, 1986. Critical evaluations.

French, J. *The Art of Distillation, or a Treatise of the Choicest Spagiricall Preparations Performed by Way of Distillation.* London, 1653.

Frick, G. F., and R. P. Stearns. *Mark Catesby. The Colonial Audubon.* Urbana: University of Illinois Press, 1961.

Friedenwald, J., and J. Ruhrah. *Diet in Health and Disease.* Philadelphia: Saunders, 1909 (and many other editions).

Friedl, J. *Health Care Services and the Appalachian Migrant.* Ohio State University, National Center for Health Services, Research Health Resources Administration, Department Health, Education and Welfare, 1978. Includes helpful review of literature.

Fries, A., ed. *Records of the Moravians in North Carolina.* Raleigh: Edwards and Broughton, 1922. Background to some of the changes considered in chapter 5.

Frik, J. V., et al. *Geschichte der Dermatologie Geographische Verteilung der Han Krankheiten Nomenklatur.* Berlin: Springer, 1928.

Fromm, E., and M. Maccoby. *Social Character in a Mexican Village.* Englewood Cliffs: Prentice-Hall, 1970.

Frost, G., and Y. Frost. *A Witch's Guide to Life.* Jerome: Luminary Press, 1985.

Fulder, S. *The Handbook of Complementary Medicine.* London: Coronet Books, 1984. A review of a wide range of alternative complementary practices; includes much documentation about recent trends in many countries.

Fulder, S., and R. Munro. *The Status of Complementary Medicine in the United Kingdom.* London: Threshold Foundation, 1982.

Furman, B. L. "Homeopathy." *Pharm. J.* 236 (1986): 70. Highlights emotive issues surrounding concepts of clinical evidence and scientific proof.

Furstenberg, A. L., and L. J. Davis. "Lay Consultation of Older People." *Soc. Sci. Med.* 18 (1984): 827–37.

Gabe, J., and P. Williams. "Rural Tranquility: Urban-Rural Differences in Tranquilliser Prescribing." *Soc. Sci. Med.* 22 (1986): 1059–66. Prompts questions about rural-urban differences.

Gábor, M. "Anti-Inflammatory Substances of Plant Origin." In *Anti-Inflammatory Drugs. Handbook of Experimental Pharmacology,* edited by J. R. Vane and S. H. Ferreira, 698–739. Berlin: Springer-Verlag, 1979.

Gaertner, E. E. "The History and Use of Milkweed (*Asclepias syriaca* L.)." *Econ. Bot.* 33 (1979): 119–23.

Galazka, S. S., and J. K. Eckert. "Clinically Applied Anthropology: Concepts for the Family Physician." *J. Fam. Pract.* 22 (1986): 159–65.

Garnier, M. *Description des Plantes, Utiles au Traitment du Cancer.* Avignon: Facquet et Jordon, 1840.

Garrison, F. H. *An Introduction to the History of Medicine.* 4th ed., rev. and enl. 1913. Reprint. Philadelphia: Saunders, 1929.

Gartrell, E. G. "Domestic Medicine in Colonial Philadelphia: The Manuscript Recipe Book of Elizabeth Coates Paschall." Paper delivered to Fifty-sixth Annual Meeting, American Association of the History of Medicine, Minneapolis, May 1983.

Gathercoal, N., and H. W. Youngken. *Check List of Native and Introduced Drug Plants in the United States Pharmacopoeia.* Prepared under the auspices of the Committee on Pharmaceutical Botany and Pharmacognosy, Division of Biology and Agriculture, National Research Council. Chicago, 1942.

Geertz, H. "An Anthropology of Religion and Magic." *J. Interdiscip. Hist.* 1 (1975): 71–89. A critique of Thomas's *Decline of Religion and Magic,* a seminal work indicating attitudinal shift during the seventeenth century away from dependence on the aid of superhuman powers.

Gendron, D. *Enquiries into the Nature, Knowledge, and Cure of Cancers.* London: Taylor, 1701.

Gentry, A. H., and K. Cook. "*Martinella* (Bignoniaceae): A Widely Used Eye Medicine of South America." *J. Ethnopharmacol.* 11 (1984): 337–43.

Gerard, J. *The Herball or Generall Historie of Plantes.* Original ed., 1597. London: T. Johnson, 1633, 1636. Reprint. New York: Dover, 1975.

Gibson, R. G., et al. "Homeopathic Therapy in Rheumatoid Arthritis: Evaluation by Double-Blind Clinical Therapeutic Trial." *J. Wholistic Med.* 5 (1983): 54–65.

Gifford, G. E. "The Charleston Physician-Naturalists." *Bull. Hist. Med.* 49 (1975): 556–74.

———. "Medicine and Natural History—Crosscurrents in Philadelphia in the Nineteenth Century." *Trans. Stud. Coll. Physicians Philadelphia* 45 (1978): 139–49.

Ginns, P. M. *Snowbird Gravy and Dishpan Pie. Mountain People Recall.* Chapel Hill: University of North Carolina Press, 1982. A collection of reminiscences.

Gledhill, D. *The Names of Plants.* Cambridge: Cambridge University Press, 1985.

Glymour, C., and D. Stalker. "Engineer, Cranks, Physicians, Magicians." *New Eng. J. Med.* 308 (1983): 960–64.

Gold, J., and W. Gates. "Herbal Abortifacients." *J. Amer. Med. Assoc.* 243 (1980): 1365–66.

Goldfrank, L., et al. "The Pernicious Panacea: Herbal Medicine." *Hosp. Physician* (October 1982): 64–75.

Goldwater, C. "Traditional Medicine in Latin America." In *Traditional Medicine and Health Care Coverage,* edited by R. H. Bannerman et al. Geneva: World Health Organization, 1983.

Good, B. J. "The Heart of What's the Matter. The Semantics of Illness in Iran." *Culture, Medicine, and Psychiatry* 1 (1977): 25–58. Notes the fragmented nature of much popular medicine.

———, and M.-J. D. Good. "The Meaning of Symptoms: A Cultural Hermeneutic Model for Clinical Practice." In *The Relevance of Social Science for Medicine,* edited by L. Eisenberg and A. Kleinman, 181–96. Dordrecht, Netherlands: Reidel, 1981.

Goode, G. B. "The Beginnings of Natural History in America." Smithsonian Institute, *Annual Report,* Jan. 30, 1897, pt. 2, 1901.

Goodwin, J. S., and J. M. Goodwin. "The Tomato Effect. Rejection of Highly Efficacious Therapies." *J. Amer. Med. Assoc.* 251 (1984): 2387–90.

Gordon, L. *A Country Herbal*. New York: Mayflower Books, 1980. Noteworthy for astrological concepts.

Goth, A. *Medical Pharmacology. Principles and Concepts*. St. Louis: Moseby, 1981.

Gottlieb, O. R. "Ethnopharmacology versus Chemosystematics in the Search for Biologically Active Principles in Plants." *J. Ethnopharmacol.* 6 (1982): 227–38.

Gowdey, C. W. "A Guide to the Pharmacology of Placebos." *Can. Med. Assoc. J.* 128 (1983): 921–25.

Gran, L. "Oxytocic Principles of *Oldenlandia affinis*." *Lloydia* 36 (1973): 174–78. A significant paper on methodology.

Gray, D. " 'Arthritis': Variation in Beliefs about Joint Disease." *Med. Anthropol.* 7, no. 4 (1983): 29–46. Australian study indicating wide range of beliefs.

Green, E. C. "A Modern Appalachian Folk Healer." *Appalachian J.* 6, no. 1 (1978): 2–15.

Green, J. R. *A History of Botany 1860–1900; Being a Continuation of Sachs' History of Botany 1530–1860*. Oxford: Clarendon Press, 1909.

———. *A History of Botany in the United Kingdom*. London: Dent, 1914.

Greenblatt, R. B., et al. "Aphrodisiacs." In *Psychopharmacology: Recent Advances and Future Prospects*, edited by S. D. Iversen, 289–302. Oxford: Oxford University Press, 1985.

Greene, E. L. *Landmarks of Botanical History*. Stanford: Stanford University Press, 1983.

Greene, S. B., et al. "Distribution of Illnesses and Its Implications in a Rural Community." *Med. Care* 16 (1978): 863–77. One conclusion is differences between black and whites.

Greene, V. W. *Cleanliness and the Health Revolution*. Soap and Detergent Association, 1984.

Greuter, W. "Floristic Studies in Greece." In *European Floristic and Taxonomic Studies*, edited by S. M. Walters, 18–37. Faringdon: Botanical Society of the British Isles, 1975.

Griffin, L. *Please Doctor, I'd Rather Do It Myself . . . with Herbs*. Salt Lake City: Hawkes, 1979. One of a number of books by this author which were having considerable influence by 1986.

Griggs, B. *Green Pharmacy: A History of Herbal Medicine*. New York: Viking Press, 1981. A chronological account of episodes in the use of medicinal plants, but the development of herbal medicine within the area of self-care is not made clear.

Grimé, W. E. *Botany of the Black Americans*. St. Clair Shores, Mich.: Scholarly Press, 1976. Includes a list of plants employed by slaves.

Gronovius, J. F., with J. Clayton. *Flora Virginica*. Leiden, Netherlands, 1739, 1743, 1762. The first edition was compiled by the Dutch botanist Gronovius, based on collections of John Clayton of Virginia. The second edition (1762) utilizes the binomial method of classification.

Grukow, H. W. "Catecholamine Activity and Infectious Disease Episodes." *J. Human Stress* 5 (1979): 11–17.

Guerra, F. "Drugs from the Indies and the Political Economy of the Sixteenth Century." *Analecta Medico-Histórica* 1 (1976): 29–54.

Gupton, O. W., and F. C. Swope. *Wild Flowers of the Shenandoah Valley and Blue Ridge Mountains.* Charlottesville: University Press of Virginia, 1979.

Guthrie, D. *A History of Medicine.* London: Nelson, 1945.

Haller, J. S. *American Medicine in Transition, 1840–1910.* Urbana: University of Illinois Press, 1981.

Halstead, F. G. "A First-hand Account of a Treatment by Thomsonian Medicine in the 1830's. Text and Notes." *Bull. Hist. Med.* 10 (1941): 680–87.

Hambridge, R. A. " 'Empiricomany, or an Infatuation in Favour of Empiricism or Quackery': The Socio-economics of Eighteenth Century Quackery." In *Literature and Science and Medicine,* edited by S. Soupel and R. A. Hambridge, 47–102. Los Angeles: William Andrews Clark Memorial Library, 1982. In part concerned with the rise of quackery.

Hamel, P. B., and M. U. Chiltoskey. *Cherokee Plants, Their Uses—A 400 Year History.* N.p., 1975.

Hamilton, A. *A Treatise on the Management of Female Complaints and of Children in Early Infancy.* New York: Campbell, 1792. Much emphasis on constitutional treatment.

Hammer, M. "Social Access and the Clustering of Personal Connections." *Soc. Networks* 2 (1980): 305–25.

———. " 'Core' and 'Extended' Social Networks in Health and Illness." *Soc. Sci. Med.* 17 (1983): 405–11.

Hand, W. D. "The Magical Transference of Disease." *North Carolina Folklore J.* 13 (1965): 83–109.

———. "Folk Medical Inhalants in Respiratory Disorders." *Med. Hist.* 12 (1968): 153–63.

———. "The Folk-Healer: Calling and Endowment." *J. Hist. Med. All. Sci.* 26 (1971): 263–75. A general discussion on the hierarchy of healers.

———. *Magical Medicine. The Folkloric Component of Medicine in the Folk Belief, Custom, and Ritual of the Peoples of Europe and America.* Berkeley: University of California Press, 1980.

Hand, W. D., et al. *Popular Beliefs and Superstitions. A Compendium of American Folklore from the Ohio Collection of Newbell Niles Puckett.* 3 vols. Boston: Hall, 1981. An invaluable collection and introductory material; folk medicine, vol. 1, pp. 255–506.

Hardin, J. W., and J. M. Arena. *Human Poisoning from Native and Cultivated Plants.* Durham: Duke University Press, 1974.

Hare, R. A. *A Text-book of Practical Therapeutics with Especial Reference to the Application of Remedial Measures to Disease and Their Employment upon a Rational Basis.* 1900. Reprint. Philadelphia: Lea and Febiger, 1909.

Harman, V. E. "A Cultural Study of a Mountain Community in Western North Carolina," Ph.D. diss., University of North Carolina, 1957.

Harper, C. "The Witches' Flying-Ointment." *Folklore* 88 (1977): 105–6.

Harris, B. C. *The Compleat Herbal. Being with Description of the Origins, the Lore, the Characteristics, the Types, and the Prescribed Uses of Medicinal Herbs, In-*

cluding an Alphabetical Guide to All Common Medicinal Plants. Barre: Barre, 1972. Reprint. New York: Bell, 1985. Notable for employing concept of doctrine of signatures.

Harrison, I. E., and S. Cosminsky. *Traditional Medicine: Implications for Ethnomedicine, Ethnopharmacology, Maternal and Child Health, Mental Health, and Public Health—An Annotated Bibliography of Africa, Latin America and the Caribbean.* New York: Garland, 1976.

Hartwell, J. L. "Plants Used Against Cancer: A Survey." *Lloydia* 30 (1967): 379–435; 31 (1967): 71–170; and others in a series. Reprinted in Hartwell, J. L. *Plants Used Against Cancer. A Survey.* Lawrence: Quarterman Publications, 1982.

―――. *Plants Used Against Cancer. A Survey.* Lawrence: Quarterman Publications, 1982.

Hartzema, A. G., and A. I. Wertheimer. "A Comparison of the 'Expectancies' of Three Different Populations about Self-Medication vs. Physician Care." *J. Soc. Admin. Pharm.* 1 (1983): 180–86.

Harvey, G. *Family Physician and House Apothecary.* London: T. R., 1676.

Harwood, A. "The Hot-Cold Theory of Disease. Implications for Treatment of Puerto Rican Patients." *J. Amer. Med. Assoc.* 216 (1971): 1153–58.

―――, ed. *Ethnicity and Medical Care.* Cambridge: Harvard University Press, 1981.

Hatcher, R. A., and M. I. Wilbert. *The Pharmacopoeia and the Physician.* Chicago: American Medical Association, 1907.

Haughton, C. S. *Green Immigrants: The Plants that Transformed America.* 1978. Reprint. New York: Jovanovich, 1980.

Hawes, L. E. *Benjamin Waterhouse, M.D.* Boston: Countway Library of Medicine, 1974.

Health Beliefs of the U.S. Population. Implications for Self-Care. Chicago: Center for Health Administrative Studies, University of Chicago, 1976.

Health from Field and Forest. Boston: W. E. Servall Company, 1917.

Hecht, A. "The Overselling of *Aloe vera.*" *FDA Consumer* (July–August 1981): 27–29.

Hedrick, U. P., ed. *Sturtevant's Notes on Edible Plants.* Albany: Lyon, 1919. Reprint. New York: Dover, 1972.

Hegnauer, R. "Arzneipflanzen Gestern, Heute und Morgen." *Planta Med.* 34 (1978): 1–25. One of many recent pleas for conservation of gene pool.

Heinerman, J. *The Science of Herbal Medicine.* Orem, Utah: BiWorld, 1980. An uncritical compilation.

Helfand, W. H., and D. L. Cowen. "Evolution of a Revolutionary Oral Dosage Form." *Pharm. Int.* 3 (1982): 393–95.

―――. "Evolution of Pharmaceutical Oral Dosage Forms." *Pharm. in Hist.* 25 (1983): 3–18.

Helman, C. G. "'Feed a Cold, Starve a Fever'—Folk Models of Infection in an English Suburban Community and Their Relation to Medical Treatment." *Culture, Medicine, and Psychiatry* 2 (1978): 107–37.

―――. "'Tonic,' 'Fuel,' and 'Food': Social and Symbolic Aspects of the Long-term Use of Psychotropic Drugs." *Soc. Sci. Med.* 15B (1981): 521–33. A strong reminder of popular concepts.

————. *Culture, Health, and Illness.* Bristol: Wright, 1984. A short textbook reviewing many topics relevant to the present account.

————. "Psyche, Soma, and Society: The Social Construction of Psychosomatic Disorders." *Culture, Medicine, and Psychiatry* 9 (1985): 1–26.

Herbert, V. *Nutrition Cultivism.* Philadelphia: Stickley, 1980.

Hertzler, A. A., et al. "Classifying Cultural Food Habits and Meanings." *J. Amer. Diet Assoc.* 80 (1982): 421–25.

Hikino, H., and K. Kiso. "Natural Products for Liver Diseases." In *Economic and Medicinal Plant Research,* edited by H. Wagner et al., 39–72. London: Academic Press, 1988.

Hill, C. E. "A Folk Medical Belief System in the American South, Some Practical Considerations." *Southern Med.* 64 (1976): 11–17.

————. "The Challenge of Comparative Health Policy Research for Applied Medical Anthropology." *Soc. Sci. Med.* 18 (1984): 861–71.

————. "Local Health Knowledge and Universal Primary Health Care: A Behavioral Case from Costa Rica." *Med. Anthropol.* 9 (1985): 11–23. Underscores some basic issues.

Hill, T. "Our Indigenous Materia Medica." *Trans. North Carolina Med. Soc.* 41 (1894): 91–94.

Hillard, J. R., and W. J. K. Rockwell. "Dysethesia, Witchcraft and Conversion Reaction. A Case Successfully Treated with Psychotherapy." *J. Amer. Med. Assoc.* 240 (1978): 1742–44. Raises issues of culture and hexing.

Hindle, B. *The Pursuit of Science in Revolutionary America, 1735–1789.* Chapel Hill: University of North Carolina Press, 1956.

Hine, F. R., et al. *Introduction to Behavioral Science in Medicine.* New York: Springer-Verlag, 1983.

Hinkle, L. E., Jr. "The Concept of 'Stress' in the Biological and Social Sciences." *Sci. Med. and Man* 1 (1973): 31–48.

————. "Stress and Disease. The Concept After 50 Years." *Soc. Sci. Med.* 25 (1987): 561–66.

Hirst, P. "Witchcraft Today and Yesterday." *Economy and Society* 11 (1982): 428–48.

Hoch, J. H. "The Legend and History of Passiflora." *Amer. J. Pharm.* 106 (1934): 166–70. Little on medical story.

————. "Bibliographic Materials in English Relating to the History of Pharmacognosy." *Amer. J. Pharm. Ed.* 23 (1959): 154–60.

Hocking, G. M. *A Dictionary of Terms in Pharmacognosy and Other Divisions of Economic Botany; A Compilation of Words and Expressions Relating Principally to Natural Medicinal and Pharmaceutical Materials and the Plants and Animals from which They Are Derived, Their Chemical Composition, Applications, and Uses.* Springfield: Thomas, 1958.

Hocking, G. M., and H. M. Burlage. "The Crude Drug Industry in North Carolina and Adjacent Areas." *Carolina J. Pharm.* 53 (1973): 29–40.

Hoffman, B. G. "John Clayton's 1687 Account of the Medicinal Practices of the Virginia Indians." *Ethnohistory* 11 (1964): 1–40.

Hoffman, G. N. "Mt. Lebanon Medicine Makers—the Shakers." *Pharm. Era* 53 (1920): 197–98, 229–31.

Hofling, C. K. "The Treatment of Depression: A Selective Historical Review." In *Depression. Clinical, Biological, and Psychological Perspectives*, edited by G. Usdin. New York: Brunner/Mazel, 1977.

Holland, J. C. "Patients Who Seek Unproved Cancer Remedies: A Psychological Perspective." *Clin. Bull.* 11 (1981): 102–5.

Hollick, F. *A Popular Treatise on Venereal Disease.* New York: Strong, 1852.

Holmstedt, B., and J. G. Bruhn. "Is There a Place for Ethnopharmacology in Our Time?" *Trends Pharmacol. Sci.* 3 (1982): 181–83. Notes, for instance, the need to deal with additive, synergistic, and antagonistic effects.

———. "Ethnopharmacology—A Challenge." *J. Ethnopharmacol.* 8 (1983): 251–56.

Horrobin, D. F. "The Role of Essential Fatty Acids and Prostaglandins in the Premenstrual Syndrome." *J. Repro. Med.* 28 (1983): 465–68.

Hort, J. A. "The Ethnobotany of the Northern Cheyenne Indians of Montana." *J. Ethnopharmacol.* 4 (1981): 1–55.

Howard, J. *Practical Observations on Cancer.* London: Hatchard, 1811.

Howe, J. W. *Excessive Venery Masturbation and Continence.* New York: Bermingham, 1884. Interesting references to use of substances (e.g., lupulin) as placebo for treatment of spermatorrhoea.

Howes, F. N. *A Dictionary of Useful and Everyday Plants and Their Common Names.* Cambridge: Cambridge University Press, 1974.

Hubbard, W. N. "The Origins of Medicinals." In *Advances in American Medicine: Essays at the Bicentennial*, edited by J. Z. Bowers and E. F. Purcell, 688–727. New York: Josiah Macy, Jr., Foundation, 1976. A chronological review from colonial times to the first effective chemotherapy.

Hudson, W. M., ed. *Hunters & Healers: Folklore Types and Topics.* Austin: Encino Press, 1971. Some examples of current usage.

Hufford, D. J. "Organic Food People: Nutrition, Health and World View." *Keystone Folklore Quarterly* 16 (1971): 179–84.

———. "Folk Healers." In *Handbook of American Folklore*, edited by R. M. Dorson, 306–13. Bloomington: Indiana University Press, 1983. Helpful for concepts of belief and disbelief.

———. "American Healing Systems, An Introduction and Exploration." Conference Booklet, Hershey Medical Center. Unpublished typescript, 1984.

Hulka, L. L., et al. "Correlates of Satisfaction and Dissatisfaction with Medical Care: A Community Perspective." *Med. Care* 13 (1975): 648–58.

Hultén, E. "The Amphi-Atlantic Plants and Their Phytogeographical Connections." In *Kungl. Svenska Vetenskapsakademiens Handlingar, Fjarde.* Bd. 7, no. 1. Stockholm: Almqvist and Wiksell, 1958.

Hultkrantz, A. "The Shaman and the Medicine-Man." *Soc. Sci. Med.* 20 (1985): 511–15.

Humphrey, H. B. *Makers of North American Botany.* New York: Ronald Press, 1961.

Hunn, E. "The Utilitarian Factor in Folk Biological Classification." *Amer. Anthropol.* 84 (1982): 830–47.

Hutchens, A. R. *Indian Herbology of North America.* Windsor: Merco, 1982. Widely quoted, but the eclecticism of sources used makes for much uncertainty.

Hutton, D. A. "Cordial Waters and Cordial Chests." *Pharm. Hist.* 3 (1973): 6–8.

Huxtable, R. J. "Herbal Teas and Toxins: Novel Aspects of Pyrrolizidine Poisoning in the United States." *Perspect. Biol. Med.* 24 (1980–81): 1–14.

Hyatt, H. M. *Hoodoo—Conjuration—Witchcraft—Rootwork.* 4 vols. Hannibal, Mo.: Alma Egan Hyatt Foundation, 1970–73.

"Inventory of Medicinal Plants: Selection and Characterization." *who Chronicle* 33 (1979): 56.

Irwin, J. R. *Alex Stewart, Portrait of a Pioneer.* West Chester: Schiffer, 1985.

Izaddoost, M., and T. Robinson. "Synergism and Antagonism in the Pharmacology of Alkaloidal Plants." In *Herbs, Spices, and Medicinal Plants*, edited by L. E. Craker and J. E. Simon, 137–58. Vol. 2 of *Recent Advances in Botany, Horticulture, and Pharmacology.* Phoenix: Oryx Press, 1987.

Jackson, B. "The Other Kind of Doctor: Conjure and Magic in Black American Folk Medicine." In *American Folk Medicine, A Symposium*, edited by W. Hand, 259–72. Berkeley: University of California Press, 1973.

Jackson, J., et al. "The Sea Islands as a Cultural Resource." *Black Scholar* 5 (March 1974): 32–39.

Jackson, S. W. "Melancholia and Mechanical Explanation in Eighteenth Century Medicine." *J. Hist. Med. All. Sci.* 38 (1983): 298–319.

Jacobs, M. L., and H. M. Burlage. *Plants of North Carolina with Reputed Medicinal Uses.* Privately published, Chapel Hill, 1958. The list does not include uses recorded in North Carolina, or the sources for the list.

Jain, S. K., et al. *Bibliography of Ethnobotany.* Delhi: Botanical Survey of India, Department of Environment, 1984. Uneven but valuable bibliography.

James, C. V. *Herbs and the Fountain of Youth.* N.p., 1969.

James, R. *A Medicinal Dictionary: Including Physic, Surgery, Anatomy, Chemistry, and Botany, in All Their Branches Relative to Medicine. Together with a History of Drugs . . . and an Introductory Preface, Tracing the Progress of Physic.* 3 vols. London: Osborne, 1743–45.

Janssen, W. F. "Cancer Quackery—The Past in the Present." *Seminars Oncology* 6 (1979): 526–36.

Jeffers, R. H. *The Friends of John Gerard (1545–1612) Surgeon and Botanist.* Falls Village: Herb Grower Press, 1967. Provides a different interpretation to the frequent criticisms of Gerard as a plagiarist.

Jefferson, T. *Notes on the State of Virginia 1781.* Edited by W. Peden. Chapel Hill: University of North Carolina Press, 1955.

Jerome, N. W. "Medical Anthropology and Nutrition." *Med. Anthropol.* 3 (1979): 339–51.

Jochle, W. "Menses-inducing Drugs: Their Role in Antique Medical and Renaissance Gynecology and Birth Control." *Contraception* 10 (1972): 425–39.

Johnson, A. T., and H. A. Smith. *Plant Names Simplified.* London: Collingridge, 1958.

Johnson, C. B. *Sixty Years in Medical Harness, or the Story of a Long Medical Life, 1865–1925.* New York: Medical Life Press, 1926.

Johnson, C. S. *Shadow of the Plantation*. Chicago: University of Chicago Press, 1934. Includes information from oral history, some on family remedies.

Johnson, C. T. *A Practical Essay on Cancer*. Philadelphia: Parker, 1811.

Johnson, J. *The Influence of the Atmosphere . . . on the Health and Functions of the Human Frame*. London: Underwood, 1818.

———. *A Treatise on Derangements of the Liver, Internal Organs, and Nervous System Pathological and Therapeutical*. Philadelphia: Clark, 1818, 1826.

Johnson, T., ed. *The Herball*. Rev. and enl. ed. 1633. (Originally by J. Gerard, 1597). Reprint. New York: Dover, 1975.

Jones, J. K. "Do Over-the-Counter Drugs Act Mainly as Placebos? Yes." In *Controversies in Therapeutics*, edited by L. Lasagna, 26–32. Philadelphia: Saunders, 1980.

Jones, L. C. "Practitioners of Folk Medicine." *Bull. Hist. Med.* 23 (1949): 480–93. A study based on an extant collection of folklore in Farmers' Museum, Cooperstown, N.Y.

Jones, M. O. "Toward an Understanding of Folk Medical Beliefs in North Carolina." *North Carolina Folklore J.* 16 (1967): 23–27.

Jones, O. L. *Peculiarities of the Appalachian Mountaineers*. Detroit: Harlo Press, 1967.

Jones, R. A., et al. "On the Perceived Meaning of Symptoms." *Med. Care* 19 (1981): 710–17.

Jones, R. K., ed. *Sickness and Sectarianism. Exploratory Studies in Medical and Religious Sectarianism*. Aldershot: Gower, 1985. A collection of essays of especial interest to the present account on exploration of similarities between medical and religious sectarianism. See, in particular, Jones's "The Development of Medical Sects," pp. 1–22.

Jones, W. H. S. "Ancient Roman Folk Medicine." *J. Hist. Med. All. Sci.* 12 (1957): 459–72.

Jones, W. I. "World Views and Asian Medical Systems: Some Suggestions for Study." In *Asian Medical Systems: A Comparative Study*, edited by A. Leslie, 383–404. Berkeley: University of California Press, 1976.

Jordan, W. C. "Voodoo Medicine." In *Textbook of Black-Related Diseases*, edited by R. A. Williams. New York: McGraw-Hill, 1975.

Jospe, M. *The Placebo Effect in Healing*. Lexington: Heath, 1978.

Josselyn, J. *New-England's Rarities Discovered*. London, 1672. Reprint with introduction and notes by E. Tuckerman. Boston: Veazie, 1865.

Justice, W. S., and C. R. Bell. *Wild Flowers of North Carolina*. Chapel Hill: University of North Carolina Press, 1979.

Kalm, P. *Travels in North America*. [1747–51]. Edited by A. B. Benson. New York: Wilson-Erickson, 1937. Reprint. Barre: Imprint Society, 1972.

Kandel, R. F., and G. H. Pelto. "The Health Food Movement. Social Revitalization or Health Maintenance System?" In *Nutritional Anthropology. Contemporary Approaches to Diet and Culture*, edited by N. W. Jerome et al., 327–63. Pleasantville, N. Y.: Redgrave, 1980.

Kapadia, G. J., et al. "Carcinogenicity of Some Folk Medicinal Herbs in Rats." *J. Nat. Cancer Inst.* 60 (1978): 683–86.

Kaposi, M. *Pathology and Treatment of Diseases of the Skin.* New York: W. Wood, 1895.

Karawya, M. S., et al. "Dephenylamine, an Antihyperglycemic Agent from Onion and Tea." *J. Nat. Prod.* 47 (1984): 775–80.

Kasl, S. V. "Pursuing the Link between Stressful Life Experiences and Disease: A Time for Reappraisal." In *Stress Research Issues for the Eighties,* edited by C. L. Cooper, 79–102. Chichester: Wiley, 1984.

Kaslof, L. J. *Wholistic Dimensions in Healing. A Resource Guide.* Garden City: Doubleday, 1978.

Kass, L. "Regarding the End of Medicine and the Pursuit of Health." *Public Interest* 40 (Summer 1975): 11–42.

Keill, J. *Essays on Several Parts of the Animal Oeconomy.* London: George Strahon, 1738.

Keith, A. *The Engines of the Human Body.* 1919. Reprint. Philadelphia: Lippincott, 1926.

Keith, B., and Company. *Revised and Enlarged Manual of the Active Principles of Indigenous and Foreign Medicinal Plants.* New York: Jersey City Evening Journal Print, 1882.

Kellogg, J. H. *Plain Facts for Old and Young.* 1882. Reprint. Buffalo: Heritage Press, 1974. Helpful for attitudes toward spermatorrhoea, etc.

Kelly, B., ed. *Southern Home Remedies.* Murfreesboro: Johnson Publishing, 1968.

Kendler, B. S. "Vegetarianism: Nutritional Aspects and Implications for Health Professionals." *J. Holistic Med.* 6 (1984): 161–72.

Kennedy, P. *Ophthalmographis; or, a Treatise of the Eye . . . to Which is Added an Appendix of Some of the Diseases of the Ear; Wherein is Observed the Communication between these Two Organs.* London: Lintoff, 1713.

Kephart, H. *Our Southern Highlanders.* New York: Outing, 1913.

Kertzer, D. J., and J. Keith. *Age and Anthropological Theory.* Ithaca: Cornell University Press, 1984.

Kett, J. F. *The Formation of the American Medical Profession.* New Haven: Yale University Press, 1968.

Kew, H. W., and H. E. Powell. *Thomas Johnson, Botanist and Royalist.* London: Longmans, 1932. Much background on Johnson's editions of Gerard's *Herbal.*

Kimata, H., et al. "Interaction of Saponin of Bupleuri Radix with Ginseng Saponin: Solubilization of Saikosaponin-a with Chikusetsusaponin V (=Ginsenoside-Ro)." *Chem. Pharm. Bull.* 33 (1985): 2849–53.

King, J. *American Eclectic Obstetrics.* Cincinnati: Wilstach, Baldwin, 1871.

———. *The American Family Physician.* Indianapolis: Douglass, 1878.

King, L. S. *The Growth of Medical Thought.* Chicago: University of Chicago Press, 1963. Pp. 111–26.

———. "The Road to Scientific Therapy, 'Signatures,' 'Sympathy,' and Controlled Experiment." *J. Amer. Med. Assoc.* 197 (1966): 250–56.

———. "Do-It-Yourself Medicine." *J. Amer. Med. Assoc.* 200 (1967): 23–29.

———. "Evidence and Its Evaluation in Eighteenth-Century Medicine." *Bull. Hist. Med.* 50 (1976): 174–90.

King-ming New, P., and R. M. Hessler. "Neighborhood Health Centers: Traditional Medical Care at an Outpost." *Inquiry* 9 (1972): 45–58.

Kirkland, J. W. "Traditional Medical Information Systems in Deep Run, North Carolina." *North Carolina Folklore J.* 30 (1982): 43–51. Argues that folk medicine remains vital and meaningful.

Kirschner, H. E. *Nature's Healing Grasses.* N.p., n.d.

Kleiman, M. B., and F. Clemente. "Support for the Medical Profession among the Aged." *Int. J. Health Services* 6 (1976): 295–99. Notes relatively low confidence in physicians among the elderly of low socioeconomic status.

Kleinman, A. "Medicine's Symbolic Reality." *Inquiry* 16 (1973): 206–13.

———. *Patients and Healers in the Context of Culture.* Berkeley: University of California Press, 1980.

Kleinman, A., and L. H. Sung. "Why Do Indigenous Practitioners Successfully Heal?" *Soc. Sci. Med.* 13B (1970): 7–26.

Kloos, H. "Food and Medicinal Plants Used by Armenian-Americans in Fresno, California." *Ethnomedicine* 5 (1978–79): 127–40. On persisting beliefs.

Kloss, J. *Back to Eden.* Santa Barbara: Woodbridge, 1972. An influential advocacy account of herbal medicine in many editions.

Knapp, D. A., and R. J. Michocki. "Placebos: Who's Being Fooled." *Amer. Pharm.*, n.s. 24 (1984): 4–5.

Koch, F. J. "We Spent the Day with Lloyd." *Eclectic Med. J.* 96 (1936): 203–10. Useful for insights into Eclectic practice.

Kolasa, K. "I Won't Cook Turnip Greens if You Won't Cook Kielbasa: Food Behavior of Polonia and Its Health Implications." In *The Anthropology of Health*, edited by E. E. Bauwens, 130–40. St. Louis: Mosby, 1978.

Kong, Y. C. "Potential Anti-Fertility Plants from Chinese Medicine." *Amer. J. Chinese Med.* 4 (1976): 105–28.

———. "*Evodia rutaecarpa*, from Pen t'sao to Action Mechanism." In *Proceedings of the 8th International Congress of Pharmacology, Tokyo.* Oxford: Pergamon Press, 1981. Pp. 239–41.

Kong, Y. C., et al. "Fertility Regulating Agents from Traditional Chinese Medicines." *J. Ethnopharmacol.* 15 (1986): 1–44.

Konturek, S. J. "Clinical Aspects of Gastric Protection." In *Proceedings of the 9th International Congress of Pharmacology, London.* Basingstoke, Hampshire: Macmillan, 1984. 3:341–44. A brief review indicating new pharmacological concepts perhaps relevant to explaining reputed herbal products.

Koos, E. L. *The Health of Regionville. What the People Thought and Did About It.* New York: Columbia University Press, 1954.

Kost, J. *Domestic Medicine. A Treatise on the Practice of Medicine.* Cincinnati: Sewell, 1859. A popular book written with sensitivity toward botanical rather than chemical medicines, and with an educational orientation.

Kramer, W. *Nature and Treatment of Diseases of the Ear.* Philadelphia: Waldie, 1838.

Kraus, M. "American and European Medicine in the Eighteenth Century." *Bull. Inst. Hist. Med.* 8 (1940): 679–93.

Krieg, M. B. *Green Medicine: The Search for Plants that Heal.* Chicago: Rand McNally, 1964.

Krieg, R. M., and P. Buchholz. "Barbiturate Misuse and Abuse. A Medical-Historical Perspective." *Illinois Med. J.* 147 (1975): 137–41. A reminder that concerns over abuse have paralleled recent growth of interest in herbs.

Krochmal, A., et al. *A Guide to Medicinal Plants of Appalachia.* Agriculture Handbook, no. 400. Washington, D.C.: Government Printing Office, 1971.

Kronenfeld, J. J. "Self Care as a Panacea for the Ills for the Health Care System: An Assessment." *Soc. Sci. Med.* 13A (1979): 263–67. Discusses self-care as a social movement and considers potentials and limitations.

Kronenfeld, J. J., and C. Wasner. "The Use of Unorthodox Therapies and Marginal Practitioners." *Soc. Sci. Med.* 16 (1982): 1119–25.

Kunitz, S. J. *Disease Change and the Role of Medicine: The Navajo Experience.* Berkeley: University of California Press, 1954. A reminder of various cultural factors at play in health care and expanding roles for the medical profession.

Kunitz, S. J., and A. A. Sorensen. "The Changing Distribution of Disease in Regionville." *Int. J. Epidemiol.* 4 (1975): 105–12. Comments on the classic study of Regionville by E. L. Koos.

Kunitz, S. J., et al. "Changing Health Care Opinions in Regionville, 1946–1973." *Med. Care* 13 (1975): 549–61.

Kuykendall, J. R., et al. *Profiles of Alabama Pharmacy.* Birmingham: Alabama Pharmaceutical Association, 1974. Provides some background to pharmacy in northeast Alabama at the time Bass was growing up and since.

Labadie, R. P. "Problems and Possibilities in the Use of Traditional Drugs." *J. Ethnopharmacol.* 15 (1986): 221–30.

Lacy, V. J., and D. E. Harnell, Jr. "Plantation Home Remedies: Medicinal Recipes from the Diaries of John Pope." *Tennessee Hist. Quart.* 22 (1963): 259–65.

Lambert, E. C. *Modern Medical Mistakes.* Bloomington: Indiana University Press, 1978.

Lamon-Havers, R. W. "Misrepresentation of Treatments of Arthritis." *Bull. Rheum. Dis.* 11 (1960): 223–26. Expresses concerns over quackery, including promotion of alfalfa tea.

Lasagna, L., ed. *Patient Compliance.* Vol. 10 of *Principles and Techniques of Human Research and Therapeutics,* edited by F. McMahon. Mount Kisco, N. Y.: Futura, 1976.

Lassek, E. V., and T. McCarthy. *Australian Medicinal Plants.* North Ryde, Australia: Methuen, 1983.

Laszlo, H. G. de. *Library of Medicinal Plants.* Cambridge: Heffer, 1958. Bibliography.

Lauterer, J. *Appalachian Profiles. Runnin' on Rims.* Chapel Hill: Algonquin, 1986.

Lawrence, C. J. "William Buchan: Medicine Laid Open." *Med. Hist.* 19 (1975): 20–35.

Lawrence, E. *Gardening for Love. The Market Bulletins.* Durham: Duke University Press, 1987. Much pertinent background, especially chapter on herb gatherers.

Lawson, J. *New Voyage to Carolina.* London, 1709. Reprint. Chapel Hill: University of North Carolina Press, 1967.

Leake, C. D. "The History of Self-Medication." *Ann. New York Acad. Sci.* 120 (1965): 815–22. One of a number of general articles which take the approach that "it is natural enough for people whenever they feel sick to try to do something for themselves."

Leighton, A. *Early American Gardens. "For Meate or Medicine."* Boston: Houghton Mifflin, 1970.

Leslie, C. "Medical Pluralism in World Perspective." *Soc. Sci. Med.* 14B (1980): 191–95.

Le Strange, R. *A History of Herbal Plants.* New York: Arco, 1977.

Levin, J. S., and J. Coreil. "'New Age' Healing in the U.S." *Soc. Sci. Med.* 23 (1986): 889–97. Suggests reasons (e.g., millenarian) that contribute to growth of interest and offers classification (mental or physical self-betterment, esoteric teachings, contemplative practice).

Levin, L. *The Hidden Health Care: Mediating Structures and Medicine.* Cambridge: Ballinger, 1981.

Levin, L., et al. *Self-Care: Lay Initiatives in Health.* New York: Prodist, 1976. Some historical perspectives.

Lewis, H. *Backways of Kent.* Chapel Hill: University of North Carolina Press, 1955.

Lewis, M. "The Antibiotic and Healing Potential of Plants Used for Teeth Cleaning." In *The Anthropology of Medicine,* edited by L. Romanucci-Ross et al., 201–30. New York: Praeger, 1982.

Lewis, R. H. *The Care of the Eyes and Ears.* Wilmington: North Carolina Board of Health, 1886.

Lewis, W. *Edinburgh New Dispensatory.* Philadelphia: Dobson, 1791.

Lewis, W. H., and M. P. F. Elvin-Lewis. *Medical Botany, Plants Affecting Man's Health.* New York: Wiley and Sons, 1977. A wide-ranging textbook with sections on herbology.

Leyel, C. E. *Herbal Delights.* 1938. Reprint. New York: Gramercy, 1986. One of a number of publications by Mrs. Lyell illustrating sustained interest in herbs in Britain during the 1920s and 1930s.

Li, H. "Floristic Relationships between Eastern Asia and Eastern North America." *Trans. Amer. Phil. Soc.* 42, pt. 2 (1952): 371–429.

Linares, E., and R. A. Bye. "A Study of Four Medicinal Plant Complexes of Mexico and Adjacent United States." *J. Ethnopharmacol.* 19 (1987): 153–83. Discusses groups and substitutes analogous to the practice of Bass.

Lindley, J. *Flora Medica: A Botanical Account of All the More Important Plants Used in Medicine.* London: Longman, 1838.

Lipkin, M. "Suggestion and Healing." *Perspect. Biol. Med.* 28 (1984): 121–26. An essay approaching placebo phenomena and medicine through a consideration of the role of suggestion.

Lipkin, M., Jr., and G. S. Lamb. "Couvade Symptoms in a Primary Care Practice: Use of an Illness without a Disease to Examine Health Care Behavior." In *The Use and Abuse of Medicine,* edited by M. W. De Vries et al. New York: Praeger, 1982.

Lloyd, G. E. R. *Science, Folklore, and Ideology. Studies in the Life Sciences in Ancient Greece.* Cambridge: Cambridge University Press, 1983. Particularly relevant because of relations between folk and scientific knowledge.

Lloyd, J. U. "Concerning the American Materia Medica." 1910. Reprinted from *Eclectic Med. J.* 94 (1934) and 95 (1935). Historical perspectives.

——. "The Eclectic Alkaloids, Resins, Resinoids, Oleo-resins and Concentrated Principles." *Bull. Lloyd Library* 12 (1910).

——. "Vegetable Drugs Employed by American Physicians." *J. Amer. Pharm. Assoc.* 3 (1912): 1228–41. Useful assessment of popularity.

——. "An American Crusade. A Phase of the Evolution of American Medicine and Pharmacy in the Struggle against Transplanted European Cruelty." Reprinted from *Eclectic Med. J.* 77 (1917).

Lloyd, J. U., and C. G. Lloyd. *Drugs and Medicines of North America*. Cincinnati: Lloyd, 1884–87.

Logan, M. H. "Anthropological Research on the Hot-Cold Theory of Disease: Some Methodological Suggestions." *Med. Anthropol.* 1 (1977): 87–112.

Long, D. "Medical Care among the North Carolina Moravians." *Bull. Med. Libr. Assoc.* 44 (1956): 271–84.

Looff, D. H. "Rural Appalachians and Their Attitudes toward Health." In *Rural and Appalachian Health*, edited by R. L. Nolan and J. L. Schwartz, 3–28. Springfield: Thomas, 1973. Much on the rural poor.

"Looking for Chinese Health Secrets." *Prevention* 28 (1976): 23–30. One of many recent popular articles contributing to growing lay interest, which by 1986 had become very conspicuous.

Loudon, I. "The Nature of Provincial Medical Practice in Eighteenth-Century England." *Med. Hist.* 29 (1985): 1–32.

Low, S. M. "The Meaning of *Nervios*: A Sociocultural Analysis of Symptom Presentation in San Jose, Costa Rica." *Cult. Med. Psychiat.* 5 (1981): 25–47.

Ludwig, A. M. " 'Nerves': A Sociomedical Diagnosis . . . of Sorts." *Amer. J. Pyschotherapy* 36 (1982): 350–57.

Ludwig, A. M., and R. L. Forrester. "The Condition of 'Nerves.' " *J. Kentucky Med. Assoc.* 79 (1981): 333–36.

——. ". . . Nerves, but Not Mentally." *J. Clin. Psychiatry* 43 (1982): 187–90.

Ludwig, E. G., and G. Gibson. "Self Perception of Sickness and the Seeking of Medical Care." *J. Health and Social Behavior* 10 (1969): 125–33.

Lynd, R., and H. Merrell. *Middletown*. New York: Harcourt Brace, 1929.

Lyon, J. L., et al. "Cancer Incidence in Mormons and Non-Mormons in Utah, 1966–1970." *New Eng. J. Med.* 294 (1976): 129–33.

Lyons, A. S., and R. J. Petrucelli. *Medicine: An Illustrated History*. New York: Abrams, 1978.

Mabry, J. H. "Lay Concepts of Etiology." *J. Chronic Dis.* 17 (1964): 371–86. Heterogeneity of symptom explanation emphasized.

McCamm, A. W. *Starving America*. New York: Doran, 1912. Basically a plea for eating food in the natural state.

McClure, S. A. "Parallel Usage of Medicinal Plants by Africans and Their Caribbean Descendents." *Econ. Bot.* 36 (1982): 291–301.

McCombe, S. C. "Folk Flu and Viral Syndrome: An Epidemiological Perspective." *Soc.*

Sci. Med. 25 (1987): 987–93. Many cases of food poisoning and reportable infectious diseases never come to the attention of disease-control specialists because laypersons and practitioners categorize the symptom sets as flu and/or viruses.

MacCormack, C. P. "Traditional Medicine, Folk Medicine, and Alternative Medicine." In Folk Medicine and Health Culture: Role of Folk Medicine in Modern Health Care, edited by T. Vaskilampi and C. P. MacCormack, i–xxv. Kuopio, Finland: University of Kuopio, 1982.

MacDonald, M. Mystical Bedlam. Cambridge: Cambridge University Press, 1981. Includes concepts seemingly relevant to some notions understood by Bass.

——. "Religion, Social Change, and Psychological Healing in England, 1600–1800." In The Church and Healing, Studies in Church History, edited by W. J. Sheils, 101–25. Oxford: Ecclesiastical History Society, 1982.

——. "Anthropological Perspectives on the History of Science and Medicine." In Information Sources in the History of Science and Medicine, edited by P. Corsi and P. Weindling, 61–80. London: Butterworth Scientific, 1983.

McElroy, A., and P. K. Townsend, eds. Medical Anthropology in Ecological Perspective. North Scituate, Mass.: Duxbury Press, 1979.

McGowen, T. A. "Assessing Appalachian Studies." Appalachian J. 9 (1982): 97–242. A useful review stressing political biases at play in interpretations of the region.

McGrary, R. "The Use of Home Medical Books in Antebellum Georgia: A Letter by John Macpherson Berrien." J. Med. Assoc. Georgia 64 (1975): 137–38.

McIntyre, M. "Herbal Medicines and Pharmacists." Pharm. J. 236 (1986): 411.

Mack, R. B. "From Grandma to Galen: Boric Acid Poisoning." North Carolina Med. J. 45 (1984): 401–2.

McLaughlin, T. If You Like It, Don't Eat It. Dietary Fads and Fancies. New York: Universe Books, 1979. Useful popular account that points out various fads.

McLean, P. S. "Conjure Doctors in Eastern North Carolina." North Carolina Folklore J. 20 (1972): 21–29.

McNair, J. B. Rhus Dermatitis from Rhus toxicodendron, radcans, and diversiloba (Poison Ivy): Its Pathology and Chemotherapy. Chicago: University of Chicago Press, 1923.

McNamara, B. Step Right Up. Garden City: Doubleday, 1976.

McQueen, D. V. "China's Impact on American Medicine in the Seventies: A Limited and Preliminary Inquiry." Soc. Sci. Med. 21 (1985): 931–35.

Maddox, G. L. "Self-Assessment of Health Status. A Longitudinal Study of Selected Elderly Subjects." J. Chron. Diseases 17 (1964): 449–60.

Maddox, G. L., et al. Introduction to Behavioral Science in Medicine. New York: Springer-Verlag, 1984. Pp. 165–76.

Maegdefran, K. Geschichte der Botanik. Stuttgart: Fischer, 1973.

Magendie, F. Formulary for the Preparation and Employment of Several New Remedies with an Appendix Containing the Experience of British Practitioners with Many of the New Remedies. Translated by Joseph Houlton. New York: Harper, 1829.

Mahoney, J. The Cherokee Physician. Asheville: Edney and Dedman, 1849. Like many Indian medicine books, much of the content is apparently white medicine.

"Mail-Order Health Frauds." In Health Quackery. Consumers Union Report of False

Health Claims, Worthless Remedies, and Unproved Theories. New York: Holt, Rhinehart, and Winston, 1980.

Major, R. H. *A History of Medicine.* Springfield: Thomas, 1954.

Malone, M. H. "The Pharmacological Evaluation of Natural Products—General and Specific Approaches to Screening Ethnopharmaceuticals." *J. Ethnopharmacol.* 8 (1983): 127–47.

Mann, R. D. *Modern Drug Use: An Enquiry on Historical Principles.* Boston: MTP Press, 1984.

Mann, R. J. "Botanical Remedies from Gene Stratton Porter's *The Harvester.*" *J. Hist. Med. All. Sci.* 30 (1975): 367–82.

Maretzki, T. W., and E. Seidler. "Biomedicine and Naturopathic Healing in West Germany. A Historical and Ethnomedical View of a Stormy Relationship." *Cult. Med. Psychiat.* 9 (1985): 383–421.

Margotta, R., and P. Lewis, eds. *An Illustrated History of Medicine.* Feltham: Hamlyn, 1968.

Marini-Bettolo, G. B. "Traditional Medicine. A World Survey on Medicinal Plants and Herbs." *J. Ethnopharmacol.* 2 (1980): 1–196. A worldwide survey of practices in many countries and discussions on methodology.

Martin, M. "Native American Medicine, Thoughts for Post-traditional Healers." *J. Amer. Med. Assoc.* 245 (1981): 141–43.

Marx, O. M. "Descriptions of Psychiatric Care in Some Hospitals during the First Half of the 19th Century." *Bull. Hist. Med.* 41 (1967): 208–14. Describes conditions rather than drug therapy.

Mason, A. "Medical Electricians—Benefactors or Quacks." *Soc. Hist. Med. Bull.* 36 (1985): 22–23.

Massey, A. B. *Virginia Flora.* Blacksburg: Virginia Agricultural Experiment Station, 1961.

Matthews, H. A. *Leaves from the Notebook of an Appalachian Physician.* Franklin: Macon Graphics, 1980. Anecdotes are helpful background to Bass's practice.

Matthews, L. G. *History of Pharmacy in Britain.* London: Livingstone, 1962.

Mattson, M. *The American Vegetable Practice.* 2 vols. in 1. Boston: Hale, 1841.

Mauries, M. *Medicines Traditionnelles.* Paris: CNRS Laboratoire d'Ethnobotanique, 1978. Helpful bibliography.

May, J. T. "The Professionalization of Neighborhood Health Centers." *Health PAC Bulletin* 12 (1981): 1–2, 6–9.

Mease, J. "An Account of the Virtues of Some American Trees, Shrubs, and Plants." *Philadelphia Med. Mus.* 2 (1806): 157–63.

Mechanic, D. "Correlates of Physician Utilization: Why Do Major Multivariate Studies of Physician Utilization Find Trivial Psychosocial and Organizational Effects?" *J. Health Soc. Behav.* 20 (1979): 387–96.

———. "Psychological Factors in the Decision to Seek Medical Care for Symptoms." *Med. Care* 19 (1981): 693–709.

Meigs, C. D. *Females and Their Diseases.* Philadelphia: Lea and Blanchard, 1848.

Mellinger, M. "The Spirit is Strong in the Root." *Appalachian J.* 4 (1977): 242–53.

Survey of Appalachian medicinal plants. Emphasis on Cherokee knowledge. No documentation and unclear how much information is firsthand. Support for the oral tradition of some of Mr. Bass's knowledge; e.g., red sassafras is better than white.

Melville, K. A., and C. R. Johnson. *Cured to Death: The Effects of Prescription Drugs.* London: Secker and Warburg, 1982.

Messer, E. "Present and Future Prospects of Herbal Medicine in a Mexican Community." In *The Nature and Status of Ethnobotany,* edited by R. I. Ford, 137–61. Anthropological Papers, no. 67. Ann Arbor: Museum of Anthropology, University of Michigan, 1978.

Metcalf, C. R. "Distribution of Latex in the Plant Kingdom." *Econ. Bot.* 21 (1967): 115–25.

Mettler, C. C., and F. A. Mettler, eds. *History of Medicine: A Correlative Text, Arranged According to Subjects.* Philadelphia: Blakiston, 1947.

Meyer, C. *American Folk Medicine.* New York: Crowell, 1973.

Meyer, D. C. *Herbal Recipes for Hair, Salves, and Liniments, Medicinal Wines and Vinegars, Plant Ash Uses.* Glenwood, Ill.: Meyerbooks, 1978.

Meyer, G. G. "On Helping the Casualties of Rapid Change." *Psychiatric Annals* 4, no. 11 (1974): 44–48.

———. "The Art of Healing: Folk Medicine, Religion, and Science." In *Folk Medicine and Herbal Healing,* edited by G. G. Meyer et al., 5–12. Springfield: Thomas, 1981.

Meyer, G. G., et al., eds. *Folk Medicine and Herbal Healing.* Springfield: Thomas, 1981. A useful collection of essays.

Meyer, J. E. *The Herbalist.* 1918. Reprint. Glenwood, 1934; Glenwood, Ill.: Meyerbooks, 1979. An influential herbal that includes Eclectic influences.

Miller, A. B. *Shaker Herbs. A History and a Compendium.* New York: Potter, 1976. Invaluable reference book that highlights variability of herb use in the various Shaker communities.

Miller, J. W. "More about Faith Healers." *North Carolina Folklore J.* 17 (1969): 97–99.

Miller, R. W. "Doctors, Patients Don't Communicate." FDA *Consumer* (July–August 1983): 6–7.

Miller, W. *A Dictionary of English Names of Plants.* London: Murray, 1884.

Milligan, W., and W. Wingrave. *A Practical Handbook of the Diseases of the Ear.* London: Macmillan, 1911.

Mills, S. "Herbal Medicine—the Physiomedical Perspectives." *J. Alt. Med.* (August 1983): 8–10. Outline of various concepts.

———. *The Dictionary of Modern Herbalism.* Wellingborough: Thorsons, 1985. This is advocatory, but with a balanced tone.

Mintz, S. W. *Sweetness and Power.* Viking: Elizabeth Sifton, 1985.

Mitchell, F. *Hoodoo Medicine, Sea Island, Herbal Remedies.* Charleston: Reed, Cannon and Johnson, 1978. A helpful source, though difficult to distinguish present from past usages, or whether or not usage was primarily by blacks or whites.

Mitchell, W. E. "Changing Others: The Anthropological Study of Therapeutic Systems." *Med. Anthropol. Newsletter* 8, no. 3 (1977): 15–20.

Mobius, M. A. J. *Geschichte der Botanik von den Ersten Anfanger bis zur Gegenweit.* Jena, East Germany: Fischer, 1937.

Modell, W. *Relief of Symptoms.* St. Louis: C. V. Mosby, 1961.

Moerman, D. E. *American Medical Ethnobotany, A Reference Dictionary.* New York: Garland, 1977.

———. "Anthropology of Symbolic Healing." *Current Anthropol.* 20 (1979): 59–80.

———. "Empirical Methods in the Evaluation of Indigenous Medical Systems." *Med. Anthropol.* 3 (1979): 525–30.

———. "General Medical Effectiveness and Human Biology: Placebo Effects in the Treatment of Ulcer Disease." *Med. Anthropol. Newsletter* (August 1979): 5–6. Challenges many assumptions.

———. "Symbols and Selectivity: A Statistical Analysis of Native America Medical Ethnobotany." *J. Ethnopharmacol.* 1 (1979): 111–19. Argues that regression analysis suggests native American medical botany is not just placebo medicine.

———. *Geraniums for the Iroquois. A Field Guide to American Indian Medicinal Plants.* Algonac, Mich.: Reference Publications, 1982. Covers mainly Indian usage.

———. *Medicinal Plants of Native America.* 2 vols. Ann Arbor: Museum of Anthropology, University of Michigan, 1986.

Mohabbat, O., et al. "An Outbreak of Veno-occlusive Disease in North-western Afghanistan." *Lancet* 2 (1976): 269–71.

Mohr, C. "Plant Life of Alabama, Montgomery." In *Contributions from the U.S. National Herbarium.* Vol. 6. Washington, D.C.: Government Printing Office, 1901. Occasional reference to medical usage is given.

Monardes, N. *Joyfull Newes out of the Newe Found Worlde.* Translated by J. Frampton 1577. Reprint. New York: Knopf, 1925. Monardes was a physician in Seville, Spain.

Montgomery, J. C. "The Value of Recent Therapeutic Literature." *North Carolina Med. J.* 37 (1896): 354–57. "We have learned how not to give medicines, rather than how to give them."

Mooney, J. *The Sacred Formulas of the Cherokees. Seventh Annual Report, B.A.E.* Washington, D.C., 1891. Reprint. Nashville: Elder, 1982.

Mooney, J., and F. M. Olbrechts. "The Swimmer Manuscript, Cherokee Sacred Formulas and Medicinal Prescriptions." *Smithsonian Inst. Bureau of Amer. Ethnol. Bull.* 99 (1932).

Moore, G. *Health Disease and Remedy. Familiarly and Practically Considered in a Few of Their Relations to the Blood.* New York: Harper, 1850.

Morantz, R. M. "The Perils of Feminist History." *J. Interdiscip. Hist.* 4 (1973): 649–60.

Morantz-Sanchez, R. M. *Sympathy and Science. Women Physicians in American Medicine.* New York: Oxford University Press, 1985. Much general background, especially chapter entitled "Doctors and Patients: Gender and Medical Treatment in Nineteenth-Century America."

"More Pressures on Herbal Medical Policy." *Pharm. J.* 23 (1985): 817. Consideration of political situations.

Morley, A. "Treating Coughs." *Pharm. J.* 236 (1986): 17–18. Ammonium chloride (no herbal preparations) only long-standing remedy still in use.

Morrell, D. C. "Symptom Interpretation in General Practice." *J. Royal Coll. Gen. Pract.* 22 (1972): 297–309.

Morris, B. "Herbalism and Divination in Southern Malawi." *Soc. Sci. Med.* 23 (1986): 367–77.

Morson, T. *A Catalogue of Drugs, Pharmaceutical Preparations, Chemical Tests, Etc., Prepared and Sold by T. Morson.* London: Morson, 1825.

Morton, A. G. *History of Botanical Science.* New York: Academic Press, 1981.

Morton, J. F. *Folk Remedies of the Low Country.* Miami: Seemann, 1974. Contains information on present and past uses, but not whether employed primarily by blacks or whites.

——— . "Economic Botany in Epidemiology." *Econ. Bot.* 32 (1978): 111–18.

——— . "Caribbean and Latin American Folk Medicine and Its Influence in the United States." *Quart. J. Crude Drug Res.* 18 (1980): 57–75. Covers herbal use in the United States by Caribbean and Latin American residents and the use by some native Americans of, for instance *Cassia reticulata* for rheumatoid arthritis.

Mossa, J. S. "A Study on the Crude Antidiabetic Drugs Used in Arabian Folk Medicine." *Int. J. Crude Drug Res.* 23 (1985): 137–45.

Motherby, G. *A New Medical Dictionary; or General Repository of Physic. Containing an Explanation of the Terms, and a Description of the Various Particulars Relating to Anatomy, Physiology, Physic, Surgery, Materia Medica, Chemistry, &c.* 2d ed. London: Johnson, 1785. Second of a number of editions. A more critical flavor toward medicinal herbs than found in James's earlier dictionary. This reflects a more conservative trend.

Moulin, D. de. *A Short History of Breast Cancer.* Boston: Nijoff, 1983.

Muenscher, W. C. *Poisonous Plants of the United States.* New York: Macmillan, 1951.

Müller-Jahncke, W. D. "Der 'Linnaeus Americanus' und seine Beziehunger zu deutschen Botanken: G. H. E. Muhlenberg." *Deutsche Apotheker-Zeitung* 177 (1977): 323–1329.

——— . "Johann David Schoepf (1752–1800): A German Physician as a Botanist and Zoologist in North America." *Pharm. Hist.* 20 (1978): 43–64.

——— . *Astrologisch-Magische Theorie und Praxis in der Heilkunde Der Fruhen Neuzeit.* Sudhoff's Archive, Monograph no. 25. Stuttgart, 1985. Helpful for background on concepts which have persisted to the present.

Mullett, C. F. "John Cook, M.D., Physician-at-Large." *Bull. Hist. Med.* 19 (1946):498–516. Insights into eighteenth-century therapy.

Mundé, P. E. *The Present Treatment of Uterine Displacement.* New York: Wood, 1895.

Murphree, A. H. "A Functional Analysis of Southern Folk Medical Beliefs Concerning Birth." In *Essays in Medical Anthropology,* edited by T. Weaver. Athens: University of Georgia Press, 1968.

Murphy, E. A. *Skepsis, Dogma and Belief: Uses and Abuses in Medicine.* Baltimore: Johns Hopkins University Press, 1981.

Murray, J. *A System of Materia Medica and Pharmacy with Notes by N. Chapman.* Philadelphia: Dobson, 1815. A critical compilation.

Mushet, W. B. "A Glance at an Obsolete Materia Medica." *Practitioner* 4 (1870): 143–51. Notes "many trivial medicines which survive amongst the vulgar."

Naisbitt, J. *Megatrends: Ten New Directions Transforming Our Lives.* New York: Warner Books, 1982.

National Analysts, Inc. *A Study of Health Practices and Opinions, Conducted for Food and Drug Administration.* Washington, D.C.: National Technical Information Service, 1972.

Nations, M. K., et al. "'Hidden' Popular Illnesses in Primary Care: Residents' Recognition and Clinical Implications." *Culture, Medicine, and Psychiatry* 9 (1985): 223–40.

"Natural Aphrodisiacs." *Lawrence Rev. Nat. Prod.* 3, no. 15 (1982): 57–59.

Ness, R. C., and R. M. Wintrob. "Folk Healing: A Description and Synthesis." *Amer. J. Psychiatry* 138 (1981): 1477–81. Argues that physicians should familiarize themselves with patients' folk-healing beliefs in order to serve them more effectively.

Neuberger, A., and T. H. Jukes. *Human Nutrition—Current Issues and Controversies.* Boston: MTP Press, 1982. Various threads of current interest explained including health quackery.

Neuburger, M. "The Doctrine of the Healing Power of Nature Throughout the Course of Time." Translated by L. J. Boyd. New York: N.p., 1932.

Neumann, A. K., and P. Lauro. "Ethnomedicine and Biomedicine Linking." *Soc. Sci. Med.* 16 (1982): 1817–24. Indicates difficulties of integration.

Newman, L. F. "Ophelia's Herbal." *Econ. Bot.* 33 (1979): 227–32.

New Sydenham Society. *The New Sydenham Society's Lexicon of Medicine and the Allied Sciences,* compiled by H. Power and L. W. Sedgwick. London: New Sydenham Society, 1899.

Nicholson, M. H., ed. *Conway Letters: The Correspondence of Ann Viscountess Conway, Henry Moore, and Their Friends.* New Haven: Yale University Press, 1930. Many insights into self-treatment during the seventeenth century.

Nissen, C. *Herbals of Five Centuries. A Contribution to Medical History and Bibliography.* Zurich: L'Art Ancien, 1958.

Nissenbaum, S. *Sex, Diet, and Debility in Jacksonian America. Sylvester Graham and Health Reform.* Westport: Greenwood, 1980.

Noble, R. L., et al. "Role of Chance Observations in Chemotherapy: *Vinca rosea.*" *Ann. New York Acad. Sci.* 76 (1958): 882–94.

Nolan, R. L., and J. L. Schwartz, eds. *Rural and Appalachian Health.* Springfield: Thomas, 1973.

Numbers, R. "The Making of an Eclectic Physician. Joseph McElhinney and the Eclectic Medical Institute of Cincinnati." *Bull. Hist. Med.* 47 (1973): 155–66.

O'Hara, M. J. *Elizabethan Dyetary of Health.* Lawrence: Coronado Press, 1977.

Ogawa, T., ed. *History of Traditional Medicine.* Osaka: Taniguchi Foundation, 1986. Symposium papers delivered 1976 and 1977.

Oliver-Bever, B., and G. R. Zahnd. "Plants with Oral Hypoglycaemic Action." *Quart. J. Crude Drug. Res.* 17 (1979–80): 139–96.

Olsen, D. M., et al. "Medical Care as a Commodity: An Explanation of the Shopping Behavior of Patients." *J. Community Health* 2 (1976): 85–91.

"On the Utility of Botany." *Med. and Phys. J.* 11 (1804): 368–72, 439–50, 526–34ff.

Ortiz de Montellano, B. R. "Empirical Aztec Medicine. Aztec Medicinal Plants Seem to Be Effective If They Are Judged by Aztec Standards." *Science* 188 (1975): 215–20.

Osler, W. *The Evolution of Modern Medicine*. New Haven: Yale University Press, 1921.

Otsuka, Y. "Comparative Study of Materia Medica." In *History of Traditional Medicine*, edited by T. Ogawa, 65–82. Osaka: Taniguchi Foundation, 1986.

Packard, F. R. *History of Medicine in the United States*. New York: Hoeber, 1931.

Page, L. G., and E. Wigginton. *Aunt Arie. A Foxfire Portrait*. New York: Dutton, Foxfire Press, 1983.

——— . *The Foxfire Book of Appalachian Cookery, Regional Memorabilia, and Recipes*. New York: Dutton, Foxfire Press, 1984.

Paine, M. *Materia Medica and Therapeutics*. New York: Wood, 1847 and 1859.

Palmer, T. *The Admirable Secrets of Physick and Chyrurgery*. Edited by T. R. Forbes. 1696. Reprint. New Haven: Yale University Press, 1984. Few references to Indian practice.

Parascandola, J. "Drug Therapy in Colonial and Revolutionary America." *Amer. J. Hosp. Pharm.* 33 (1976): 807–9.

Parente, P. P., ed. *The Regimen of Health of the Medical School of Salerno*. New York: Vantage Press, 1967.

Parker, R. C., Jr., and A. A. Sorenson. "The Tides of Rural Physicians: The Ebb and Flow or Why Physicians Move out of and into Small Communities." *Med. Care* 16 (1978): 152–66.

Parsons, E. *Folk-lore of the Sea Islands, South Carolina*. Cambridge: American Folklore Society, 1923.

Peacock, J. L. *Consciousness and Change*. Oxford: Blackwell, 1975.

Pearsall, M. *Little Smoky Ridge*. Birmingham: University of Alabama Press, 1959.

——— . "Communicating with the Educationally Deprived." *Mountain Life and Work* 42, no. 1 (1966): 8–11. A short but salutary discussion.

Pellegrino, E. D. "The Healing Relationship: The Architectonics of Clinical Medicine." In *The Clinical Encounter. The Moral Fabric of the Physician-Patient Relationship*, edited by E. E. Shelp, 153–72. Dordrecht, Netherlands: Reidel, 1983.

Penso, G. "The Role of WHO in the Selection and Characterization of Medicinal Plants (Vegetable Drugs)." *J. Ethnopharmacol.* 2 (1980): 183–88.

Percival, T. *Medical Ethics*. Manchester: Russell, 1803. Medical ethics play a key role in defining quackery.

Perman, S. "Curing Beliefs and Practices in the Outer Hebrides." *Folklore* 88 (1977): 107–9.

Perry, J. W. *Spices*. New York: Chemical Publishing, 1969.

Peterson, G. "Boone's Wilcox Drug Company: A Family Business for Five Generations." *Watauga County Times . . . Past* 11 (1983): 3–10.

Peterson, W. L., et al. "Healing of Duodenal Ulcer with an Antacid Regimen." *New Eng. J. Med.* 297 (1977): 341–45.

Petiver, J. "Some Attempts Made to Prove that Herbs of the Same Make or Class for the Geneality, Have the Same Virtue and Tendency to Work the Same Effects." *Phil. Trans.* 21 (1969): 289–94.

Petkov, V. "Bulgarian Traditional Medicine: A Source of Ideas for Phytopharmacological Investigations." *J. Ethnopharmacol.* 15 (1986): 121–32.

Pfaff, D. W., ed. *Taste, Olfaction, and the Central Nervous System.* New York: Rockefeller University Press, 1985. Background to discussions on determining medicinal actions from sensory properties.

Phillips, W. R. "Patients, Pills, and Professionals: The Ethics of Placebo Therapy." *Pharos* 44 (Winter 1981): 21–25.

Phillipson, J. D. "The Pros and Cons of Herbal Remedies." *Pharm. J.* 227 (1981): 387–92.

———. "A Small Cog in a Big World." *Pharm. J.* 235 (1985): 334–40.

Pickard, M. E., and R. C. Buley. *The Midwest Pioneer: His Ills, Cures, and Doctors.* Crawfordsville, Ind.: Banta, 1945.

Pickering, G. "Medicine on the Brink: The Dilemma of a Learned Profession." *Perspect. Biol. Med.* 21 (1978): 551–60.

Pickstone, J. V. "Establishment and Dissent in Nineteenth-Century Medicine: An Exploration of Some Correspondence and Connections between Religious and Medical Belief Systems in Early Industrial England." In *The Church and Healing,* edited by W. J. Sheils, 165–89. Oxford: Ecclesiastical History Society, 1982.

Pierce, R. V. *The People's Common Sense Medical Adviser.* Buffalo: World's Dispensary Print, 1883 and numerous later editions.

Pierpoint, W. S. "Phenolics in Food and Foodstuffs: The Pleasures and Perils of Vegetarianism." In *The Biochemistry of Plant Phenolics,* edited by C. F. van Sumere and P. J. Lea, 427–51. Oxford: Clarendon, 1985.

Pisani, J. M. "Are Most Over-the-Counter Medicines Really Placebos?" In *Controversies in Therapeutics,* edited by L. Lasagne, 33–39. Philadelphia: Saunders, 1980.

Plowden, C. C. *A Manual of Plant Names.* London: Allen and Unwin, 1970.

Podell, R. N. *Physician's Guide to Compliance in Hypertension.* Rahway, N.J.: Merck, 1975.

Porcher, F. P. *Resources of the Southern Fields and Forests, Medical, Economical, and Agricultural.* Charleston: Evans and Cogswell, 1863.

Porkert, M. *The Theoretical Foundations of Chinese Medicine, Systems of Correspondence.* Cambridge: MIT Press, 1974.

Porteous, A. *Forest Folklore, Mythology and Romance.* London: Allen and Unwin, 1928.

Porter, R. "Lay Medical Knowledge in the Eighteenth Century: The Evidence of the Gentleman's Magazine." *Med. Hist.* 29 (1985): 138–68.

Postell, W. D. *The Health of Slaves on Southern Plantations.* Baton Rouge: Louisiana State University Press, 1951.

Potter, S. O. L. *Therapeutics, Materia Medica, and Pharmacy.* Philadelphia: Blakiston, 1913.

Poynter, F. N. L., and W. J. Bishop. "A 17th Century Doctor and His Patients: John Symcotts, 1592?–1662." *Beds. Hist. Rec. Soc. Pubs.* 31 (1951).

Press, I. "Problems in the Definition and Classification of Medical Systems." *Soc. Sci. Med.* 14B (1980): 45–57.

Price, E. T. "Root Digging in the Appalachians. The Geography of Botanical Drugs." *Geog. Rev.* 50 (1960): 1–20.

Primack, A. "Cultural Background and Medicinal Care." *Urban Health* (January 1984): 22–28.

Prior, R. C. A. *Popular Names of British Plants: Their Origin and Meaning.* London: Williams and Norgate, 1870. Traces the vernacular names of most plants to Anglo-Saxon, Latin, and in some cases Greek origins.

Puckett, N. N. *Folk Beliefs of the Southern Negro.* Chapel Hill: University of North Carolina Press, 1926.

Pusey, W. A. *The History of Dermatology.* Springfield: Thomas, 1933.

Quick, J. "Integration or Co-optation: Bringing Traditional Medicinal Plants into Public Health Programs." In *The Use and Abuse of Medicine,* edited by M. W. De Vries et al., 254–64. New York: Praeger, 1982.

Radford, A. E., et al. *Manual of the Vascular Flora of the Carolinas.* Chapel Hill: University of North Carolina Press, 1968.

Rafinesque, C. S. *Medical Flora; or Manual of the Medical Botany of the United States of North America.* Philadelphia: Atkinson and Alexander, 1828–30.

Raine, J. W. *The Land of Saddle-bags. A Study of the Mountain People of Appalachia.* New York: Council of Women for Home Missions and Missionary Education Movement of the United States and Canada, 1924.

Ranney, M. H. "The Medical Treatment of Insanity." *Amer. J. Insanity* 14 (1857): 64–68.

Raper, A. F. *Preface to Peasantry, A Tale of Two Black Belt Counties.* Chapel Hill: University of North Carolina Press, 1936.

Raphael's Medical Astrology or the Effects of the Planets and Signs upon the Human Body. London: Foulsham, 1910. Much of the information is known to Bass.

Rather, L. J. *The Genesis of Cancer: A Study in the History of Ideas.* Baltimore: Johns Hopkins University Press, 1978.

———. " 'The Six Things Non-Natural' A Note on the Origins and Fate of a Doctrine and a Phrase." *Clio. Med.* 3 (1978): 337–47.

Rea, M.-A. F. "Early Introduction of Economic Plants into New England." *Econ. Bot.* 29 (1975): 333–56.

Reed, H. S. *A Short History of the Plant Sciences.* Waltham, Mass.: Chronica Botanica, 1942.

Reed, L. S. *The Healing Cults, A Study of Sectarian Medical Practice: Its Extent, Causes, and Control.* Committee on the Costs of Medical Care, no. 16. Chicago: University of Chicago Press, 1932.

"The Religious Component in Southern Folk Medicine." *Conch* 8 (1976): 26–51.

Relman, A. S. "The New Medical Industrial Complex." *New Eng. J. Med.* 303 (1980): 963–70.

Remington, J. P. *The Practice of Pharmacy.* Philadelphia: Lippincott, 1894.

Renbourn, E. T. "The History of Sweat and Prickly Heat, 19th–20th Century." *J. Invest. Derm.* 30 (1958): 249–59.

Rexrode, C. R. "Take Moonshine According to Age: Healing in Pendelton County, West Virginia, 1900–1940," B.A. thesis, Harvard University, 1980.

Rhee, K. S., and A. C. Stubbs. "Health Food Uses in Two Texas Cities." *J. Amer. Diet Assoc.* (1976): 542–45.

Rhode, E. S. *The Old English Herbals*. London: Longmans, 1922.

Rhodes, L. A. "'This Will Clear Your Mind': The Use of Metaphors for Medication in Psychiatric Settings." *Cult. Med. Psychiat.* 8 (1984): 49–70.

Richardson, J. D., and F. D. Scutchfield. "Priorities in Health Care: The Consumer's Viewpoint in an Appalachian Community." *Amer. J. Pub. Health* 63 (1973): 72–82.

Riddle, J. M. *Dioscorides on Pharmacy and Medicine*. Austin: University of Texas Press, 1985.

Rieff, D. *The Triumph of the Therapeutic: Uses of Faith After Freud*. New York: Harper and Row, 1966.

Rietbrock, N., and B. G. Woodcock. "Two Hundred Years of Foxglove Therapy." *Trends Pharmacol. Sci.* 6 (1985): 267–69. Covers significant differences in action according to method of application.

Ring, E. F. J., and S. Trotman. "Techniques for Measuring Skin Temperature and Blood Flow." *Pharm. J.* 231 (1983): 270–71.

Rinzler, C. A. *The Dictionary of Medical Folklore*. New York: Crowell, 1979. A reminder of the development of "new" beliefs.

Rippere, V. "Some Historical Dimensions of Common Sense Knowledge about Depression and Antidepressive Behaviour." *Behav. Res. and Therapy* 18 (1980): 373–85.

———. "The Survival of Traditional Medicine in Lay Medical Views: An Empirical Approach to the History of Medicine." *Med. Hist.* 25 (1981): 411–14.

Risse, G. B. "Calomel and the American Medical Sects during the Nineteenth Century." *Mayo Clin. Proc.* 48 (1973): 57–64.

———. "Transcending Cultural Barriers: The European Reception of Medicinal Plants from the Americas." *Veröff. Int. Gesell. Gesch. Pharm.* 53 (1984): 31–39.

———. "'Typhus' Fever in Eighteenth-Century Hospitals: New Approaches to Medical Treatment." *Bull. Hist. Med.* 59 (1985): 176–95.

Rivers, W. H. R. *Medicine, Magic, Religion*. New York: Harcourt, 1924.

Robinson, V. *The Story of Medicine*. New York: Tudor Publishing, 1931.

"J. I. Rodale [1891–1971] in Memoriam." *Prevention* 23, no. 8 (1971): 14–18. Insights into a major figure behind the popularization of many health foods.

Rodale, R. "The Evaluation of the Quality of Health Care. A Lay Perspective." *Eval. and Health Prof.* 6 (1983): 143–48.

Rodnan, G. P. "Growth and Development of Rheumatology in the United States—A Bicentennial Report." *Arthritis and Rheumatism* 20 (1977): 1149–68.

Roe, D. A. "Attempts at the Eradication of Pellagra. A Historical Review." In *Aspects of the History of Epidemiology. Times, Places, and Persons*, edited by A. M. Lilienfeld, 62–83. Baltimore: Johns Hopkins University Press, 1980.

———. *A Plague of Corn. A Social History of Pellagra*. Ithaca: Cornell University Press, 1981.

Roe, D. A., and T. C. Campbell, eds. *Drugs and Nutrients: Their Interactive Effects*. New York: Dekker, 1984. A reminder of possible ramifications of long-term ingestion of pharmacologically active substances.

Roemer, M. I., and B. Foulkner. "The Development of Public Health Services in a Rural County 1838–1949." *J. Hist. Med. All. Sci.* 6 (1951): 22–43.

Rogers, A. D. *Liberty Hyde Bailey: A Story of American Plant Science.* Princeton: Princeton University Press, 1949.

Rogers, E. G. *Early Folk Medical Practices in Tennessee.* Murfreesboro: Mid-South Publishing, 1941.

Rogers, F. B. "Dr. Lyman H. Luce (1842–92). Physician-Naturalist of Martha's Vineyard, Massachusetts." *J. Hist. Med.* 32 (1977): 423–27.

Rogers, J. "Talking Out Fire." *North Carolina Folklore J.* 16 (1968): 46–52.

Rogers, S. L. *The Shaman. His Symbols and His Healing Power.* Springfield: Thomas, 1982.

Rolleston, J. D. "Ophthalmic Folk-lore." *Brit. J. Ophthalmol.* 26 (1942): 481–502.

Rook, A., and J. Savin, eds. *Recent Advances in Dermatology.* Vol. 5. Edinburgh: Churchill Livingstone, 1980.

Rosch, P. J., and H. M. Kearney. "Holistic Medicine and Technology: A Modern Dialectic." *Soc. Sci. Med.* 21 (1985): 1405–9. The dialectic discussed is illustrated in Bass's transition to promoting health foods.

Rosen, G. *Preventive Medicine in the United States 1900–1975. Trends and Interpretations.* New York: Science History Publications, 1975.

Rosenau, M. J. *Preventive Medicine and Hygiene.* New York: Appleton, 1918. Pp. 522–23.

Rosenberg, C. E. "The Place of George M. Beard in Nineteenth-Century Psychiatry." *Bull. Hist. Med.* 36 (1962): 245–59. Argues that Beard's ideas were a mosaic of fashionable and controlling ideas of his time.

———. "Medical Text and Social Context: Explaining William Buchan's Domestic Medicine." *Bull. Hist. Med.* 57 (1983): 22–42.

Rosenberg, C., and E. J. Smith. "Public Preferences and Medical Care in the Provinces: Seventeenth-Century New England." Paper presented at the Fifty-sixth Annual Meeting of the American History of Medicine Association, Minneapolis, May 1983.

Rosenblatt, R. A., and I. S. Moscovice. *Rural Health Care.* Chichester: Wiley and Sons, 1982.

Rosengarten, F., Jr. "A Neglected Mayan Galactogogue—Ixbut (*Euphorbia lancifolia*)." *J. Ethnopharmacol.* 5 (1982): 91–112.

Rosengarten, T. *All God's Dangers. The Life of Nate Shaw.* New York: Knopf, 1974.

Russell, P. A. *Man's Mastery of Malaria.* London: Oxford University Press, 1955. One of a number of accounts listing folklore remedies.

Rydén, M. "The English Plant Names in Gerard's *Herbal* (1597)." In *Stockholm Studies in English Philology, Linguistics and Literature.* 1978. Pp. 142–50. Indicates value of Gerard's *Herbal* as source of English vernacular names (some noted as very local names) published for the first time, some coined by Gerard.

———. *Shakespearean Plant Names, Identifications and Interpretations.* Stockholm Studies in English, no. 18. 1978.

———. "English Plant-Name Research." In *Papers from the First Nordic Conference for English Studies,* edited by S. Johansson and B. Tysdahl, 374–83. Oslo: University of Oslo Press, 1981. Indicates some ramifications of paying attention to vernacular names.

———. *The English Plant Names in the Grete Herbal (1526); A Contribution to the Historical Study of English Plant-Name Usage.* Stockholm Studies in English, no. 61. 1984.

Saegert, J., and E. A. Young. "Nutrition Knowledge and Health Food Consumption." *Nutrition and Behavior* 1 (1983): 103–13.

Salan, R., and T. Maretzki. "Mental Health Services and Traditional Healing in Indonesia: Are the Roles Compatible?" *Culture, Medicine, and Psychiatry* 7 (1983): 377–412.

Salber, E. J., et al. "Access to Health Care in a Southern Rural Community." *Med. Care* 14 (1976): 971–86. Notes fewer visits to physicians among blacks.

Sandner, D. *Navaho Symbols of Healing.* New York: Harcourt Brace Jovanovich, 1979. Raises questions about the extent of symbolism in other cultures.

Sankar, A. " 'It's Just Old Age': Old Age as a Diagnosis in American and Chinese Medicine." In *Age and Anthropological Theory,* edited by D. J. Kertzer and J. Keith, 250–80. Ithaca: Cornell University Press, 1984.

Saunders, L., and G. W. Hewes. "Folk Medicine and Medical Practice." *J. Med. Educ.* 28, no. 9 (1953): 43–46.

Savitt, T. L. *Medicine and Slavery. The Diseases and Health Care of Blacks in Antebellum Virginia.* Urbana: University of Illinois Press, 1978.

Scarborough, J. "Theophrastus on Herbals and Herbal Remedies." *J. Hist. Bio.* 11 (1978): 353–86.

———. "On Medications for Burns in Classical Antiquity." *Clin. Plastic Surg.* 10 (1983): 603–10.

Scarborough, J., and V. Nutton. "The Preface of Dioscorides' Materia Medica: Introduction, Translation, and Commentary." *Trans. Stud. Coll. Phys. Philadelphia* 4, ser. 5 (1982): 187–27.

Scarpa, A. "Pre-Scientific Medicines: Their Extent and Value." *Soc. Sci. Med.* 15A (1981): 317–26. Argues for more studies on traditional medicines.

Scarpa, A., and Guerci, A. "Depigmenting Procedures and Drugs Employed by Melanoderm Populations." *J. Ethnopharmacol.* 19 (1987): 17–66.

Schanenberg, P., and F. Paris. *Guide to Medicinal Plants.* Translated by M. P. Jones. Guildford: Lutterworth Press, 1977.

Schedler, P. W. "Folk Medicine in Denton County Today: Or, Can Dermatology Displace Dishrags?" in *Hunters and Healers: Folklore Types and Topics,* edited by W. M. Hudson, 11–17. Austin: Encino Press, 1971.

Schiffman, S. S. "Taste and Smell in Disease." *New Eng. J. Med.* 308 (1983): 1275–79. Various reasons considered for taste disorders.

Schipochliev, T. "Extracts from a Group of Plants Enhancing Uterine Tonus." *Vet-MedNanki* 18 (1981): 87–94.

Schleiffer, H., ed. *Sacred Narcotic Plants of the New World Indians, An Anthology of Texts from the 16th Century to Date.* New York: Hafner, 1973.

Schneider, A. *Literature on Medicinal Plant and Drug Plant Culture.* Milwaukee: Pharmaceutical Review, 1908. Useful bibliography.

Schoepf, J. *Materia Medica Americana*. 1787. Reprint. *Bull. Lloyd Library*, Reproduction Series, 1903.

Schoonover, S. G. "Alabama Public Health Campaign, 1900–1919." *Alabama Rev.* 28 (1975): 218–33.

Schultes, R. E. "Hallucinogens of Plant Origin." *Science* 163 (1969): 245–54.

———. "Solanaceous Hallucinogens and Their Role in the Development of New World Cultures." In *The Biology and Taxonomy of the Solanaceae*, edited by J. G. Hawkes et al. London: Academic Press, 1979.

"Scientific Evaluation of Complementary Medicine." *Lancet* 1 (1986): 158. Raises question of spiritual healing dissociating pain.

Scott, S. C. "The Relationship between Beliefs About the Menstrual Cycle and Choice of Fertility Regulating Methods within Five Ethnic Groups." *Int. J. Gynaecol. Obst.* 13 (1975): 105–9. Concepts about the body are among the major factors which influence women in their rejection or choice of contraceptives. One of many publications on this topic where cultural factors at play are relatively easy to determine.

Scroggs, A. A. "Report of the Medicinal Plants." MS. North Carolina State Archives, 1871.

Secrest, A. J. "Contemporary Folk Medicine." *North Carolina Med. J.* 25 (1964): 481–82.

Seidler, E., ed. *Medizinische Anthropologie Beiträge für eine Theoretische Pathologie*. Berlin: Springer-Verlag, 1984.

Seijas, H. "An Approach to the Study of the Medical Aspects of Culture." *Current Anthropol.* 14 (1973): 544–45.

Selye, H. "The Stress Concept: Past, Present and Future." In *Stress Research Issues for the Eighties*, edited by C. L. Cooper, 1–20. Chichester: Wiley, 1984.

"Shamen and Endorphins." *Ethos* 10 (1982): 119–22, 299–343. Possibility that endorphins might be involved in the frequently reported analgesia (and euphoria) associated with shamanic rituals.

Shanmugasundaram, K., et al. "Plasma Cholesterol and Lipoprotein Lowering Effect of Anna Pavala Sindhorrma." *J. Ethnopharmacol.* 8 (1983): 19–34.

Shapiro, A. K., and E. Shapiro. "The Placebo Effect: Art or Science?" *Medical Times* (June 1982): 45s–50s.

Shapiro, A. K. "The Placebo Effect." In *Principles of Psychopharmacology*, edited by W. G. Clark and J. Del Guidice. New York: Academic Press, 1978.

Shapiro, A. K., and L. Morris. "The Placebo Effect in Healing." In *Handbook of Psychotherapy and Behavior Change*, edited by S. L. Garfield and A. E. Bergin, 477–536. New York: Aldine, 1978.

Shapiro, A. K., and E. Shapiro. "The Placebo Effect: Art or Science." *Medical Times* (June 1982): 45s–50s.

Shapiro, A. K., et al. "Reliability and Validity of a Placebo Test." *J. Psychiat. Res.* 15 (1980): 253–90.

Sharma, P. V. *Introduction to Dravyaguna (Indian Pharmacology)*. Varanesi, Chankhamba: Orientatia, 1976.

Shaw, C. "Memories of a Folk Doctor: Dr. Cicero West." *North Carolina Folklore J.* 28 (1980): 22–41.

Shealy, C. N. "Holism, Science or Mysticism? or How Scientific is Medicine?" *J. Holistic Med.* 3 (1981): 30–37. Contains many popular arguments against regular medicine.

Sheils, W. J., ed. *The Church and Healing.* Oxford: Ecclesiastical History Society, 1982. A collection of essays which includes much of tangential relevance to Bass's practice.

Shellard, E. J. "A History of British Pharmacognosy." *Pharm. J.* (1981): 680–83 and subsequent articles.

———. "Some Pharmacognostical Implications of Herbal Medicine and Other Forms of Medicine Involving Plants." *Royal Soc. Health J.* 102 (1982): 218–21. Expresses concern over lack of quality control.

———. "Medicines from Plants with Special Reference to Herbal Products in Great Britain." *Planta Med.* 53, no. 2 (1987): 121–23.

Sheridan, R. B. *Doctors and Slaves. A Medical and Demographic History of Slavery in the British West Indies, 1680–1834.* Cambridge: Cambridge University Press, 1985. Some information on relations between professional and folk medicine.

Sherman, H. C. *Chemistry of Food and Nutrition.* New York: Macmillan, 1941. Sherman's many influential writings seem to contradict the assertion of a separation of nutrition from clinical medicine during the first half of the nineteenth century, but Sherman was a professor of chemistry.

Sherman, J. A. *The Complete Botanical Prescriber.* Cornwallis: Cornwallis Naturopathic Clinic, 1979.

Sherman, J. F. "Challenges to the Use of Animal Models in Research, Education, and Teaching." *Trans. Stud. Coll. Phys. Philadelphia* 7 (1985): 253–60.

Sherman, M., and T. Henry. *Hollow Folk.* New York: Crowell, 1923.

Shi, D. E. *The Simple Life, Plain Living and High Thinking in American Culture.* New York: Oxford University Press, 1985.

Shimkin, M. B. *Contrary to Nature. Being an Illustrated Commentary on Some Persons and Events of Historical Importance in the Development of Knowledge Concerning Cancer.* Washington, D.C.: Department of Health, Education, and Welfare, 1977.

Shortt, S. E. D. "Physicians, Science and Status: Issues in the Professionalization of Anglo-American Medicine in the Nineteenth Century." *Med. Hist.* 27 (1983): 51–68.

Shryock, R. H. *American Medical Research Past and Present.* New York: Commonwealth Fund, 1947.

———. *The Development of Modern Medicine: An Interpretation of the Social and Scientific Factors Involved.* New York: Knopf, 1947.

———. *Medicine and Society in America 1660–1860.* New York: New York University Press, 1960.

———. *Medicine in America: Historical Essays.* Baltimore: Johns Hopkins University Press, 1966.

Sibley, E. *Culpeper's English Physician and Complete Herbal.* London: Lewis and Roden, 1805.

Sicherman, B. "The Uses of a Diagnosis: Doctors, Patients, and Neurasthenia." *J. Hist. Med. All. Sci.* 32 (1977): 33–54.

Siegel, R. K. "The Natural History of Hallucinogens." In *Hallucinogens: Neurochemi-*

cal, Behavioral, and Clinical Perspectives, edited by B. L. Jacobs, 1–18. New York: Raven Press, 1984.

Sigerest, H. E. "Rise and Fall of the American Spa." *Ciba Symposium* (1946): 313–26.

———. "Towards a Rennaissance of the American Spa." *Ciba Symposium* (1946): 327.

Simon, J. E., et al. *Herbs. An Indexed Bibliography 1971–1980. The Scientific Literature on Selected Herbs, and Aromatic and Medicinal Plants of the Temperate Zone.* Hamden, Conn.: Archon Books, 1984.

Simon, R. M. "Regions and Social Relations: A Research Note." *Appalachian J.* 11 (1983–84): 23–31. If Appalachia is not a class or region, what is it?

Simpson, W. "The Names of Medicinal Plants of Commercial Value Gathered in North Carolina: Their Value, and Relative Amount Sold in This Country and Exported." *Proc. Amer. Pharm. Assoc.* 42 (1894): 210–20.

Singer, C., with E. Ashworth Underwood. *A Short History of Medicine.* 2d enl. ed. 1928. Oxford: Oxford University Press, 1962.

Singer, M., et al. "Hypoglycemia: A Controversial Illness in U.S. Society." *Med. Anthropol.* 8 (1984): 1–35.

Singer, P. "From Anthropology and Medicine to Therapy and Neo-Colonialism." *Conch* 8 (1976): 1–25.

Slack, P. "Mirrors of Health and Treasures of Poor Men: The Uses of Vernacular Medical Literature of Tudor England." In *Health, Medicine, and Mortality in the Sixteenth Century*, edited by C. Webster, 237–73. Cambridge: Cambridge University Press, 1979.

Small, J. K. *Manual of the Southeastern Flora.* Chapel Hill: University of North Carolina Press, 1933.

Smallwood, M. S. C. *Natural History and the American Mind.* New York: Columbia University Press, 1941.

Smith, A. G., and J. H. Young. "Folk Medicine at the Indian Trading Post." *Medicine at Emory* (1973): 42–47.

Smith, G. "Prescribing the Rules of Health: Self-Help and Advice in the Late Eighteenth Century." In *Patients and Practitioners. Lay Perceptions of Medicine in Pre-Industrial Society*, edited by R. Porter, 249–82. Cambridge: Cambridge University Press, 1985.

Smith, M. C. "Lay Periodical Coverage of the Minor Tranquilizers—The First Quarter Century." *Pharm. in Hist.* 25 (1983): 131–36.

Smith, P. *The Indian Doctor's Dispensatory. Being Father Smith's Advice Respecting Diseases and Their Cure.* Cincinnati, 1813. Reprint. *Bull. Lloyd Library.* Reproduction Series, no. 2, 1901.

Smith, T. "Herbs from Private Resources in the Community." In *Folk Medicine and Herbal Healing*, edited by G. G. Meyer et al., 197–212. Springfield: Thomas, 1981.

Smith, W. H. Y., et al. "Intestinal Parasite Survey in Alabama." *Amer. J. Pub. Health* 27 (1937): 471–75.

Smithe, B. R. *Killing Cancer. The Jason Winters Story.* Boulder: Vinton, 1980.

Snow, L. F. "Folk Medical Beliefs and Their Implications for Care of Patients: A Review Based on Studies among Black Americans." *Ann. Int. Med.* 81 (1974): 82–96.

———. " 'High Blood' Is Not High Blood Pressure." *Urban Health* (June 1976): 54–56.

————. "Sorcerers, Saints, and Charlatans: Black Folk Healers in Urban America." *Culture, Medicine, and Psychiatry* 2 (1978): 69–106.

————. "Con Men and Conjure Men: A Ghetto Image." In *Images of Healers, Literature and Medicine*, edited by A. H. Jones, 45–78. Albany: State University of New York Press, 1983.

Snow, L. F., and S. M. Johnson. "Modern Day Menstrual Folklore. Some Clinical Implications." *J. Amer. Med. Assoc.* 237 (1977): 2736–39. Highlights many nonscientific concepts.

Snyder, P. "The Use of Nonprescribed Treatments by Hemodialysis Patients." *Culture, Medicine, and Psychiatry* 7 (1983): 57–76.

Sonnedecker, G. "The Rise of Drug Manufacture in America." *Emory Univ. Quart.* 21 (1965): 73–87. Discusses a major force changing medicine.

————. "Home Medication on the American Frontier (1804)." *Veröff. Int. Ges. Gesch. Pharm.* 38 (1972): 259–71.

————. *Kremers and Urdang's History of Pharmacy.* Philadelphia: Lippincott, 1976.

Sontag, S. *Illness and Metaphor.* London: Allen Lane, 1977.

Spector, R. E. *Cultural Diversity in Health and Illness.* Norwalk: Appleton-Century-Crofts, 1985. A general textbook with an apt title.

Spiegeberg, O. *A Textbook of Midwifery.* 2 vols. London: New Sydenham Society, 1887–88.

Spiers, C. H. "The Drug Suppliers of George Washington and Other Virginians." *Pharm. Hist.* 7 (1977): 1–3.

Spillane, J. D. *The Doctrine of the Nerves: Chapters in the History of Neurology.* Oxford: Oxford University Press, 1981.

Spinelli, W. B. *The Primitive Therapeutic Use of Natural Products. A Bibliography.* Pittsburgh: N.p., 1971.

Spjut, W., and R. E. Perdue. "Plant Folklore: A Tool for Predicting Sources of Antitumor Activity?" *Cancer Treatment Reports* 60 (1976): 979–85. Suggests a correlation between plants used in folklore and those with anticancer activity.

Spykerboer, J. E., et al. "Parental Knowledge and Misconceptions about Asthma: A Controlled Study." *Soc. Sci. Med.* 22 (1986): 553–58. Yet another reminder of popular beliefs and fairly widespread popularity of herbs for asthma.

Stabler, C. V. "The History of the Alabama Public Health System," Ph.D. diss., Duke University, 1945.

Stacey, B. F. "On the Medicinal Agents of Indians: 'What Medicinal Articles Are in Popular Use among the Indian Tribes, and What Properties Ascribed to Such as Are Unknown to Commentaries?'" *Proc. Amer. Pharm. Assoc.* 21 (1873): 616–21.

Stage, S. *Female Complaints. Lydia Pinkham and the Business of Women's Medicine.* New York: Norton, 1979.

Stalker, D., and D. Glymour, eds. *Examining Holistic Medicine.* Buffalo: Prometheus, 1985. Generally critical surveys.

Stall, S. *What a Young Man Ought to Know.* Toronto: Briggs, 1897.

Stannard, J. "Early American Botany and Its Sources." In *Bibliography and Natural History*, edited by T. R. Buckman, 73–102. Lawrence: University of Kansas Libraries, 1964.

———. "P. A. Mattioli. Sixteenth Century Commentator on Dioscorides." *Bibliogr. Contrib.* 1 (1969). Lawrence: University of Kansas Libraries. Draws attention to list of synonyms.

———. "Medicinal Plants and Folk Remedies in Pliny, *Historia Naturalis.*" *Hist. Philo. Life Sci.* 24 (1982): 3–23.

———. "Medieval Arzneitaxe and Some Indigenous Plant Species." In *Orbis Pretus. Kultur- und Pharmaziehistorische Studien*, edited by W. Dressendörfer and W.-D. Müller-Jahnke, 267–72. Frankfurt am Main: Govi-Verlag, 1985.

———. "The Theoretical Bases of Medieval Herbalism." *Med. Heritage* (May–June 1985): 186–98.

Starr, P. *The Social Transformation of American Medicine.* New York: Basic Books, 1982.

Stearn, W. T. "From Theophrastus and Dioscorides to Sibthorpe and Smith: The Background and Origin of the *Flora Graeca.*" *Bio. J. Linn. Soc.* 8 (1976): 285–98.

Stearns, R. P. *Science in the British Colonies of America.* Urbana: University of Illinois Press, 1970.

Steedly, M. M. "The Evidence of Things Not Seen: Faith and Tradition in a Lumbee Healing Practice," Master's thesis, University of North Carolina, 1979.

Steele, G. *Maternity and Infant Care in a Mountain County in Georgia.* Washington, D.C.: Government Printing Office, 1923.

Steele, I. K., ed. *Atlantic Merchant-Apothecary Letters of Joseph Cruttenden 1710–1717.* Toronto, University of Toronto Press, 1977.

Steiner, R. P., ed. *Folk Medicine. The Art and the Science.* Washington, D.C.: American Chemical Society, 1986. A wide-ranging collection of essays.

Stekert, E. J. "Focus for Conflict. Southern Mountain Medical Beliefs in Detroit." *J. Amer. Folklore* 83 (1970): 115–56. Highlights such characteristics of mountain people as seeking to be "average" in urban northern settings. Especially relevant is the section on self-diagnosis and the persistence of folk medicine and the effects of urbanization (e.g., use of baby aspirin).

Stephenson, J. B. *Shiloh: A Mountain Community.* Lexington: University of Kentucky Press, 1968.

Stevens, W. *Observations on the Healthy and Diseased Properties of the Blood.* London: Murray, 1832.

Stevenson, D. R. "Intervillage Preference of High Blood Pressure Medicinal Plants on St. Kitts, West Indies." *Med. Anthropol.* 3 (1979): 503–24.

———. "High Blood Pressure. Medicinal Plant Use and Arterial Blood Change." In *Plants in Indigenous Medicine and Diet. Biobehavioral Approaches*, edited by N. L. Etkin, 252–65. Bedford Hills, N.Y.: Redgrave, 1986.

Stitt, V. J., Jr. "Root Doctors as Providers of Primary Care." *J. Nat. Med. Assoc.* 75 (1983): 719–21.

Stoeckle, J. D. "Medical Advice Books: The Search for the Healthy Body." *Soc. Sci. Med.* 18 (1984): 707–12.

Stoeckle, J. D., and G. A. White. *Plain Pictures of Plain Doctoring. Vernacular Expression in New Deal Medicine and Photography.* Cambridge: MIT Press, 1985.

Stoffer, S. S., et al. "Advice from Some Health Food Stores." *J. Amer. Med. Assoc.* 244 (1980): 2045–46. Concerns over such advice.

Strader, C. "A Winston-Salem Herbalist." *North Carolina Folklore J.* 27 (1979): 20–25.

Strausbaugh, P. D., and E. L. Core. *Flora of West Virginia*. Silver Spring, Md.: Seneca Books, 1978.

Strong, P. M. *The Ceremonial Order of the Clinic*. London: Routledge and Kegan Paul, 1979.

Sturtevant, W. C. *Bibliography on American Indian Medicine and Health*. Washington, D.C.: Smithsonian Institution, Bureau of American Ethnology, 1962.

Sugarman, J., and R. R. Butters. "Understanding the Patient: Medical Words the Doctor May Not Know." *North Carolina Med. J.* 46 (1985): 415–17.

Sullivan, G. "Herbs Available to the Public." In *Folk Medicine and Herbal Healing*, edited by G. G. Meyer et al., 179–96. Springfield: Thomas, 1981.

Sure, B. *The Vitamins in Health and Diseases*. Baltimore: Williams and Wilkins, 1933.

Sussman, L. K.; L. N. Robins; and F. Earls. "Treatment-Seeking for Depression by Black and White Americans." *Soc. Sci. Med.* 24 (1987): 187–96. Perspectives and differences between blacks and whites.

Swados, F. "Negro Health on Antebellum Plantations." *Bull. Hist. Med.* 10 (1941): 460–72.

Swain, G. Letter in Controller Papers, Southern Historical Collection, University of North Carolina, Chapel Hill.

Taberner, P. V. *Aphrodisiacs, The Science and the Myth*. Philadelphia: University of Pennsylvania Press, 1985.

Talbot, C. H. "America and the European Drug Trade." In *First Images of America*, edited by F. Chiappelli, 833–44. Berkeley: University of California Press, 1976. A useful review.

———. "Folk Medicine and History." In *American Folk Medicine*, edited by W. Hand, 7–10. Berkeley: University of California Press, 1976. Suggests that folklorists are overly concerned with diffusion rather than origins.

Taylor, N. *Plant Drugs that Changed the World*. London: Allen and Unwin, 1966.

Taylor, R. G. *Sharecroppers: The Way We Really Were*. Wilson: Mark, 1984.

Teeling-Smith, G. "Safer Medicines from Better Science Rather than Stricter Regulation." *Pharm. J.* 231 (1983): 237–39.

Teigen, P. M. "This Sea of Simples—The Materia Medica in Three Early English Receipt Books." *Pharm. in Hist.* 22 (1980): 104–8.

———. "Taste and Quality in Late Galenic Pharmacology." Paper presented at Fifty-sixth Annual Meeting of the American Association History of Medicine, Minneapolis, May 1983.

———. "Taste and Quality in 15th- and 16th-Century Galenic Pharmacology." *Pharm. in Hist.* 29 (1987): 60–68.

Temkin, O. "The Dependence of Medicine upon Basic Scientific Thought." In *The Historical Development of Physiological Thought*, edited by C. McBrooks and P. F. Cranefield. New York: Hafner, 1959. Highlights problems of definition and issues of scientific and practical medicine.

———. "Historical Aspects of Drug Therapy." In *Drugs in Our Society*, edited by P. Talalay. Baltimore and London: Johns Hopkins University Press, 1964.

———. *Galenism: Rise and Decline of a Medical Philosophy*. Ithaca: Cornell University Press, 1973.

Thomas, D. L., and L. B. T. Thomas. *Kentucky Superstitions*. Princeton: Princeton University Press, 1920.

Thomas, G. *A Practical Treatise of the Diseases of Women*. Edited by P. F. Munde. Philadelphia: Lea Brothers, 1891.

Thomas, K. *Religion and the Decline in Magic*. New York: Scribner's Sons, 1971. Thomas argues that magic declined in the eighteenth century not because technological progress eliminated the need for ritual magic but because society had moved to new ideas of self-reliance and self-confidence.

Thomas, R. *The Grosset Encyclopedia of Natural Medicine*. New York: Grosset and Dunlap, 1980. Some useful definitions.

Thompson, R. C. "Whatever Happened to Camphorated Oil?" *Consumer* 17, no. 6 (1983): 4–5.

Thompson, S. *Motif Index of Folk-Literature*. Bloomington: Indiana University Press, 1955–58.

Thomson, S. "Samuel Thomson's Autobiography." In his *New Guide to Health or Botanic Family Physician*. Boston: Adams, 1835. Reprint. *Bull. Lloyd Library* 11 (1909).

Thomson, W. A. R., ed. *Medicines from the Earth; a Guide to Healing Plants*. New York: McGraw-Hill, 1978.

Thorndike, L., ed. *The Herbal of Rufinis*. Chicago: University of Chicago Press, 1946.

Tilhagen, C.-H. *Papers on Folk-Medicine*. Stockholm: Nordic Museum. Reprinted from *ARV Journal of Scandinavian Folklore* 18–19 (1962–63).

Tisserand, R. B. *The Art of Aromatherapy*. New York: Destiny Books, 1977.

Tissue, T. "Another Look at Self-Rated Health Care." *J. Gerontology* 27 (1972): 91–94. Highlights problems of self-rated health care data.

Tonkin, R. D. "Role of Research in the Rapprochement between Conventional Medicine and Complementary Therapies: Discussion Paper." *J. Royal Soc. Med.* 80 (1987): 362–64.

A Touchstone for Physick, Directing by Evident Marks and Characters to Such Medicines, as without Purgers, Vomiters, Bleedings, Issues, Mineral or Any Other Disturbers of Natures May Be Securely Trusted for Care in All Extremities, and Be Easily Distinguished by Such as Are Hazardous or Dangerous. London: J. W., 1667.

Tournefort, J. *Materia Medica or a Description of Simple Medicines Generally Used in Physick*. London: J. H., 1708.

Traling, D. C. "Voodoo, Rootwork, and Medicine." *Psychosomatic Med.* 29 (1967): 483–91.

Trease, G. *Pharmacy in History*. London: Bailliere Tindall, 1964.

Trotter, R. T. II. "Folk Remedies Are Indicators of Common Illnesses: Examples from Old United States–Mexico Border." *J. Ethnopharmacol.* 4 (1981): 207–21.

Trotter, R. T. II., and J. A. Chavira. *Curanderismo. Mexican American Folk Healing*. Athens: University of Georgia Press, 1981.

Trotter, R. T. II, and M. H. Logan. "Informant Consensus: A New Approach for Identifying Potentially Effective Medicinal Plants." In *Plants in Indigenous Medicine and Diet: Biobehavioral Approaches*, edited by N. Etkin, 91–112. Bedford Hills, N.Y.: Redgrave, 1986.

Trotter, R. T. II, et al. "Ethnography and Bioassay: Combined Methods for a Preliminary Screen of Home Remedies for Potential Pharmacological Activity." *J. Ethnopharmacol.* 8 (1983): 113–19.

Trotter, R. T. II, et al. "Ethnopharmacology and Epidemiology: New Directions for Ethnomedical Research." *J. Ethnopharmacol.* 8 (1983): 245–46.

Trumpington, Baroness. "Alternative Medicines and Therapies and the DHSS." *J. Royal Soc. Med.* 80 (1987): 336–38. Raises significant points such as patients' freedom of choice and the notion of keeping the best of both worlds.

Truswell, A. S. "Food Sensitivity." *Brit. Med. J.* 291 (1985): 951–55. Some perspective on food allergies often considered to be widespread by practitioners of alternative medicine (sometimes called pseudo food allergy).

Tucker, L. "Herbal Medicine Revisted: Science Looks Anew at Ancient Chinese Pharmacology." *Amer. Pharm.* 19, no. 10 (1979): 16–28.

Tullos, A. "Tommie Bass: A Life in the Ridge and Valley Country," Master's thesis, University of North Carolina, 1976.

Turner, N. J. "Counter-Irritant and Other Medicinal Uses of Plants in Ranunculaceae by Native Peoples in British Columbia and Neighbouring Areas." *J. Ethnopharmacol.* 11 (1984): 181–201.

Turner, V. W. *The Forest of Symbols*. Ithaca: Cornell University Press, 1967. A seminal work on the role of symbols, including health.

Turner, W. *Libellus de Re Herbaria 1538 and the Names of Herbes, 1548*. London: Ray Society edition, 1965.

Twemlow, S. W., and G. O. Gabbard. "The Illusion that Heals: A Tentative Explication of the Placebo Response." *J. Holistic Med.* 7 (1985): 89–96.

Twigg, J. "Food for Thought, Purity and Vegetarianism." *Religion* 9 (1979): 13–35.

Tyler, V. E. *The Honest Herbal.* 1982. Reprint. Philadelphia: Stickley, 1987.

———. "Three Proprietaries and Their Claim as American Indian Remedies." *Pharm. in Hist.* 26 (1984): 146–49.

———. "Plant Drugs in the Twenty-first Century." *Econ. Bot.* 40 (1986): 279–88.

———. "Herbal Medicine in America." *Planta Med.* 1 (1987): 1–4.

Ullrich, A. C. "Traditional Healing in the Third World." *J. Holistic Med.* 6 (1984): 200–212.

Underwood, E. J. *Trace Elements in Human and Animal Nutrition*. New York: Academic Press, 1977.

Urdang, G., ed. *Pharmacopoeia Londinensis of 1618*. Reprint. Madison: State Historical Society of Wisconsin, 1944.

The Use of Essential Drugs. World Health Organization Technical Report Series, no. 722. 1985.

Vaillancourt, P. M. *Bibliographic Control of the Literature of Oncology*. Metuchen, N.J.: Scarecrow Press, 1969.

Vanderpoof, H. Y. "The Holistic Hodgepodge: A Critical Analysis of Holistic Medicine and Health in America Today." *J. Fam. Pract.* 19 (1984): 773–81.

Vaseline: Its History and Therapeutical Value. New York: N.p., 1884.

Vaskilampi, T., and C. P. MacCormack. *Folk Medicine and Health Culture; Role of Folk Medicine in Modern Health Care.* Kuopio, Finland: University of Kuopio, 1982.

Veith, I. "English Melancholy and American Nervousness." *Bull. Menninger Clinic* 32 (1968): 301–17.

Velimirovic, B., ed. *Modern Medicine and Medical Anthropology in the United States–Mexico Border Populations.* Washington, D.C.: Pan American Health Organization, 1978.

Verbrugge, L. M. "Triggers of Symptoms and Health Care." *Soc. Sci. Med.* 20 (1985): 855–76.

Viney, L. L. *Images of Illness.* Malabar, India: Kriger, 1983.

Vogel, G. "Natural Substances with Effects on the Liver." In *New Natural Products and Plant Drugs with Pharmacological, Biological, or Therapeutical Activity,* edited by H. Wagner and P. Wolff, 249–65. Berlin: Springer-Verlag, 1977.

Vogel, V. J. *American Indian Medicine.* Norman: University of Oklahoma Press, 1970.

———. "American Indian Foods Used as Medicine." In *American Folk Medicine, A Symposium,* edited by W. Hand, 125–42. Berkeley: University of California Press, 1976.

———. "American Indian Influence on the American Pharmacopoeia." In *Folk Medicine and Herbal Healing,* edited by G. G. Meyer et al., 103–12. Springfield: Thomas, 1981.

Voigts, L. E. "Anglo-Saxon Plant Remedies and the Anglo-Saxons." *Isis* 70 (1979): 250–68. Stresses the practical aspect of Anglo-Saxon writings.

von Sachs, J. *History of Botany 1530–1860.* Translated by H. E. F. Garnsey. Oxford: Clarendon Press, 1980.

Vuori, H. "WHO and Traditional Medicine." In *Folk Medicine and Health Culture: Role of Folk Medicine in Modern Health Care,* edited by T. Vaskilampi and C. P. MacCormack, 165–89. Kuopio, Finland: University of Kuopio, 1982.

Waddell, G., et al. "Symptoms and Signs: Physical Disease or Illness Behaviour." *Brit. Med. J.* 289 (1984): 739–41. One of many reminders of the clinical value in distinguishing symptoms and signs of physical disease from those of illness behavior.

Wallace, D. J. "Thomsonians: The People's Doctors." *Clio Medica* 14 (1980): 169–86.

Waller, T., and G. Killion. "Georgia Folk Medicine." *Southern Folklore Quart.* 36 (1972): 71–91. Lists of remedies, many nonnatural.

Wallis, R. "Betwixt Therapy and Salvation: The Changing Form of the Human Potential Movement." In *Sickness and Sectarianism,* edited by R. K. Jones, 23–51. Aldershot: Gower, 1985.

Walsh, J. J. *Psychotherapy.* New York: Appleton, 1912. One of a number of works appearing at the time which encouraged the trend to view all therapy outside professional medicine as psychotherapy.

Walshe, W. H. *The Anatomy, Physiology, Pathology, and Treatment of Cancer, with Additions by J. Mason Warren.* Boston: Ticknor, 1844.

Walton, A. H. *Aphrodisiacs: From Legend to Prescription*. Westport: Associated Booksellers, 1958. Study of aphrodisiacs through the ages with sections on foods.

Ware, G. W. *Southern Vegetable Crops*. New York: American Book, 1937.

Waring, E. J. *Bibliotheca Therapeutica*. 2 vols. London: New Sydenham Society, 1879. Valuable bibliography covering much continental literature.

Waring, J. I. *A History of Medicine in South Carolina 1670–1825*. Columbia: South Carolina Medical Association, 1964.

Warner, J. H. "The Nature-Trusting Heresy: American Physicians and the Concept of the Healing Power of Nature in the 1850's and 1860's." *Perspect. Amer. Hist.* 11 (1978): 291–324.

———. "Physiological Theory and Therapeutic Explanation in the 1860s: The British Debate on the Medical Use of Alcohol." *Bull. Hist. Med.* 54 (1980): 235–57.

———. *The Therapeutic Perspective*. Cambridge: Harvard University Press, 1986.

Warren, J. *View of the Mercurial Practice in Febrile Diseases*. Boston: Wait, 1813.

Wassén, S. H. "The Anthropological Outlook for Amerindian Medicinal Plants." In *Plants in the Development of Modern Medicine*, edited by T. Swain, 2–65. Cambridge: Harvard University Press, 1972.

———. "On Concepts of Disease among Amerindian Tribal Groups." *J. Ethnopharmacol.* 1 (1979): 285–93.

Watson, R. R. *Nutrition, Disease Resistance, and Immune Function*. New York: Dekker, 1984.

Watson, W. H. "Folk Medicine and Older Blacks in Southern United States." In *Black Folk Medicine*, ed. W. H. Watson, 54–66. New Brunswick: Transaction Books, 1984.

———, ed. *Black Folk Medicine. The Therapeutic Significance of Faith and Trust*. New Brunswick: Transaction Books, 1984.

Watson, W. N. B. "The Scotch Fiddle." *Scottish Stud. Vol.* 15 (1971): 141–45.

Watt, J. M. "Magic and Witchcraft in Relation to Plants and Folk Medicine." In *Plants in the Development of Modern Medicine*, edited by T. Swain. Cambridge: Harvard University Press, 1972.

Webster, C., ed. *Health, Medicine and Mortality in the Sixteenth Century*. Cambridge: Cambridge University Press, 1979. Contains papers relevant to popular traditions and background to our early story.

Weil, A. T. *Health and Healing. Understanding Conventional and Alternative Medicine*. Boston: Houghton Mifflin, 1983.

Weil, A. T. "Botanical vs. Chemical Drugs: Pros and Cons." In *Folk Medicine and Herbal Healing*, edited by G. G. Meyer et al., 287–312. Springfield: Thomas, 1981.

Wells, C. M. M. "A Small Herbal of Little Cost, 1762–1778: A Case Study of a Colonial Herbal as a Social and Cultural Document," Ph.D. diss., University of Pennsylvania, 1980.

Welsh, S. O., and R. M. Marston. "Review of Trends in Food Use in the United States, 1909–1980." *J. Amer. Diet Assoc.* 81 (1982): 120–25. Highlights changing food sources of energy.

Werner, R. "Traditionelle Medizin und Moderne Medizin—Kontradiktio oder Symbiose?" *Veröff. Gesundh. Wesen.* 40 (1978): 347–60. One of a number of pleas for a rapprochement: "We should respectfully open our mind to the great importance of 'belief' in the mighty supernatural powers curing sickness."

Wesley, J. *Primitive Physick: Or an Easy and Natural Method of Curing Most Diseases.* London: Trye, 1747.

Westberg, G. E., ed. *Theological Roots of Wholistic Health Care.* Hindale: Wholistic Health Centers, 1979.

Wheelwright, E. G. *Medicinal Plants and Their History.* 1935. Reprint. New York: Dover, 1974.

Whisnant, D. E. *All That Is Native & Fine.* Chapel Hill: University of North Carolina Press, 1981.

White, B. L., et al. *Placebo. Theory, Research, and Mechanisms.* New York: Guilford Press, 1985.

White, S. "Medicine's Humble Humbug: Four Periods in the Understanding of the Placebo." *Pharm. in Hist.* 27 (1985): 51–60.

Whitener, R. "Selections from Folk-ways and Folk Speech. Poison Oak Cures." *North Carolina Folklore J.* 29 (1981): 55.

Whorton, J. C. *Crusaders for Fitness. The History of American Health Reformers.* Princeton: Princeton University Press, 1982. Topics include vegetarianism and Rodale; pertinent to the present account.

Whorton, J. C. "Traditions of Folk Medicine in America." *J. Amer. Med. Assoc.* 257 (1987): 1632–35. Distinctions between traditional and sectarian medicine not made as by most authors.

Wigginton, E. "Two Faith Healers Tell Exactly How It's Done." *North Carolina Folklore J.* 16 (1968): 163–65.

Wigginton, E., and M. Bennett, eds. *Foxfire.* Garden City: Doubleday, 1984.

Wilder, A. *History of Medicine. A Brief Outline of Medical History and Sects of Physicians, from the Earliest Historic Period; with an Extended Account of the New Schools of the Healing Art in the Nineteenth Century and Especially a History of the American Eclectic Practice of Medicine.* New Sharon: New England Eclectic Publishing, 1901. Survey of nineteenth-century Eclectic practice.

Williams, A. *Textbook of Black-Related Diseases.* New York: McGraw-Hill, 1975.

Williams, B. T. "Are Public Health Education Campaigns Worthwhile?" *Brit. Med. J.* 288 (1984): 170–71.

Wilson, E. *Diseases of the Skin.* Philadelphia: Blanchard and Lea, 1852.

Wilson, G. " 'Store-Bought' Remedies in the Mammoth Cave Region." *North Carolina Folklore J.* 29 (1981): 58–62.

Wisswaesser, C. "Roots and Ramifications of Medicinal Herbs in Eighteenth-Century North America." *Trans. Stud. Coll. Phys. Philadelphia* 44 (1976): 194–99.

Withington, E. T. *Medical History from the Earliest Times: A Popular History of the Healing Art.* 1894. Reprint. London: Scientific Press, 1964.

Wolfe, R. J. *Jacob Bigelow's American Medical Botany.* 1817–21. Reprint. Boston: Bird and Bull Press, 1979.

Wolff, B. B., and S. Langley. "Cultural Factors and the Response to Pain: A Review." *Amer. Anthropol.* 70 (1968): 494–501.

Wolff, J. *Die Lebre von der Krebskrankheiten von den altesten Zeiten biz zur Gegenwort.* 4 vols. Jena, East Germany: Fischer, 1914–29. Many valuable historical sources considered.

Wood, G. B. "Introductory Lecture to the Course of Materia Medica in the University of Pennsylvania." *Amer. J. Pharm.* 184 (1838): 298–322.

Wood, G. B., and F. Bache. *The Dispensatory of the United States of America.* Philadelphia: Lippincott, 1836 (and 1847, 1868, 1870).

Wood, H. C. *A Treatise on Therapeutics, Comprising Materia Medica and Toxicology.* Philadelphia: Lippincott, 1874 (and 1877, 1882).

World Health Organization. *The Promotion and Development of Traditional Medicine.* World Health Organization Technical Report Series, no. 622, 1978.

Worthington-Roberts, B., and M. Brekin. "Fads or Facts? A Pharmacist's Guide to Controversial 'Nutrition' Products." *Amer. Pharm.*, n.s. 23 (1983): 410–22.

Wundt, W. *Grundzüge der Physiologische Psychologie.* Leipzig: Engelmann, 1893.

Wynter, W. E. *Minor Medicine. A Treatise on the Nature and Treatment of Common Ailments.* New York: Appleton, 1908. Helpful for some perspectives on minor ailments and self-treatment.

Xiao, P.-G. "Traditional Experience of Chinese Herb Medicine. Its Application in Drug Research and New Drug Searching." In *Natural Products as Medicinal Agents,* edited by J. L. Beal and F. Reinhard, 351–94. Stuttgart: Hippocratic Verlag, 1982.

Yamaguchi, M. *World Vegetables. Principles, Production, and Nutritive Values.* Westport: Avi, 1983.

Yoder, D. "Folk Medicine." In *Folklore and Folklife: An Introduction,* edited by R. Dorson, 141–215. Chicago: University of Chicago Press, 1972.

———. "Hohman and Romanus. Origins and Diffusion of the Pennsylvania German Powwow Manual." In *American Folk Medicine, A Symposium,* edited by W. Hand, 235–48. Berkeley: University of California Press, 1976.

Young, A. "When Rational Men Fall Sick: An Inquiry into Some Assumptions Made by Medical Anthropologists." *Culture, Medicine, and Psychiatry* 5 (1981): 317–35.

———. "The Anthropologies of Illness and Sickness." *Ann. Rev. Anthropol.* 11 (1982): 257–85.

Young, J. H. *The Medical Messiahs.* Princeton: Princeton University Press, 1967.

———. *American Self-Dosage Medicines. An Historical Perspective.* Lawrence: Coronado Press, 1974. A review with much attention to legislative restraint.

———. "The Agile Role of Food: Some Historical Reflections." In *Nutrition and Drug Interrelations,* edited by J. N. Hathcock and J. Coon, 1–18. New York: Academic Press, 1978.

———. "The Footmaster Who Fooled Them." *Yale J. Biol. Med.* 53 (1980): 555–56. Young's writings, widely quoted, reveal a philosophical orientation toward protection: "Both philosophical currents and the impact of events in the twentieth century revealed human nature as harboring the potential for stubborn blindness and for great evil. Progress, which many in the nineteenth century came to deem inevitable, had slowed if not reversed itself."

———. "Self-Dosage Medicine in America, 1906–1981." *South Atlantic Quart.* 80 (1981): 379–90. Argues in favor of protective regulations.

————. "Nutritional Quackery." *Assoc. Food and Drug Officials* (1983): 3–11. An account indicating recent trends in "quackery" and opposing trends.

————. "Sulfanilamid and Diethylene Glycol." In *Chemistry and Modern Society: Historical Essays in Honor of Aaron J. Ihde*, edited by J. Parascandola and J. C. Whorton, 105–25. ACS Symposium Series, no. 228. Washington, D.C.: American Chemical Society, 1983.

————. "Three Southern Food and Drug Cases." *J. Southern Hist.* 49 (1983): 3–36.

————. "Laetrile in Historical Perscpectives." In *Politics, Science, and Cancer: The Laetrile Phenomenon*, edited by G. E. Markle and J. C. Peterson. AAS Selected Symposium, no. 46. Boulder: Westview Press, 1980.

Zabrowski, M. "Cultural Components in Response to Pain." *J. Social Issues* 8 (1952): 16–30.

Zamula, E. "Of Pills that Pack Too Much Punch." *FDA Consumer* (1984): 38–40. Warning about Chinese herbal remedies contaminated with phenylbutazone.

Zirkle, C. "John Clayton and Our Colonial Botany." *Virginia Mag.* 67 (1959): 284–94.

Zwinger, T. *Theatrum Botanicum.* 1696. Revised edition. Basel: Bischoffs, 1744.

Index

John K. Crellin, the John Clinch Professor of History of Medicine at Memorial University of Newfoundland, is a physician, pharmacist, and historian. He is the author of many books including *Medical Ceramics in the Wellcome Institute, Home Medicine: The Newfoundland Experience* and is coeditor of *Alternative Health Care in Canada: Nineteenth and Twentieth Century Perspectives.* He served as editor of Tommie Bass's *Plain Southern Eating* (Duke University Press, 1988), and has also published two children's books and numerous articles in pharmaceutical and medical journals.

Jane Philpott was, until her death in 1997, Professor Emerita in the Department of Botany and in the School of Forestry and Environmental Studies at Duke University. She also served as Dean and Marshall of the university, was a visiting botanist at Kew Gardens, and an adviser to Encyclopedia Britannica Films on Plants. She contributed to *Botanical Gazette* and *McGraw-Hill Encyclopedia of Science and Technology.*

Library of Congress Cataloging in Publication Data
Crellin, J. K.
Trying to give ease : Tommie Bass and the story of herbal medicine / John K. Crellin and Jane Philpott.
p. cm.
Previously published in 1990 by Duke University Press under the title: Herbal medicine past and present. Volume 1: Trying to give ease.
Includes bibliographical references and index.
ISBN 0-8223-0877-0 (cloth : alk. paper). —
ISBN 0-8223-2017-7 (paper : alk. paper)
1. Bass, A. L. Tommie — Interviews.   2. Materia medica, Vegetable — Appalachian Region.   3. Medicinal plants — Appalachian Region.
4. Herbs — Therapeutic use — Appalachian Region.   I. Philpott, Jane.   II. Bass, A. L. Tommie.   III. Title.
RS164.B324C74   1997
615'.321'0974 — dc21   97-15490   CIP